Charitable Knowledge explores the interconnections among medical teaching, medical knowledge, and medical authority in eighteenth-century London. The metropolis lacked a university until the nineteenth century, so the seven major voluntary hospitals – St. Bartholomew, St. Thomas, Guy, the Westminster, St. George, the Middlesex, and the London – were crucial sites for educating surgeons, surgeon–apothecaries, and visiting physicians.

Lawrence explains how charity patients became teaching objects, and how hospitals became medical schools. She demonstrates that hospital practitioners gradually gained authority through their clinical teaching, research, and social status in London's urban medical culture, transforming the old tripartite structure into a loosely unified group of de facto general practitioners dominated by hospital men. As hospital physicians and surgeons became the new elite, they profoundly shaped what counted as "good" knowledge among medical men, both in the construction of clinical observations and in the proper use of science.

Charitable knowledge

Cambridge History of Medicine

Edited by

CHARLES ROSENBERG, Professor of History and Sociology of Science, University of Pennsylvania

Other titles in the series:

Continued on page following the Index

Charitable knowledge
Hospital pupils and practitioners in eighteenth-century London

SUSAN C. LAWRENCE
The University of Iowa

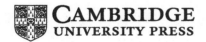

CAMBRIDGE
UNIVERSITY PRESS

PUBLISHED BY THE PRESS SYNDICATE OF THE UNIVERSITY OF CAMBRIDGE
The Pitt Building, Trumpington Street, Cambridge, United Kingdom

CAMBRIDGE UNIVERSITY PRESS
The Edinburgh Building, Cambridge CB2 2RU, UK
40 West 20th Street, New York NY 10011–4211, USA
477 Williamstown Road, Port Melbourne, VIC 3207, Australia
Ruiz de Alarcón 13, 28014 Madrid, Spain
Dock House, The Waterfront, Cape Town 8001, South Africa

http://www.cambridge.org

First published 1996
First paperback edition 2002

A catalogue record for this book is available from the British Library

Library of Congress Cataloguing in Publication data
Lawrence, Susan C.
Charitable knowledge: hospital pupils and practitioners in eighteenth-
century London / Susan C. Lawrence.
          p.   cm. – (Cambridge history of medicine)
Includes index.
ISBN 0 521 36355 1 (hardback)
1. Medicine – England – London – History – 18th century.
2. Teaching hospitals – England – London – History – 18th century.
3. Medical education – England – London – History – 18th century.
I. Title.   II. Series.
[DNLM: 1. Medical Staff, Hospital – education.   2. Hospitals,
Voluntary – history – London.   3. History of Medicine, 18th Cent. –
London. WX 18 1996]
R488.L8L38   1996
610′.942′09033–dc20
DNLM/DLC
for Library of Congress   95-17710   CIP

ISBN 0 521 36355 1 hardback
ISBN 0 521 52518 7 paperback

*In memory of
my father
and my brother*

CONTENTS

Contents   ix

TABLES AND FIGURES

PREFACE

"Charitable knowledge," I have been told, is a rather peculiar conjunction of words. *People* are benevolent, generous, lenient, merciful, or philanthropic, giving of their time, compassion, or money; *knowledge* – well, knowledge, qua knowledge, is not. Yet "charitable knowledge" captures the major arguments in this book. Practitioners in eighteenth-century London hospitals used their medical knowledge and skills for charitable ends. They spent hours voluntarily attending to the sick poor. They tried to help ill men and women to get better, whether or not they were particularly successful with their cures or especially kind to the poor folk under their care. During the eighteenth century, hospital physicians and surgeons made teaching pupils on the wards integral to hospitals' charitable duties. In order to do that, they had to make the daily presence of large numbers of pupils on the wards fit into the meaning of charity for the lay governors whose time and money supported the hospitals. Using hospital patients as teaching objects had to become a *good* thing to do, a valuable contribution to social betterment for all people, not just a useful experience for a very small number of apprentices and personal assistants.

The modern teaching hospital exists because we – as a culture if not as individuals – in a fundamental sense value the moments when an experienced clinician instructs a medical student using the body and responses of a hospital patient. (This is, of course, sometimes valued more in the abstract than when one is the patient.) What is enshrined here is not the patient's "gift" of his condition and cooperation, although that may be appreciated, but rather the clinician's benevolence and generosity in sharing her knowledge and skills with a neophyte, *whatever* the patient may feel about the experience. Clinical teaching could only become – and remain – institutionalized in hospitals because even if we see it exploiting patients for purposes other than care, we understand that it serves a higher good – producing qualified doctors for other people, including ourselves. Hospital practitioners had to make this argument in the eighteenth century. That they did so successfully explains our comfortable belief that it is true.

The second point that "charitable knowledge" offers arises from the first. The knowledge that eighteenth-century medical men made, deployed, and taught on – and off – the wards was itself configured by the rituals and meaning of charity practice in the major London hospitals. The lay and medical men who built, ran, and supported the voluntary hospitals envisioned that respectable, even eminent, practitioners would volunteer to serve them. In London, this meant physicians and surgeons who knew the customs suited to practice among the well-to-do. I argue that hospital physicians and surgeons always used their charity work to display behavior appropriate for elite practitioners, no matter what else they did with it. Practicing on the poor was all about practicing among the rich, *not* in the sense of providing the same remedies, operations, and attention, but in the more fundamental sense that having a hospital post distinguished a man with prestige, learning, and expertise from the common run of ordinary practitioners. In much of this volume, I present the complex implications of this perspective. It has allowed me to connect the social context of hospital practice with the ways that eighteenth-century medical men wrote about their clinical experiences; to intertwine the meaning of gentlemanly manners with the meaning of science within medicine; to explain the persistence of two visions of the body and its diseases – the physician's constitutional one and the surgeon's anatomical one – into the nineteenth century; and to explore the powerful ways that hospital men's teaching both created the general practitioner and kept him subordinate to them.

Charitable Knowledge, then, is a book about medical authority constructed in and through the voluntary hospitals of eighteenth-century London. As such, it is about the transformation of the traditional medical occupations – physician, surgeon, and apothecary – into the modern medical profession before the advent of organic chemistry, systematic microscopy, or anesthesia, indeed, before all of the changes that we now believe give medicine authority through correct science and efficacious practice. By the early nineteenth century, all sorts of medical students, ordinary practitioners, lay patients, politicians, and booksellers recognized that they were supposed to pay attention to the physicians and surgeons who staffed London's well-known charities for the sick poor. During the eighteenth century, the practitioners and pupils at St. Bartholomew's, St. Thomas's, Guy's, the Westminster, St. George's, the London, and the Middlesex hospitals made these institutions into sites for the production and legitimization of both reliable doctors and good medical knowledge. They still do.

I began this project over a decade ago and with each passing year the number of those who contributed time, inspiration, support, criticism, and even well-meaning impatience has grown substantially. Many of my students, colleagues, and friends at the University of Toronto, Ball State University, and the University of Iowa have given more than most of them will ever know to the final shape of this book. I regret that I cannot thank all of them individually in this Preface.

Financial support for research travel made this work possible. I am extremely grateful to the University of Toronto for support during my graduate program; to the American Philosophical Society for a summer research grant; to the National Endowment for the Humanities for a Travel to Collections grant (FE-20881–87); to Ball State University for a Faculty Research Grant; and the University of Iowa for international travel funds.

I could not have contemplated, carried out, or finished this study without access to eighteenth-century hospital records, manuscripts, and publications. I deeply appreciate the time and effort that the staff men and women of many libraries and archives not only took to provide me with helpful suggestions and material, but also continue to take to preserve and to catalogue the collections entrusted to them. In particular, I want to thank the librarians and archivists of the Bodleian Library of the University of Oxford, the British Library, the Corporation of London Record Office, the Greater London Record Office, the Guildhall Library, the Norfolk Record Office, the Royal College of Surgeons of England, the Royal College of Physicians of London, the Royal Society of London, the University of Edinburgh Library, the London Hospital Medical School Library, St. George's Hospital Medical School Library, St. Thomas's Hospital Medical School Library, the Wills Library at Guy's Hospital Medical School, and the Wellcome Institute for the History of Medicine in London. I owe a special debt of gratitude to Mr. Bompas, former Secretary of Guy's Hospital, for permission to study the student registers in his office; to the late Mr. Ralph Winterton, for access to the Middlesex Hospital archives; to Mr. Hugh Anderson, former Honorary Archivist to St. George's Hospital Archives, for access to St. George's Hospital archives; to Sue Palmer, when Archivist of the Guy's Hospital records at the Greater London Record Office, for information from material unfit for consultation; to Janet Foster, when District Archivist for the St. Bartholomew's Hospital Archives, for bringing me Ludford Harvey's diary; and to Claire Daunton, when District Archivist for the London Hospital archives, for her help with dozens of dusty volumes. They all went out of their way to let me work for long hours on the hospitals' boards of governors records.

For permission to reproduce Fielding's 1786 map of London, I acknowledge the Westminster City Archives; Michael Wilcox provided the graphics expertise to label the hospitals' locations.

On this side of the Atlantic, the staff of the Science and Medicine Library, John Robart's Library, and the Thomas Fisher Rare Book Library of the University of Toronto were endlessly patient with my requests. On my research trips to the National Library of Medicine, I always found the staff of the Historical Division generous with their kindness and expertise. I thank the University of Iowa's library staff for their assistance over the last few years, as I have written and rewritten this book. Additional noteworthy support from the University of Iowa came with the enthusiasm and skill of two graduate research assistants, Gail Hutchison and Louisa Starr Mack, and from Melanie DeVore, who has been a calm source of secretarial expertise and patience during the final year it has taken to prepare the manuscript. Thank you all.

This book went through many versions during a decade of increasingly abundant work on eighteenth-century medicine, science, and culture, and I owe many thought-provoking moments to the scholars whose work I acknowledge in my notes. Excellent work continues to appear, such as *Medicine in the Enlightenment,* edited by Roy Porter (Amsterdam: Rodopi, 1995), published since the manuscript went to the Press in July 1994 and so not included in my analysis or references. For their considerable intellectual stimulation and challenge, my deep gratitude goes out to Toby Gelfand, my doctoral dissertation adviser, Cathy Crawford, Andy Federer, Jan Golinski, Henry Horwitz, Roy Porter, and John Harley Warner. Harold Cook, Charles Rosenberg, Daniel Goldstein, and Gail Zlatnik read and offered insightful and helpful comments on large portions of my manuscript; for their efforts to make this book better, I am enormously grateful. All the remaining flaws are entirely my own. A workgroup at the University of Iowa kept me going throughout all the ups and downs of academic life: Sally Kenney, Teresa Mangum, and Gita Patel, you did it. Lastly, Mary Fissell has done all of the above, and more. Her support, reading, criticism, enthusiasm – and long conversations about eighteenth-century medicine, culture, science, and poverty – always helped me to shape and to refine my arguments. That we sometimes disagreed reminded me at crucial moments that writing a book can be fun.

A note on quotations and dates: I have remained faithful to the spelling and grammar of eighteenth-century sources in all quotations, except that I have written superscripted abbreviations, such as w^{ch}, as "wch." I use [*sic*], therefore, only when the peculiarities of the author's prose have convinced readers of the manuscript that there must be a mistake in the quotation. All dates before 1752 are given new style, with the calendar year beginning on January 1, unless otherwise noted.

1

Introduction: Hospital medicine in eighteenth-century London

> Were I to guess at the most probable future improvements in physic, I should say, that they would arise from a more general, and more accurate examination of diseases after death. And were I to place a man of proper talents on the most direct road for becoming truly *great* in his profession, I would choose a good, practical Anatomist, and put him into a large hospital to attend the sick, and dissect the dead.[1]

So wrote William Hunter, surgeon turned physician, in an introductory lecture for his London anatomy class in the early 1780s.[2] Hunter made a nicely prescient guess about the direction of progress in medicine. Read with the benefit of hindsight, his comment evokes the juncture of three paths into the "direct road" to medical modernity. First, Hunter pointed to an empirical methodology for "improvements in physic" that detached the investigation of disease from patients' experiences of illness and from direct concern for treating it. A newly conceptualized medicine started at death, when the bedside-practitioner gave up and the scientist-practitioner took over – and these were the same person. Second, Hunter placed his man in a hospital where he had equal power "to attend the sick" and to "dissect the dead." Casting the hospital as an institution where practitioners deployed new methods to produce new knowledge transformed an expres-

---

1 William Hunter, *Two Introductory Lectures, delivered . . . to his last course of Anatomical Lectures at his Theatre in Windmill-Street* (London: J. Johnson, 1784), 73; emphasis original. Published a short time after his death, the extended title of his work promised that this text was "as . . . left corrected for the press by himself." Running to over one hundred pages, however, the text probably had quite a number of authorial embellishments – either that or his students sat through an extremely lengthy performance.
2 At this point in his career, William Hunter was a wealthy and well-known man. He had worked his way to financial success through his lucrative practice as a man-midwife to well-off London families, and to professional fame through his anatomical investigations and years as a lecturer. Samuel Foart Simmons and John Hunter, *William Hunter, 1718–1783: A Memoir*, ed. C. Helen Brock (Glasgow: University of Glasgow Press, 1983); Roy Porter, "William Hunter: A Surgeon and a Gentleman," and C. Helen Brock, "The Happiness of Riches," in *William Hunter and the Eighteenth Century Medical World*, ed. W.F. Bynum and Roy Porter (Cambridge: Cambridge University Press, 1985), 7–56.

sion of charitable care and social concern into a foundation for professional medical authority. Third, Hunter linked a man's acquisition of such knowledge to "becoming truly *great* in his profession." Besides the obvious implication that men, not women, were the ones with such talents, Hunter's assertion depended upon the existence of a "profession" in which "a good, practical Anatomist" *could* improve "physic."[3] Herein lay a conjunction of traditionally distinct areas of occupational expertise: the surgeon's skill in practical anatomy, necessary for operating and treating traumas and wounds (the realm of "external" disorders), with the physician's mastery over the subtle signs of fevers, nervous diseases, and digestive upsets (the region of "internal" disorders), treated with drugs and an appropriate regimen. His remark, too, implies a sense of "greatness" defined and valued by professional peers, one based upon a meritocracy of insider knowledge taking precedence over lay standards for social and intellectual success. Hunter – popular practitioner, successful lecturer, gentleman, and man of science – thrived under the penumbra of hospital medicine and articulated its potential power. Understanding the construction and meaning of that authority is the main purpose of this book.

In this chapter I lay out the outlines of my arguments, starting with an overview of the broad trends in eighteenth-century English culture that are crucial for my claims about continuity and change within London medicine. I then discuss two issues that have dominated scholarly understanding of eighteenth-century medicine for the past thirty years: first, the change in Western medical perceptions associated with "the birth of the clinic" and, second, the transformation of medical occupations into a single medical profession in early-modern to modern England. The rest of the chapter concentrates on the meaning of "hospital medicine."

In researching and writing this book, I have come to see and to articulate a new vision of hospital medicine, one that binds culture, the clinic, and the notion of "profession" inextricably together. I firmly believe that no explanation of how medical power is constructed, established, and perpetuated is satisfactory unless it works at ground level, where ordinary people – patients, neighborhood practitioners, newspaper readers, medical students – lived and made choices. This book is thus a synthesis of historical scholarship on eighteenth-century medicine, science, and culture; a contribution to historical knowledge of the hospitals, medical education, and

---

3 Throughout the book, I use "physic" to refer to the area of medicine that learned physicians practiced. "Surgery" refers specifically to the surgeons' realm of expertise and practice. I use "medicine" to refer to all medical activities, including both physic and surgery, and "medical practitioners" to encompass physicians, surgeons, and apothecaries. The only exceptions to this usage occur when I use "medical" instead of the archaic "physical" to modify certain forms of ward-walking and lectures in explicit contrast to "surgical."

medical community in London; and a long conversation about medical authority. I think that medical practitioners always depend upon many intertwining factors – social, intellectual, economic, literary, political, institutional – for their authority at the bedside and among themselves. No single position or characteristic, be it high social status or strong claims to scientific knowledge, grants a medical man the power to define a person's experience with illness and to be obeyed when trying to control it. Only when several attributes work in concert, with some of them more or less invisible to both the patient and her practitioner, does a medical man or woman achieve compliance. In the eighteenth century (and, I would argue, ever afterward), hospitals became crucial sites for various elements of medical authority to come together and become embodied in the hospital practitioner himself, in his language, behavior, public appearances, and private consultations.

Studying London's hospitals, practitioners, and pupils in the years between 1700 and 1820 reveals the relationships among institutions, medical training, and medical publications that created medical practitioners with different degrees of occupational and social power based more and more upon access to certain kinds of hospital knowledge. For this argument, looking at only one or two institutions would have been woefully inadequate. I have examined all seven of London's general hospitals – St. Thomas's, St. Bartholomew's, Guy's, the Westminster, St. George's, the Middlesex and the London – together for the first time. Using material from their governors' minute books, student notes, and pupil registers, I frequently stress the characteristics shared by these urban charities, while appreciating the puzzling and quixotic differences among them. These were not the discrete, independent institutions often pictured in the histories devoted to their individual developments. As people moved between the hospitals, moreover, traveling around London for governors' meetings, lectures, or ward-walking, "hospital medicine" gained a level of conceptual abstraction within the urban medical community. The sense that hospital medicine transcended any particular institution significantly increased the status granted to hospital teaching and hospital men's claims to good knowledge. Historians must compare and contrast the work done in multiple sites in an urban center in order to produce a workable analysis of institutional medicine within a larger social context. Thus I move among London's hospitals for my evidence and examples precisely because I need to convey both their commonalities and their revealing peculiarities. To submerge the seven hospitals under more convenient generalizations, admittedly an important task for the historian, would undermine my conceptual point: the hospitals solved similar problems with different means, each indicative of the *range* of responses within a common set of values about charity, the poor, and standards for medical practice. And it is this range, not one particular reaction, that defined and supported hospital medicine.

Just as no one hospital was the site of hospital medicine, no single individual – or easily definable group of individuals – stands out as key to its intellectual construction and professional development. Certainly a handful of men associated with London hospitals in the eighteenth century, such as William Cheselden, Percivall Pott, John Hunter, and Matthew Baillie, acquired both contemporary and historical reputations as individuals who contributed new practices, observations, and theories to medical knowledge. Scholars have written biographies for these luminaries and, for a few, have subjected their work to analytic study; I have relied upon these texts with both gratitude and caution. To date it has been next to impossible to know how representative or unique such individuals were in contemporary terms. And it has been all too easy to make heroes (especially of John Hunter) by dismissing those around them as backward or short-sighted. To remedy my own unease with such characterizations, I collected information on all of the physicians and surgeons who served one of the general hospitals between 1700 and 1820 (see Appendix I.A for a list). This information provided a base for rough generalizations, particularly on how many hospital men lectured or published on medical topics. As a consequence of this approach, this book is full of obscure people. And rightly so, for they are the ones who really constructed the mundane rituals and expectations surrounding hospital medicine, the meat-and-potatoes routines of taking students onto the wards, treating charity and private patients, and discussing their ideas with their pupils and peers. The men who acquired a place in the historical lists of contributors to medical knowledge derived the ways that they used science to further medical questions, their appropriation of hospital patients for teaching and detached clinical observations, and the means to communicate their ideas to medical audiences from a much broader community of medical men. I name practitioners, sometimes many of them, deliberately to evoke the extent and complexity of the networks making up that diffuse community.

In stressing the formation of accepted practices among hospital men, from the convention of taking pupils on ward rounds to the custom of publishing accounts of patients' cases in medical journals, I have confronted one of the more unexpected challenges of this project. To me, one of the most interesting problems in the history of science and medicine is to understand precisely how new knowledge and methods become boring, such fundamental aspects of daily life that they are not only unquestioned, but also scarcely worth mentioning or even thinking about.[4] To appreciate

4 The notion of the importance of accepted routine in science harks back to Thomas Kuhn's points about "normal" science in his *The Structure of Scientific Revolutions* (Chicago: University of Chicago Press, 1962). Recent work on the anthropology of scientific practice,

the potency of standard methods of inquiry and, more importantly, of *uncontroversial* knowledge, demands that these be investigated and explained closely just when they seem to have the least active roles in prompting new insights. The very insignificance of the routine, the undisputed, and the stable is vitally significant for the construction of authority. I argue, for example, that hospital medical men primarily took up "safe" science – that well established, heavily descriptive and undertheorized sort of science which avoided overt philosophical, religious, or social issues – precisely because it carried the appearance of consensus about the natural world into medical knowledge. The force of such beliefs and customs inheres less in the convictions or rituals themselves than in their implicit acceptance. It is this force that I have sought to track as it moved and shifted during the construction of hospital medicine in eighteenth-century London.

THE SETTING

Scholars have given the eighteenth century many labels to identify it as a period in the broad sweep of historical time. Every label has its champions and critics. This was, for instance, the Age of Enlightenment – but did England have an Enlightenment?[5] The Industrial Revolution, too, began in eighteenth-century England, but questions about where, when, and why continue to fuel discussion of this tendentious historical concept.[6] For the purposes of this book, I have eschewed these traps by following Roy Porter's sense of the "long" eighteenth century in England and Wales (and, to a certain extent, Scotland). This encompasses the decades between the Glorious Revolution of 1688 and the end of the wars with Napoleonic France in 1815. Although bounded by major political events, the long eighteenth century draws its thematic strengths from a wide variety of perspectives on economic, social, and intellectual history. I rely on this rich historiographical tradition because the medical world of eighteenth-century London was inextricably caught up in the gradual transformation of eco-

---

especially that by Bruno Latour (see his *Science in Action* and *Laboratory Life*), has developed and nuanced the ways that scientific knowledge becomes embedded – and unquestioned – in practice. I believe that historians of science and medicine have a great deal to gain from asking critical questions about the origin and continuity of "routine" knowledge and practice. We still do not understand the construction of the obvious, especially when "obvious" information and methods have continued into the present.

5 Roy Porter, "The Enlightenment in England," in *The Enlightenment in National Context,* ed. Roy Porter and Michael Teich (Cambridge: Cambridge University Press, 1981), 1–18; J. G. A. Pocock, "Clergy and Commerce: The Conservative Enlightenment in England," in *L'Età dei Lumi,* vol. 1 [Storia e Diritto, Studi 16] (Napoli: Jouene Editore, 1985), 525–62.

6 See, for example, J. Hoppitt, "Understanding the Industrial Revolution," *Historical Journal* 30 (1987): 211–24; A. E. Musson and Eric Robinson, *Science and Technology in the Industrial Revolution* (Manchester: Manchester University Press, 1969).

nomic conditions, social relationships, and ideas that made life in 1815 at once continuous with, and yet quite different from, life in 1688.[7]

Among the panoply of trends detailed in the literature on eighteenth-century England, three provide the overarching characterizations of English society and London culture most germane to my account of how hospital governors, medical practitioners, and pupils wrote and acted during the eighteenth century. First, English men and women participated in "the birth of a consumer society," part of the long story of the rise of capitalism and material prosperity.[8] The marketplace, where cash bought an increasing number of goods and services, from necessities to luxuries, crept into more and more aspects of metropolitan and provincial life. Banking, manufacturing, and trade expanded, sometimes within long-established structures and institutions, such as a few of the City of London's centuries-old guilds and companies, but more often in and around recent establishments, from major corporations, such as the Bank of England (1694), to small shops, like John Senex's London store for precision instruments (ca. 1706).[9] The catch-all operations of supply, demand, and market price which have become major explanatory forces for the dynamics of change during this century apply as well to the "medical marketplace."[10] People bought and sold medical goods, from drugs to books and

7 Roy Porter, *English Society in the Eighteenth Century*, 2nd. ed. (New York: Penguin Books, 1990); Roy Porter, "English Society in the Eighteenth Century Revisited," in *British Politics and Society from Walpole to Pitt 1742–1789*, ed. J. Black (New York: St. Martin's Press, 1990); Joanna Innes, "Jonathan Clark, Social History and England's 'Ancien Regime,' " *Past and Present* no. 115 (1987): 165–200; Jonathan Clark, "On Hitting the Buffers: The Historiography of England's Ancien Regime," *Past and Present* no. 117 (1987): 194–207.

8 Neil McKendrick, John Brewer, and J. H. Plumb, *The Birth of a Consumer Society: The Commercialization of Eighteenth-Century England* (Bloomington: Indiana University Press, 1982); John Brewer and Roy Porter, eds., *Consumption and the World of Goods* (London: Routledge, 1993).

9 Larry Stewart, *The Rise of Public Science: Rhetoric, Technology and Natural Philosophy in Newtonian Britain, 1660–1750* (Cambridge: Cambridge University Press, 1992), 173.

10 Dorothy Porter and Roy Porter, *Patient's Progress: Doctors and Doctoring in Eighteenth-Century England* (Stanford: Stanford University Press, 1989), and Roy Porter, *Health for Sale: Quackery in England, 1660–1850* (Manchester: Manchester University Press, 1989), provide a clear articulation of the marketplace model for medical practice in the eighteenth century. This model has increasingly appeared throughout the literature in the history of medicine (see, for example, Nancy Siraisi, *Medieval and Renaissance Medicine* [Chicago: University of Chicago Press, 1990]), primarily to emphasize the unregulated conditions of most medical practice in the past. Danger now lurks in seeing the "marketplace" everywhere, for it becomes a potent metaphor for other kinds of exchanges and values in social and medical relationships. Status, for example, or access to wealthy patients, or effective control over the laboring poor become the figurative commodities in high demand and obtaining them the marks of successful manipulation of the social market. Motives reduce to the social analogues of economic interests, and market-driven competition between individuals and groups the springs of action. Overuse of this metaphor already suggests that it needs to be revised and contained.

medical services, from a local woman's nursing care, to an elite physician's advice or a practitioner's course of lectures, as cash commodities.

Second, more and more English men and women belonged to the middling classes, the individuals and families living between the obviously poor, who lacked the land, movable goods, education, steady income and relative independence needed for security and respectability, and the gentry and aristocracy, who had the birth, marriages, manners, objects, and (usually) land on which to rest gentility and political power. The expansion of the middling ranks and literal marketplaces had gone hand in hand for centuries since middling sorts were the ones organizing the money, trade, and manufacturing that fueled the cycles of economic growth and contraction. While closely connected to material prosperity, the expansion of the middle classes in this century had as much to do with changing social relationships and values as with money to purchase goods and services. Social and cultural historians emphasize that the choices the middling sorts made to be secure, to belong to the "haves" rather than the "have-nots," led them to construct and conform to the rituals of a newly polite, urban-oriented society. They merged customs of the monied bourgeoisie, for example, the practical training of their sons in business and their daughters in housewifery, with the manners, education, and conspicuous consumption of the gentry and aristocracy.[11]

The search for upward mobility and the gradual formation of middle-class cultures, however, were by no means a process of slavish imitation and adaptation of elite values and styles. That is a major reason why the notion of a single middle class in the eighteenth century is such a slippery and untenable concept. The dynamics of social relationships constantly worked through exchanges of beliefs and opinions about appropriate behavior between groups and individuals for whom political patronage, family ties, religious faith, and other significant loyalties tempered economic distinctions and modified crude economic interests.[12] The funds that supported London's charity hospitals, for instance, paid for the buildings,

11 For detailed discussions of these generalizations, see Porter, *English Society,* and Penny Corfield, "Class by Name and Number in Eighteenth-Century Britain," *History* 72 (1987): 38–61; Peter Earle, *The Making of the English Middle Class: Business, Society and Family Life in London, 1660–1730* (London: Methuen, 1989); Nicholas Rogers, *Whigs and Cities: Popular Politics in the Age of Walpole and Pitt* (Oxford: Clarendon Press, 1989); Paul Langford, *A Polite and Commercial People: England, 1727–1783* (Oxford: Clarendon Press, 1989), and *Public Life and the Propertied Englishman, 1689–1798* (Oxford: Clarendon Press, 1991).

12 For recent discussions of "class" and social hierarchy in our understanding of eighteenth-century culture, see Corfield, "Class by Name and Number"; Jonathan Clark, *English Society 1688–1832* (Cambridge: Cambridge University Press, 1985); Innes, "Jonathan Clark"; Clark, "On Hitting the Buffers"; as well as the classic by E. P. Thompson, "Eighteenth-Century English Society: Class Struggle without Class," *Social History* 3 (1978): 133–65.

goods, and services intended to provide shelter and treatment for the deserving sick poor throughout the eighteenth century. Why people made charitable contributions, and what economic, social, or spiritual benefits they thought might accrue from their generosity varied considerably, however. The *display* of doing good united hospital donors, but their motives and goals arose from a range of values and social relationships.

The same point applies to notions of knowledge. Over the past two decades, scholars have probed the changing distinctions between patrician and plebeian beliefs, between the "polite" and the "vulgar" in social expressions and behaviors, and between "elite" and "popular" cultures in early modern society.[13] Baldly stated, in the conscious – or unconscious – search for ways to define their increasing status, the middling sorts put as much effort into distinguishing themselves from the lower orders as they did in adopting watered-down versions of elite life-styles to show their identification with the upper orders. Obtaining a patina of elite culture, of course, could help. But where most middling sorts had no hopes of actually joining elite circles, they had daily experience with the lower ones, in their servants, their work people, their neighbors, and even their relatives. The pervasive concern in eighteenth-century life to identify and to shun superstitions, irreligion, vulgar phrases, coarse manners, and offensive amusements belonged to the middle classes, not to the established elite or to the happily common, whose very ranks meant they could do pretty much what they pleased.

Seeing the social connotations associated with the display of certain kinds of knowledge has become a critical theme in the history of science, medicine, and health care. Patrick Curry, in his work on astrology, and Mary Fissell, in her discussions of popular medicine, for example, have persuasively argued that when the middle and upper classes rejected certain beliefs and practices they did so in part because common folk held them, not because they were inherently less rational or scientific than those the upper folk believed and applied.[14] Nearly all formally educated medical practitioners belonged to the middling sorts, from provincial surgeon–apothecaries to hospital physicians, as did many of their paying patients and pupils.[15] As these people collectively defined "good" medical knowledge and determined suitable ways to learn it, display it, and apply it, they

13 Porter, *English Society*; Peter Burke, *Popular Culture in Early Modern Europe* (London: Temple Smith, 1978); Mary Fissell, *Patients, Power and the Poor in Eighteenth Century Bristol* (Cambridge: Cambridge University Press, 1991); Patrick Curry, *Prophecy and Power: Astrology in Early Modern England* (Princeton, NJ: Princeton University Press, 1989).
14 Curry, *Prophecy and Power*, 109–117; Fissell, *Patients, Power and the Poor* and "Readers, Texts and Contexts: Vernacular Medical Works in Early Modern England," in *The Popularization of Medicine, 1650–1850*, ed. Roy Porter (London: Routledge, 1992), 72–96.
15 Irvine Loudon, *Medical Care and the General Practitioner: 1750–1850* (Oxford: Clarendon Press, 1986), esp. 100–25.

continuously reflected and responded to the changing mores of the middling ranks. In this sense, then, whether or not London's hospital practitioners taught pupils "better" medical theories and treatments, I believe that they certainly taught them securely middle-class medicine.

The third broad trend apparent in eighteenth-century England draws directly upon the expansion of the marketplace and the rise of the middle classes. Several historians have contended that, while printing with movable type heavily influenced scholarship, education, ideas, and ideologies in the sixteenth and seventeenth centuries, only in the eighteenth century did a print "culture" start to emerge in parts of Europe, London among them. Following the deliberate lapse of the Licensing Act in 1695, which had legalized censorship and restricted the number of presses in Britain, the printing trades took off. Texts, pamphlets, periodicals, and – most emblematic of the new urban life in this period – novels and newspapers, rolled off the presses in increasing numbers. Sold, circulated, and read, in private or out loud, relatively inexpensive and accessible printed materials extended what middling sorts could know, and when, and how.[16] Historians of the Enlightenment have long stressed that eighteenth-century men and women did not come up with hordes of brand-new ideas about politics, or social life, or the natural world that made them create revolutions in government or industry. Instead, they had more sweeping access to and debates over "old" ones, transforming classical and medieval concepts, such as "natural law," "equality," or the Galenic humors, into new ones, with different implications and applications.[17] Print in the eighteenth century created newly expanding public audiences, moving more information into the marketplace for that nameless and increasingly undefinable "reader."

The expansion of print culture undermined the status of oral traditions, the medium of common folk. As more and more people started to elevate the authority of the printed word over mere hearsay, they began to trust

16 Alvin Kernan, *Samuel Johnson and the Impact of Print* (Princeton, NJ: Princeton University Press, 1987), esp. chapters 2, 3, and 5; Terry Belanger, "Publishers and Writers in Eighteenth-Century England," in *Books and Their Readers in Eighteenth-Century England,* ed. Isabel Rivers (New York: St. Martin's Press, 1982), 5–26; Jon P. Klancher, *The Making of English Reading Audiences, 1790–1832* (Madison: University of Wisconsin Press, 1987), 3–17, provides a useful introduction to the making of literary audiences at the end of the eighteenth century.

17 The transformation of both Greco-Roman metaphysics and political ideologies in the seventeenth and eighteenth centuries into "modern" (revolutionary) forms has received extensive analysis. See, for example, Gary Hatfield, "Metaphysics and the New Science," in *Reappraisals of the Scientific Revolution,* ed. David C. Lindberg and Robert S. Westman (Cambridge: Cambridge University Press, 1990), 93–166; P. M. Heimann, "Voluntarism and Immanence: Conceptions of Nature in Eighteenth-Century Thought," *Journal of the History of Ideas* 39 (1978): 271–83; Isaac Kramnick, *Republican and Bourgeois Radicalism: Political Ideology in Late-Eighteenth-Century England and America* (Ithaca, NY: Cornell University Press, 1990), 71–98, 163–99.

universalized information over mere local wisdom. Samuel Johnson put together his marvelous *Dictionary* at midcentury, for instance, to instruct the literate in "polite" versus "vulgar" words, pinning down meanings and standards of usage for – whom else? – middling readers.[18] Medical authors prepared texts in English for practitioners, pupils, and patients, who proceeded to buy them for the same reasons – because in the context of a print culture the secrets and skills passed from a single master to his apprentice appeared as a liability, an overly narrow and personal basis for practice. The growth of the medical press, like the growth of the press in general, subtly shifted what counted as "good" knowledge, who made it, and where it could be found.

As primarily urban phenomena, all three of these sweeping changes shaped London. One of the largest cities in Europe, London, by demographers' estimates, consistently held about 10 percent of the population of England and Wales during the eighteenth century, with roughly 500,000 inhabitants in 1700 and close to a million in 1801. An even larger proportion (one-sixth, according to one historian's modest guess) experienced the metropolis during their lives, and a great many more received goods and news from the capital.[19] In the early eighteenth century, most of London's residents lived outside the City of London proper, the medieval town with its own charter, government, and remnants of fortifications, and outside the City of Westminster, the location of Parliament. Greater London had already expanded to connect these two areas, and in the eighteenth century it moved outward into neighboring villages and fields in Middlesex, Surrey, and Essex. It stretched along the Thames and the major roads that linked the capital to its provincial hinterlands.[20]

The Cities of London and Westminster provide contrasting symbols for greater London's significance as the nation's center of wealth, power, and influence. The City of London stood for commerce, for the center of trade and finance, with its manufacturing, banking, and monied companies that managed the circulating wealth of goods and credit. To the east of the City spread the docks and warehouses and warrens of the East End, housing merchant marines, lightermen, porters, and sea captains. In contrast, the City of Westminster represented national politics, landed wealth, and their appendages. Home to the House of Lords and the House of Commons, to several Royal residences and secondary Households, Westminster and its surrounding West End squares and streets were the Town and the Crown. The aristocracy, the gentry, and the country families resident during the social season from fall to spring lived there with the attorneys, tradespeo-

18 Kernan, *Samuel Johnson and the Impact of Print*, 152–203.
19 George Rudé, *Hanoverian London, 1714–1808* (London: Secker & Warburg, 1971), ix.
20 Rudé, *Hanoverian London*, 1–19; E. A. Wrigley, "A Simple Model of London's Importance in Changing English Society and Economy," *Past and Present* no. 37 (1967): 44–70.

ple, servants, day laborers, actors, and purveyors of virtuous entertainment and illicit pleasures the upper folk needed for comfort and amusement. Various areas and neighborhoods throughout the metropolis had particular reputations and status, in part due to concentrations of artisans, such as weavers in Spitalfields, in part stemming from the efforts of developers to create up-scale spots, such as the spacious arrangement of Hanover Square.[21]

A mecca for actors, artists, authors, and other people with belief in their talents and aspirations for fame, London had a considerable claim on the nation's cultural and professional riches. While Oxford and Cambridge, small towns housing England's illustrious universities, held pride of place for stuffy scholarship and occasional brilliance, serious, witty and pseudo intellectuals thrived in London's coffeehouses, clubs, societies, and dinner parties. The Royal Society of London, founded in 1662, was one of London's more formal institutions for learning and debate. It became a major literal and symbolic place for gatherings of men interested in the natural world.[22]

For medical practitioners, London also had three corporate groups that, in principle, provided sites for some medical instruction and technical conversation, along with supervision over metropolitan practice. The Worshipful Society of Apothecaries, the Barber–Surgeon's Corporation (to 1745), and its successor body, the Company of Surgeons (1745–1800), were City companies, akin to craft guilds. They registered their members' apprentices and saw to these young men's botanical excursions and attendance at anatomical demonstrations, respectively. The third group, the Royal College of Physicians, had been chartered by the Crown in the sixteenth century. In the eighteenth century, it was still a "college" in the Renaissance sense, a group of elite urban physicians who monitored entry into learned practice in the capital, not a place to educate aspiring physicians.

All of the other major cities that historians have scrutinized, such as Padua, Leiden, Vienna, Edinburgh, and Paris, had universities that dominated instruction of the medical elite, the learned physicians, and that passed judgments (whether anyone paid attention or not) on the training of the lower orders, the apothecaries and surgeons. Efforts to grasp how

21 A. L. Beier and Roger Finlay, eds. *The Making of the Metropolis, 1500–1700* (London and New York: Longman, 1986); Max Byrd, *London Transformed: Images of the City in the Eighteenth Century* (New Haven, CT: Yale University Press, 1978); Lawrence Stone, "The Residential Development of the West End of London in the Seventeenth Century," in *After the Reformation: Essays in Honor of J. H. Hexter*, ed. Barbara C. Malamente (Philadelphia: University of Pennsylvania Press, 1980), 167–212; L. D. Schwarz, "Social Class and Social Geography: The Middle Classes in London at the End of the Eighteenth Century," *Social History* 7 (1982): 167–85.
22 Porter, *English Society*, 161–2; Larry Stewart, *The Rise of Public Science*.

hospitals served as sites for clinical training in these cities have nearly always had an eye on when and how these institutions developed relationships with a university and its students and professors.[23] London provides a notable comparison and contrast: plenty of hospitals, but no university until the nineteenth century. No formally appointed professors, no set curricula, no public disputations of scholarly queries and theses, no degree-granting ceremonies cast their reminders of traditional academic medicine over London's medical circles.

London thus provides a remarkable case study of the formation of a medical community around decentralized hospital teaching. Over the course of the century, independent lecturers and hospital men in London devised alternate routes for acquiring "academic" medical knowledge and clinical experience. For run-of-the-mill eighteenth-century practitioners, peer approbation increasingly depended on having, supporting, or promoting certain kinds of medical theory, methods, and practice. Indeed, the university medical degree, apprenticeship indentures, or entry into physicians' colleges, surgeons' companies, or apothecaries' corporations obviously had had both social and occupational significance for centuries precisely because such public signals marked distinctive knowledge and experience. London's informal, ad hoc system of private lectures and hospital ward-walking, however, at once supplemented and subtly undermined university study and apprenticeship as sufficient ways to gain medical expertise. Accessible medical lectures, medical societies, and a prolific medical press generated a newly articulate rank and file. And, as both prominent and lowly practitioners participated in defining "good" knowledge and practice, they further constructed claims to medical authority based upon their specialized training in and around London's hospitals. Such claims were not new. But their ultimate success was.

TRANSFORMATIONS

Anyone writing on the history of Western medicine between 1750 and 1850 deals, in one way or another, with the initial transition from early modern to modern medicine. It is unavoidable. While early modern beliefs about health and disease, early modern patterns of practice, and early modern hierarchies of authority certainly carried on into the nineteenth and twentieth centuries, such older ideas and structures became the hangover

23 Guenter Risse, *Hospital Life in Enlightenment Scotland* (Cambridge: Cambridge University Press, 1986); Lisa Rosner, *Medical Education in the Age of Improvement* (Edinburgh: Edinburgh University Press, 1991); Laurence Brockliss, "Medical Teaching at the University of Paris," *Annals of Science* 35 (1978): 221–51; Erna Lesky, "The Development of Bedside Teaching at the Vienna Medical School from Scholastic Times to Special Clinics," in *The History of Medical Education,* ed. Charles D. O'Malley (Berkeley: University of California Press, 1970), 217–34.

effects of the past, increasingly connected to uneducated lay knowledge, unreformed professional behavior, and ongoing inequities in social and economic status. Developments in the biological and physical sciences, especially through experimental methods in physiology, pharmacology, and chemistry, constructed modern scientific medicine hand in hand with the gradual emergence of these modern sciences themselves in the later eighteenth century. Technological inventions extended practitioners' diagnostic, conceptual, and therapeutic access to disease in patients' living bodies. The stethoscope (1816), for instance, is the quintessential symbol of practitioners' ability to discern what was previously hidden. During the late eighteenth and early nineteenth centuries, surgeons and physicians expanded their activities within hospitals, embedding medical training and clinical investigations in these institutions. Inside and outside hospitals and nascent laboratories, medical practitioners sought to reform standards for education and training and demanded the umbrella of state authority for increasing collective autonomy. Such changes are the standard fare of surveys in the history of Western medicine, and for good reason – they happened.[24] Precisely how, why, where, and when these changes occurred, and with what immediate and gradual effects on medical knowledge, care, and power, however, have spurred much research and debate.

Historians have agreed for quite some time that central conceptual and institutional changes first took place – at least most clearly and most decisively – in Paris between the 1780s and 1830s, not in Leiden or Vienna, nor in Edinburgh or London. In Paris during the late eighteenth and early nineteenth centuries, the old medicine of classical texts, of a language of symptoms and humors, and of complex individualism finally started to lose its persuasive power to describe and to account for most sicknesses. The old methods of formal clinical instruction and interpretation, in which physicians merely used a handful of patients to illustrate the intersection of constitutions, illnesses, the environment and therapies, ultimately became seen as sterile demonstrations of traditional rituals. On the cusp of the nineteenth century, French medical authors wrote about illnesses and death in new ways, embedding disease in the body's organs and, with a newly powerful vocabulary of localization, in tissues. Hospitals, with ward after ward of the sick and dying, became central medical institutions for physicians and their students to probe the unknown.[25]

24 Richard Shryock, *The Development of Modern Medicine: An Interpretation of the Social and Scientific Factors Involved* (Madison: University of Wisconsin Press, 1974), 57–78, 151–210; Erwin Ackerknecht, *A Short History of Medicine* (Baltimore: Johns Hopkins University Press, 1982).
25 Shryock, *Modern Medicine*, 151; Ivan Waddington, "The Role of the Hospital in the Development of Modern Medicine: A Sociological Analysis," *Sociology* 7 (1973): 211–5; Charles Rosenberg, *The Care of Strangers: The Rise of America's Hospital System* (New York: Basic Books, 1987), 82–5; See also: Malcolm Nicolson, "The Introduction of

Two of the core texts firmly establishing that modern medicine started in Paris came from scholars with radically different agendas in the 1960s. Michel Foucault's *La Naissance de la Clinique* (1963, 2nd ed. 1972) marks one of the philosopher's early forays into understanding medicine as a system of power constituted by, and deployed within, certain kinds of knowledge about the body. His analysis displayed contemporary concern over the deep structures of human thought, over the relationships among language, experience, and epistemology that literally and metaphorically allowed certain things to be known and other things to remain unknowable.[26] His later work on prisons and sexuality extended this profound critique of the ways that knowledge and power intimately intersect and has offered scholars in many fields a model and a language for theorizing and debating relationships between control and modernity.[27] In decided contrast, Erwin Ackerknecht, in his *Medicine at the Paris Hospital 1794–1848* (1967), situated the birth of the "new" medicine within the "political and technological revolution" in France after 1789.[28] A more conventional historian, Ackerknecht argued that the political and social changes associated with the French Revolution underlay the fundamental philosophical and intellectual transformation in medicine that allowed it finally to put neo-Hippocratism and Galenism aside.

Despite their quite different aims and interpretations, Foucault, in his vision of the "birth of the clinic," and Ackerknecht, in his invention of "hospital medicine," focus on the same shift in medical methods and concepts. For both, as for scholars before and after their seminal works, modern medicine meant the new epistemological foundations for clinical study and teaching that the Paris hospitals made possible. It was in these institutions that medical men of science discovered a numerous and sequestered population of the sick poor whose illnesses they watched, whose treatments they controlled, whose bodies they autopsied, and whose cases they counted. In the Paris hospitals, physicians correlated pathological anatomy with clinical symptoms and subtle signs elicited through touch and internal sounds, as well as by vision and verbal interrogation. By the 1820s, they had begun to count cases, revitalizing the use of numerical methods as clinical tools. Champions of the new science of clinical medi-

Percussion and Stethoscopy to Early Nineteenth-Century Edinburgh," in *Medicine and the Five Senses*, William Bynum and Roy Porter, ed. (Cambridge: Cambridge University Press, 1993), 134–5; Fissell, *Patients, Power and the Poor*; Risse, *Hospital Life*; John Harley Warner, *The Therapeutic Perspective: Medical Practice, Knowledge and Identity in America, 1820–1885* (Cambridge, MA: Harvard University Press, 1986).

26 Michel Foucault, *The Birth of the Clinic: An Archeology of Medical Perception*, trans. A. M. Sheridan Smith (New York: Pantheon Books, 1975).

27 Patricia O'Brien, "Michel Foucault's History of Culture," in *The New Cultural History*, ed. Lynn Hunt (Berkeley: University of California Press, 1989), 25–46.

28 Erwin Ackerknecht, *Medicine at the Paris Hospital 1794–1848* (Baltimore: The Johns Hopkins University Press, 1967), xi, 3–58.

cine increasingly detached disease from what the patient experienced to what the practitioner knew was hidden in the patient's body, encoded in physical signs and producing specific symptoms. And students flocked to the Paris hospitals to learn these new methods and concepts through their own experience of hospital patients and cadavers.[29]

"Paris medicine" and "the clinic" have served long and well as symbolic moments for the expansion of objectification, standardization, and quantification central to modern medicine. Indeed, "Paris medicine" has taken on such stature in the history of medicine that the changes in medical perceptions and power ascribed to its physicians have recently spurred a wave of much needed revisionism.[30] Some scholars have contested the centrality of Paris as *the* site for both the new clinicoanatomical method and the new numerical approach to case histories.[31] More importantly, trying to unpack the meaning of Paris medicine has stimulated questions about just what it meant to localize disease in the body, about just what went on in hospitals that allowed practitioners to gain seemingly boundless power over patients and their corpses, and about the enormous attraction that the French capital had for medical students.[32] What happened to medical perceptions in Paris between the 1780s and 1820s clearly raises important questions about medi-

29 Russell Maulitz, *Morbid Appearances: The Anatomy of Pathology in the Early Nineteenth Century* (New York: Cambridge University Press, 1987). Maulitz has a detailed and sophisticated discussion of these points; see his work, and his notes, for references to the extensive literature on the clinicoanatomical method and the Paris hospitals.

30 Caroline Hannaway and Ann LaBerge, "Reinterpreting Paris Medicine," unpublished plenary session paper, American Association for the History of Medicine meeting, 14 May 1993.

31 Othmar Keel, "The Politics of Health and the Institutionalisation of Clinical Practices in Europe in the Second Half of the Eighteenth Century," in *William Hunter and the Eighteenth Century Medical World,* ed. Bynum and Porter, 207–58; Othmar Keel, "John Hunter et Xavier Bichat: les rapports de leurs travaux en pathologie tissulaire," *Actas XXVII Congreso Internacional de Historia de la Medicina* (Barcelona: Acadèmia de ciències Mèdiques, 1981), 535–49; Ulrich Tröhler, "Quantification in British Medicine and Surgery, 1750–1830, with Special Reference to Its Introduction into Therapeutics," Ph.D. dissertation, University of London, 1978; Andrea Rusnock, "The Quantification of Things Human: Medicine and Political Arithmetic in Enlightenment England and France," Ph.D. dissertation, Princeton University, 1990.

32 Toby Gelfand, *Professionalizing Modern Medicine: Paris Surgeons and Medical Science and Institutions in the 18th Century* (Westport, CT: Greenwood Press, 1980); idem, "Gestation of the Clinic," *Medical History* 25 (1981): 169–80; Karl M. Figlio, "The Metaphor of Organization: An Historiographical Perspective on the Bio-Medical Sciences of the Early Nineteenth Century," *History of Science* 14 (1976): 17–53; Pauline Mazumdar, "Anatomical Physiology and the Reform of Medical Education," *Bulletin of the History of Medicine* 57 (1983): 230–46; Stephen J. Cross, "John Hunter, the Animal Economy, and Late Eighteenth Century Physiological Discourse," *Studies in History of Biology* 5 (1981): 1–110; Geoffrey Sutton, "The Physical and Chemical Path to Vitalism: Xavier Bichat's Physiological Researches on Life and Death," *Bulletin of the History of Medicine* 58 (1984): 53–71; Colin Jones, *The Charitable Imperative: Hospitals and Nursing in Ancien Régime and Revolutionary France* (London: Routledge, 1989); Maulitz, *Morbid Appearances,* 134–60; John Harley Warner, "Remembering Paris: Memory and the American Disciples of French Medicine in the 19th Century," *Bulletin of the History of Medicine* 65 (1991): 301–25.

cal ideas in London, but Parisian physicians did not simply set unproblematic standards which Londoners somehow failed to meet. In order to assess the deep connections between changes in medical perceptions and the articulation of certain kinds of medical knowledge, in Paris or elsewhere, scholars must scrutinize the ways that medical men interacted with each other, with their patients, and with their students.

While much remains to be done to understand these elements in the shift to modern medicine, considerable scholarship on the medical professions in Britain has laid a foundation for investigating these relationships, especially because this material highlights the constant tension between quite different sources of medical authority. Until fairly recently, a good deal of the work on eighteenth-century British medicine evinced a respectful preoccupation with great men, great ideas, and unproblematic descriptions of progress. In this literature, scholars more or less assumed that the modern medical profession ultimately gained power to direct education, licensing, and practice because medical science finally started to get things right, at which point professional authority obviously became appropriate. In the 1970s, however, a flurry of interest in the history of professionalization in medicine inspired a series of sociological–historical works that dealt in part with the late-eighteenth- and early-nineteenth-century movements for medical reform in England and Wales. A rich pamphlet literature, numerous failed Parliamentary Bills, a Select Committee on Medical Education (1834), and, finally, the Medical Act of 1858 all seemed to beg for analysis of practitioners' strategies to control their own work and standards, excluding the unqualified from treating the sick, well before medical science started to work its miracles on diagnosis, prognosis, rational therapy, and surgical interventions.[33]

In the past ten years, historians have eloquently pointed out that exposing the roots of a "profession" in early modern England misrepresents contemporary expectations about medical occupations and medical practice. Margaret Pelling, Irvine Loudon, and Roy Porter, among others, have sensibly replaced the search for nascent professions with a richer historical vision of a range of medical practitioners operating in a nearly unregulated marketplace for medical services. Eighteenth-century medical occupations make a great deal more sense when placed along a spectrum from local healers and shopkeepers to carriage-owning surgeons and university-educated physicians, from "irregulars" to "regulars." Roughly

---

33 Charles Newman, *The Evolution of Medical Education in the Nineteenth Century* (London, New York: Oxford University Press, 1957); Bernice Hamilton, "The Medical Professions in the Eighteenth Century," *Economic History Review*, 2nd ser., 4 (1951): 141–69; Eliot Friedson, *Profession of Medicine* (New York: Dodd, Mead, 1972); Noel Parry and José Parry, *The Rise of the Medical Profession* (London: Croom Helm, 1976); M. Jeanne Peterson, *The Medical Profession in Mid-Victorian London* (Berkeley: University of California Press, 1978).

defining "regular" practitioners as those who sought formal training through apprenticeship or university study and tried to make a living from practice, and "irregulars" as those who picked up medical knowledge through ad hoc experience and attended the sick alongside their other occupations and avocations, emphasizes the fluid boundaries between these groups. In London, as in other cities with separate corporate bodies for physicians, surgeons, and apothecaries, members tended to rally around their colleagues primarily to battle with other medical occupations, while competing – publicly and sometimes nastily – with their corporate brethren.[34] Among the regulars, then, the strength of collective agreement about good medical knowledge and techniques varied according to who attacked whom, a vital point to remember when seeking hints of nascent professional solidarity.

Ill people up and down the social scale treated themselves, consulted quacks, or went to formally licensed surgeons and physicians, with fine disregard for notions of "professional" standards. Elite patients, as Nicholas Jewson argued in 1974, not only had the power to choose whatever practitioner suited their own notions of appropriate medical knowledge, care, and polite behavior, but in the process literally shaped that knowledge by expecting that a practitioner's theories and treatment conform to their own views of disease, health and nature.[35] Generalizing this insight to other groups and other cultural values in the marketplace suggests that gender, family connections, political views, religious beliefs, neighborhood mores, along with a patient's education and desperation, were all elements shaping medical authority in any particular clinical encounter. Yet a practitioner's influence over patients – or lack of it – must not be conflated with his or her influence *among* practitioners. How, when, and why lay people, whether as patients, hospital governors or Members of Parliament, accepted various practitioners' claims for expertise are thus slightly different problems from how, when, and why such claims were grounded in specific kinds of knowledge among practitioners. Different, but not distinct: practitioners relied heavily on broader cultural and intellectual criteria for producing acceptable evidence and arguments on issues of contemporary medical concern; lay people did look for signs of peer-approved expertise when accepting medical care.

34 For discussion of professional rivalries and disputes, see David Harley, "Honour and Property: The Structure of Professional Disputes in Eighteenth-Century English Medicine," in *The Medical Enlightenment of the Eighteenth Century*, ed. Andrew Cunningham and Roger French (Cambridge: Cambridge University Press, 1990), 138–64; Harold J. Cook, *The Decline of the Old Medical Regime in Stuart London* (Ithaca, NY: Cornell University Press, 1986).
35 Margaret Pelling, "Medical Practice: Trade or Profession?" in *Professions in Early Modern England*, ed. W. Prest (London: Croom Helm, 1987), 90–128; Irvine Loudon, *Medical Care*; Porter, *Health for Sale*; Nicholas Jewson, "Medical Knowledge and the Patronage System in Eighteenth-Century England," *Sociology* 8 (1974): 369–85.

The recent focus on fragmentation, individual competition, and intra-occupational rivalries has served as a vital corrective to stories of the march toward professionalization. Now that historians have firmly established the blurry lines between regulars and irregulars, and have revealed the force of individual practitioners' self-interest as a check on occupational loyalty, however, I return attention to the formation of a medical community in eighteenth-century London.[36] In some respects, my interest harks back to that earlier search for the modern medical profession, in that I discuss the ways that practitioners sought legitimacy through collective claims to have good knowledge. This is the same old struggle at the core of defining a profession – how to separate the insiders from the outsiders according to the insiders' criteria and through the insiders' autonomous control. Yet, instead of looking at the overt movements for professional power, seen when medical men took up reforming activism within and against the traditional medical corporations, I concentrate on the underlying trends creating shared medical identities and values.[37]

In my view, scholars still underestimate the significance of medical education in shaping appropriate professional behavior as well as in conveying a body of knowledge and a set of therapeutic practices. Medical education in eighteenth-century London blended the apothecary's, surgeon's, and physician's expertise into a body of core knowledge and a single set of practices for the de facto general practitioner. This shared knowledge included anatomy, surgery, pharmacy, and physic and was the basis for the demarcation of the regular surgeon–apothecary–man-midwife from the uneducated irregular. It was visibly expressed and affirmed from the 1770s, when practitioners participated in medical societies and wrote for medical journals. These societies and journals, in turn, offered alternate intellectual outlets for medical men from those aimed at the generally literate and educated, such as *Gentleman's Magazine,* the *Philosophical Transactions of the Royal Society,* and even many medical monographs. As medical men offered their ideas and experiences primarily to their peers, they began the process of claiming autonomy for their medical practice, distinct from the

---

36 Hilary Marland, *Medicine and Society in Wakefield and Huddersfield, 1780–1870* (Cambridge: Cambridge University Press, 1987); Ian Inkster, "Marginal Men: Aspects of the Social Role of the Medical Community in Sheffield, 1790–1850," in *Health Care and Popular Medicine in Nineteenth Century England,* ed. John Woodward and David Richards (New York: Holmes and Meier, 1977), 128–63.

37 I am indebted to much recent work on the ways that ideas of medical "identity" intersect with cultural values and claims to specialized knowledge. See, in particular: Harold J. Cook, "Good Advice and Little Medicine: The Professional Authority of Early Modern English Physicians," *Journal of British Studies* 33 (1994): 1–31; John Harley Warner, "The Fall and Rise of Professional Mystery: Epistemology, Authority and the Emergence of Laboratory Medicine in Nineteenth Century America," in *The Laboratory Revolution in Medicine,* ed. Andrew Cunningham and Perry Williams (Cambridge: Cambridge University Press, 1992), 110–41.

views of patients, irregular competitors, and past practitioners. Turning to other medical men for approval of medical methods and theories created the possibility for professional reputations separate from those defined by successful practice among the socially respectable or by acceptance among natural philosophers and natural historians.

Whether medical men in 1815 belonged to a "profession" more than did those in 1700 is still a moot point, one bound to raise more questions about what defines a profession than to help us appreciate how differently practitioners behaved after a century of changes in urban medical culture. Hence, while I often use "occupation" as a term less loaded with possible dispute than "profession," the latter word still serves to evoke an occupation surrounded by a set of beliefs about knowledge and practice dear to those trying to exclude outsiders, and having some success with it. By exploring the relationships between the individualized medical marketplace and the development of a medical community, I balance the sorts of claims that medical men made about themselves, their work, and their knowledge with what other evidence suggests that they actually did, or could do.

It was one thing for certain eighteenth-century medical men to *say* they had new knowledge or better methods, but quite another to have other practitioners, pupils, or patients pay any attention to them. That pupils, practitioners, and at least some patients increasingly followed what hospital physicians and surgeons in London said and did returns me to the medical institution that has figured prominently in both the Paris model and discussions of professionalization in Britain. The eighteenth- and early-nineteenth-century hospital was at once a concrete place, full of pain, death, and human struggle, and an ongoing metaphor for transformations in practitioners' ability to understand disease and to deal with it. I believe that these meanings are inseparable.

HOSPITAL MEDICINE

As long as there have been hospitals, specific structures devoted to treating sick people who resided in them during periods of illness or injury, there has been hospital medicine. But it looked rather different in the sixth, twelfth, fifteenth, and eighteenth centuries, as the cultural expectations and rituals concerning care, appropriate healers, and authority varied across time and space. In broad terms, I see "hospital medicine" as a set of relationships among people, institutions, and knowledge. During the eighteenth century, as I argue from different perspectives throughout this book, the relationships between science and medicine, between social context and cultural change, between practitioners and hospital governors, and between practitioners and their patients all constructed hospital medicine. Throughout the century, hospital relationships were always as concerned with morality as they were with efficient or effective medical practice; with practitioners' social status as much as their science; and with patients' role as objects of charity as much as their role as possible objects for clinical observation. The hospital medicine emerging in the early-nineteenth century was a culmination of ongoing relationships through which medical men established control over their work and their patients, and by which they gained the authority to define "good" knowledge coming to – and from – institutional bedsides.

My conceptualization of hospital medicine as a network of relationships both grows out of and contributes to much recent work on the history and anthropology of science, especially that by Steven Shapin, Simon Schaffer, Jan Golinski, and Bruno Latour.[38] These scholars have stressed that "science" is what "scientists" *do*, not an abstract body of knowledge separate from those who create it, use it, and pass it on to others. These scholars' thoughtful analyses of texts in the history of science, moreover, have demonstrated the ways that language and rhetorical style worked in the past to establish an author's credibility.[39] I have adopted both of these perspectives. Hospital men, their pupils, and their colleagues constructed medical knowledge in the eighteenth century through their behavior, what they said about health and disease, and what they wrote about themselves. By practicing, teaching, experimenting, and writing, they engaged in a never-ending process of making and deploying knowledge through personal experience, observations, and interpretations.

The hospital men interested in "advancing" medical knowledge regularly used the assumptions and styles of contemporary science to guide their

38 Joseph Rouse, "What Are Cultural Studies of Scientific Knowledge?" *Configurations* 1 (1992): 1–22; Steven Shapin, "Discipline and Bounding: The History and Sociology of Science as Seen Through the Externalism–Internalism Debate," *History of Science* 30 (1992): 333–69; Steven Shapin and Simon Schaffer, *Leviathan and the Air-Pump: Hobbes, Boyle, and the Experimental Life* (Princeton, NJ: Princeton University Press, 1985); Steven Shapin, "The House of Experiment in Seventeenth Century England," *Isis* 79 (1988): 373–404; Jan Golinski, *Science as Public Culture: Chemistry and Enlightenment in Britain, 1760–1820* (Cambridge: Cambridge University Press, 1992); Bruno Latour, *Science in Action: How to Follow Scientists and Engineers Through Society* (Milton Keynes, UK: Open University Press, 1987); Adrian Desmond, *The Politics of Evolution: Morphology, Medicine and Reform in Radical London* (Chicago: University of Chicago Press, 1989); Kathryn M. Hunter, *Doctors' Stories: The Narrative Structure of Medical Knowledge* (Princeton, NJ: Princeton University Press, 1991).

39 Peter Dear, ed., *The Literary Structure of Scientific Argument* (Philadelphia: University of Pennsylvania Press, 1991); Peter Dear, " 'Totius in Verba': Rhetoric and Authority in the Early Royal Society," *Isis* 76 (1985): 145–61; Andrew E. Benjamin, Geoffrey Cantor, and John R. R. Christie, eds., *The Figural and the Literal: Problems of Language in the History of Science and Philosophy: 1630–1800* (Manchester: Manchester University Press, 1987); Marcello Pera and William R. Shea, eds., *Persuading Science: The Art of Scientific Rhetoric* (Canton, MA: Science History Publications, 1991); Hunt, *The New Cultural History*. The role of language in the construction of knowledge itself has a vast literature. I have been particularly stimulated by George Lakoff, *Women, Fire and Dangerous Things: What Categories Reveal about the Mind* (Chicago: University of Chicago Press, 1987).

questions, methods, and interpretations. They chose to adopt and extend what I call "safe" science, with "safe" serving as a potent metaphor for ways to think about and to practice inquiries into nature that conformed to the cultural sensibilities of the lay elite. Hospital physicians and surgeons, already part of the medical elite at the beginning of the eighteenth century in London, were among those who conveyed "safe" science from gentlemanly circles – especially the Royal Society – to ordinary medical men through their lecturing, hospital practice, and writing. As elite interest in science changed – with the emergence of a new chemistry at the end of the eighteenth century, for instance – so too did hospital men's research projects. They shaped both what passed for routine, unproblematic knowledge and, as important, what counted as appropriate ways to approach new questions. Thus, in order for hospital men to establish themselves as a professional elite in the second half of the eighteenth century, they had to construct new medical ideas and methods all the while paying careful attention to the nuances of knowledge in lay society.

I do not wish to imply that hospital men were merely following the whims of fashionable knowledge and cynically imitating the latest in scientific and political opinions. Quite the contrary: from their perspective hospital physicians and surgeons behaved with sensible circumspection and dignity. Caution about the word "experiment" when applied to clinical experience, for example, displayed elite practitioners' concern to balance appropriate conservatism in practice – one does *not* experiment on patients – with a properly innovative spirit – one *does* experiment judiciously on patients – or else how would medicine advance? Hospital men negotiated this tension quite carefully, deploying a rhetoric of "observation" and "judgment" that supported their status as men of good character as well as good science.

At a deeper level, I argue that hospital men practiced safe science by avoiding explicit comment on ideas about nature – such as materialism – that challenged contemporary orthodoxy. They participated in the ongoing construction of the belief that "good" science was apparently impartial accounts of matters of fact perceived and discussed by the right people with the right training in the right places, with "right" defined, in turn, within their own networks, lecture rooms, and ward rounds. Those who published case accounts, autopsy observations, or reports on experiments promoted a descriptive, understated style that implicitly denied – by omission – that such knowledge rested upon any social, moral, or metaphysical assumptions open to debate or dispute. The power of their work rested, indeed, not on what they said about how to do science or how to reach responsible interpretations of phenomena in the abstract, since they mostly avoided any such conscious introspection, but how they practiced and wrote about science for lay and medical audiences. In the process of doing safe science hospital men participated in making science the sine qua non of neutral knowledge: objective, undisputable, effective, and, ultimately, modern. And they took this sense of detached, benign science into the hospitals, reinforcing the gradual shift from individual narratives of illness to dry, dispassionate clinical accounts, where descriptions of patients sound more and more like reports of laboratory experiments.

Doing medicine in a hospital did not make it hospital medicine; nor was hospital medicine practiced only in hospitals. Hospitals are never self-contained worlds. On the one hand, since the care, therapies, and social relationships between practitioners and patients in a hospital replicated those outside it, historians need to be cautious about presuming that an institution's walls necessarily created special conditions within them. On the other hand, when hospital practitioners and pupils took the knowledge and experience acquired on the wards to meetings of the Royal Society or the Medical Society of London, to medical lectures, to their private patients, or to their writing tables when composing case notes, articles, and books, they constructed hospital medicine for many different audiences well away from the wards. Hospitals thus provided specific sites where interactions occurred, where relationships formed, and where people localized knowledge, without meaning that any particular set of experiences, beliefs, or behavior belonged only to these institutions. I see hospitals as a focus for change in eighteenth-century medicine, then, not simply because their structures, rules, and rituals presented opportunities for new relationships among practitioners, pupils, and patients, but because those practitioners and pupils wrote about hospitals as significant places for clinical consultations, observations, and training. The value of knowledge gained from texts, from apprenticeship or university study remained – but the belief that following only these routes gave a medical man sufficient expertise declined.

I distinguish investigations into what Guenter Risse called "hospital life" from explorations, like this one, into what pupils and practitioners made of their hospital work.[40] Reconstructing a hospital's nosology, epidemiology, and treatment protocols, as Risse has through his examination of clinical case notes from the Infirmary in Edinburgh, highlights the patterns of disease among the poor admitted into the institution and hospital practitioners' responses.[41] My aim, in contrast, has been to tease out the range

40 For work on the patient's point of view in general, see Roy Porter, ed., *Patients and Practitioners: Lay Perceptions of Medicine in Pre-Industrial Society* (Cambridge: Cambridge University Press, 1985); for eighteenth-century hospital experiences in particular, see Mary Fissell, *Patients, Power and the Poor*, 148–70.
41 Guenter Risse, *Hospital Life*; Guenter Risse and John Harley Warner, "Reconstructing Clinical Activities: Patient Records in Medical History," *Social History of Medicine* 5 (1992): 183–205.

of interactions among patients, pupils, and practitioners on the wards; to illuminate the processes involved in connecting abstract medical ideas to bedside observations, apart from what ailed a sick person and what practitioners did about it. Few manuscript clinical notes for London's hospital patients exist, yet practitioners' published accounts of hospital medicine provide valuable information for understanding the cultural meaning of these clinical encounters. Practitioners' case histories and commentaries, written for various purposes and audiences, reveal medical men's assumptions and priorities about what they needed to remember and how they needed to argue, whatever the "real" experiences of diseases and injuries were on the wards. For outsiders, be they provincial apothecaries or twentieth-century historians, the relationships constituting hospital medicine were both made, and made visible, primarily when those involved in it wrote about them.

During the eighteenth century, hospital medicine became, in a fundamental sense that my book explores, *public* medicine.[42] While I shall explore the complex relationships between "public" and "private" in the following chapters, my basic point is quite straightforward: lots of people with no emotional or familial connection to the sick – pupils, practitioners, governors, other patients – all observed them on the wards, talked about them, and wrote about them. People saw what hospital physicians, surgeons, other pupils, other staff, other patients did, and they heard what they said. Others, in medical lectures and during meetings of medical societies, heard about the hospital sick and their treatment. Still others read about these experiences in medical journals and monographs. Of course "private" patients, the ones seen in the intimacy of their homes, among their relatives and friends, perhaps with an apprentice at hand, or subjected to consultations of various practitioners, also had multiple observers. They, too, had accounts of their conditions gossiped about, discussed at medical meetings, and written up for others to read. But the hospital provided an arena for witnessed interactions – especially through the expansion of ward-walking – that constantly opened up to inspection the connections among illness, interpretations, and elite practitioners' behavior. Here, pupils and other practitioners regularly saw staff men deploying their authority over knowledge and interacting with each other.

These senses of public and private resonate, moreover, with the gender divisions of work and power in early modern and modern British society. While sometimes critiqued as overly simplistic, the dichotomy between

---

42 Historians of science have explored the idea of "public" knowledge in the early modern period. See, in particular, William Eamon, "From the Secrets of Nature to Public Knowledge: The Origins of the Concept of Openness in Science," *Minerva* 23 (1985): 321–47; Golinski, *Science as Public Culture*; Stewart, *The Rise of Public Science*.

men's ability to act in public spaces and middle-class women's increasing confinement to the home in the eighteenth and nineteenth centuries applies to London's hospital world. Throughout the entire period covered in my analysis, hospital physicians and surgeons, their lecturing colleagues, and their fellow medical society members were men. So too were the vast majority of their pupils, with a few exceptions of female pupils studying midwifery at midcentury.[43] Within the hospitals, women served as matrons, which were respectable positions for middle-aged widows, and as nurses, laundresses, and other hospital servants drawn from the lower orders. Ladies donated money to some of these charities, and hence held governors' privileges to recommend patients, but did not attend hospital meetings. Women on the wards, in short, were poor patients, or patients' relatives and friends, or equally marginal servants. The hospital medicine constructed during the eighteenth century excluded women from ward-walking – the means to becoming well-educated regular medical practitioners – even though women still trained as midwives through apprenticeship. This process both reflected and augmented the larger social movements that restricted educated women's paid work.[44] Public hospital medicine thus contrasted overtly with private domestic medicine, in a way that reinforced the dominant place of male practitioners as those in charge not only of what happened to the sick and injured, but also of how that experience appeared in the medical literature.

I use the "public" notion of hospital practice, furthermore, to ground the relationships between physicians and surgeons that underlay the ways they understood disease, practiced medicine, and investigated both clinical and scientific problems over the course of the century. Certainly elite physicians and surgeons consulted on private patients, taking their own theoretical perspectives to the bedsides of the well-to-do. In the hospitals, however, the basic organization of these charitable institutions *required* that physicians and surgeons regularly consult with one another, from the initial moment when they decided whether a new patient was a medical or surgical case, to routine conversations about patients whose problems blurred the usual demarcations between internal and external conditions. In fulfilling their public duties, physicians and surgeons constantly negotiated the boundaries between their areas of expertise. Physicians often expe-

43 Only the Middlesex Hospital records contain references to female pupils, and then only in connection with the lying-in ward. No female pupils appear in any of the formal pupil registers of the eighteenth-century general hospitals in London. Middlesex Hospital, Minutes of the Weekly Board, Court of Governors, 17 Apr. 1770, 5 Nov. 1771.
44 Earle, *The Making of the English Middle Class*, 158–74; Porter, *English Society*, 22–34, 84; Porter and Porter, *Patient's Progress*, 173–85; Leonore Davidoff and Catherine Hall, *Family Fortunes: Men and Women of the English Middle Class, 1780–1850* (Chicago: University of Chicago Press, 1987).

rienced the "surgical point of view" at work in these encounters, and, just
as significantly, surgeons experienced the physicians' points of view on
how to conceptualize and to treat internal disorders. While watching each
other week after week, staff men thus shaped a hospital medicine that drew
their basic physiological and pathological principles together for a broad
notion of "medicine" encompassing both physic and surgery.

At the very same time, however, hospital staff men reinscribed the
differing ways that physicians and surgeons practiced both on the wards
and among their well-to-do private patients. As much as they constructed
shared concepts, they strove to maintain the distinctions between their
areas of expertise because these were vital for elite practice. Elite physicians
did not *do* surgery; elite surgeons – with some important qualifications that
I discuss in later chapters – did not do physic. They held to their separate
spheres not only while making their daily clinical rounds and consultations,
but also when they took up investigative projects in the medical sciences.
Physicians did chemistry, which had traditional connections to learned
medicine, because it enhanced their mastery of the language and processes
of internal constitutional disorders. Surgeons pursued questions in anatomy, morbid anatomy, and experimental physiology because these areas
displayed their mastery of anatomical language and surgical skills.

Hospital men's dual public roles – blurring the conceptual distinctions
between physic and surgery while holding on to the differences between
elite physicians and surgeons – transformed the traditional hierarchy of
London's medical occupations (physicians, surgeons, and apothecaries) into
the modern hierarchy of hospital consultants and general practitioners.
Pupils attending ward rounds, listening to hospital lectures, and reading
the medical literature learned that they shared a fundamental body of
knowledge with their hospital teachers, knowledge that drew them all into
a common medical community. But common knowledge did not confer
equal status, either within the medical community among other practitioners or outside it among paying patients. Hospital physicians and
surgeons, by absorbing and displaying behavior appropriate to the traditional elites at clinical bedsides and when doing research, subtly converted
older forms of social and intellectual dominance into modern professional
authority.

Teaching, especially public hospital teaching, was central to the construction of hospital knowledge. Hospitals had been used for training
medical men ever since London surgeons took their apprentices with them
into the wards, probably from the foundation of St. Thomas's and St.
Bartholomew's in the twelfth century. On the Continent, a few university
physicians had used carefully chosen hospital patients to demonstrate disease since at least the sixteenth century, a practice that a few London

physicians may have offered informally in the seventeenth century.[45] Ward teaching changed dramatically in the eighteenth century, however, when the pupils who entered the London hospitals ceased needing personal connections to hospital staff and instead paid to spend a few months or a year walking through the wards observing all sorts of the sick and injured. At the same time, the number of ward-walking pupils increased considerably.[46] Both the detachment from a single mentor's supervision and the increasing number of pupils meant that a few individual pupils became groups of students, collections of men always present during rounds but with ever-changing faces.

Ward teaching first opened charity patients to medical inspection for purposes other than their basic care and individual treatment. The gradual, sometimes almost imperceptible process by which the hospital patients became teaching objects to men passing through the wards altered the charitable relationships among patrons, practitioners, and the poor. To the poor person's duty to behave properly in the hospital, to follow its rules for decorum and piety, hospital staff men added the obligation to let his or her symptoms, verbal accounts, and interactions with drugs and operations instruct practitioners whom she or he might never see again. This new obligation, it seems to me, was not about poor patients' becoming depersonalized objects – they already were the objects of charity, incarnate lessons in social goodness and moral renewal, for hospital visitors to observe and interrogate. But it nevertheless made a hospital patient a multiply useful object, subject to medical as well as moral scrutiny.[47] Over time, as more pupils observed patients more often for medical information without participating in the care of the sick, hospital men claimed that, indeed, the very purposes of these charitable institutions included teaching medical students. The fact that eighteenth-century hospital governors and staff men actually agreed that teaching served the interests of Christian charity was essential to the construction of hospital medicine.

Teaching during ward-rounds subjected the patient *and the hospital practitioner* to medical inquiries detached from the direct delivery of physical, emotional, or spiritual care. Since the notion of detached observation underlies what it means for a human being to become an "object" in the first

---

45 Jerome Bylebyl, "The School of Padua: Humanistic Medicine in the Sixteenth Century," in *Health, Medicine and Mortality in the Sixteenth Century*, ed. Charles Webster (Cambridge: Cambridge University Press, 1983), 335–70; G. A. Lindeboom, "Medical Education in the Netherlands, 1575–1750," in *The History of Medical Education*, 201–16; R. Kondratas, "The Medical Ideas and Clinical Practice of Joseph Frank (1771–1842)," *Acta Congressus Internationalis XXIV Historiae Artis Medicinae* (Budapest, 1976), 425–32.
46 For parallel developments in Edinburgh, see Rosner, *Medical Education*.
47 Nicholas Jewson, "The Disappearance of the Sick-Man from Medical Cosmology, 1770–1870," *Sociology* 10 (1976): 225–44, summarizes the "medicalization" of hospital patients as objects; see also Fissell, *Patients, Power and the Poor*, 126–47, 171–95.

place, hospital teaching deepened and legitimized the transformation of the individual patient into an object of clinical investigation.[48] When a hospital practitioner treated a sick person and talked about her or him to an audience of other medical men, he made the patient into a public object. At those moments, the practitioner acted upon accepted medical theories, whether he articulated them or not, and defined appropriate medical practice. The interaction crucial to making medical knowledge then shifted from the practitioner and his patient to the practitioner and his observers, men with no investment in the therapeutic relationship between the practitioner and the ill person. The practitioner himself thus became an object of scrutiny, and watching and hearing him, as much as seeing the patient, became the way to acquire medical expertise.

Of course hospital relationships per se neither created clinical detachment nor invented the clinical significance that patients had for medical observers. Such attitudes were as old as systematic medical practice itself. Yet hospital teaching underlay a new sort of hospital medicine in the eighteenth century because it made seeing hospital patients as the objects of detached clinical observations part of *routine* hospital experience for practitioners and large numbers of transient pupils. The detachment fostered in ward-walking reinforced the clinical detachment that practitioners needed in order to see patients as objects of clinical inquiries, and vice versa. When hospital physicians and surgeons used charity patients to study the effects of new drugs, to try new operations, and to probe into the causes of disease and death, paying pupils learned that these displays were appropriate to certain clinical relationships. All of these acts gave patients' verbal responses and physical reactions significance outside the basic, conventional duty the practitioner had to treat the ill and injured. Through hospital work and the London lectures associated with it, medical men and their students took the ways that private patients had always served as sources for clinical knowledge and, whether knowingly or not, enlarged their mastery over how, when, and why a charity patient's case contained information useful to practitioners. And they took this mastery home with them, to the bedsides of private patients, where they perceived cases valuable to other medical men, and conveyed this knowledge to their brethren at medical society meetings and in print.

I have constructed a vision of hospital medicine that casts it as a complex set of social, medical, and intellectual relationships literally and figuratively located in and around institutions designed to care for the sick poor. In the hospitals, cheap medications and standard institutional diets were substituted for expensive and individualized treatments deemed suitable for the upper ranks at home, yet pupils learned the rituals of professional consulta-

---

48 Hunter, *Doctors' Stories*, 25–6, 58–63, 132–47; Jewson, "The Disappearance of the Sick-Man."

tions proper for practice among the well-to-do. On the wards, students experienced their own middling status, as socially distant from the poor in their beds as they were from the noblemen in the boardrooms. Immersion in the records of eighteenth-century London hospitals, in the publications of medical practitioners, and in manuscript notes about lectures, medical society meetings, patients' cases, and postmortem appearances, has taught me at least one thing. Having the power to determine what, out of all a sick person's experiences and corporeal remains, had conceptual significance lies at the heart of medical authority among practitioners. Locating that power in hospital men and in medical men of science made modern medicine. Just how that happened in London is the subject of this book and the strength of its arguments. Getting and keeping such power were neither obvious nor inevitable when hospital physicians and surgeons entered the wards in 1700, ready to serve the poor with their charitable knowledge.

I close this introduction with a brief outline of the following chapters, each of which elaborates on facets of the interwoven connections among medical knowledge, medical practice, and the charitable impulses of eighteenth-century English men and women. I have divided this book into two parts in order to focus on different aspects of the changing construction of hospital medicine in eighteenth-century London. The four chapters in the first part cover the entire period from 1700 to 1815, highlighting the gradual, cumulative effects of small shifts in organizational structures, professional politics, and the medical marketplace on medical education in the metropolis. In Part II, I discuss the relationships among science, medical knowledge, medical societies, and the medical press in shaping the urban medical community that hospital ward-walking and medical lectures both produced and depended upon for their increasing significance. For this part of my account, I use 1760 as a rough dividing point between two periods in London's medical culture. I contrast the years before 1760 with the later half of the century, when the number of lectures and ward-walking pupils in London increased significantly, medical societies proliferated, and medical journals started to appear regularly. Parts I and II thus work together to interweave the stability of institutions and ideas throughout the long eighteenth century with the sources of change that transformed them.

Chapters 2 and 3 provide the institutional contexts for the entire volume. In Chapter 2, I concentrate upon hospitals as institutions displaying complex values and social purposes. St. Thomas's, St. Bartholomew's, the Westminster, Guy's, St. George's, the London, and the Middlesex all served as emblems of charitable care for the sick poor as well as places for certain physicians and surgeons to practice, to teach, and to collect clinical observations. I discuss how the lay governors at these various charities elected staff men and what sorts of practitioners succeeded in the ballots. In Chapter 3, I turn to London's three medical corporations, the Royal College of Physicians, the surgeons' body in its three forms – the Barber–Surgeons' Company (to 1745), the Corporation of Surgeons (1745–1800) and the Royal College of Surgeons (1800–   ) – and the Worshipful Society of Apothecaries. I focus particularly on the role that each of these groups had in providing medical training to aspiring practitioners, either directly through in-house lectures and demonstrations, or, more importantly, indirectly through their criteria for membership and licensing. Medical reform movements in the late eighteenth and early nineteenth centuries then serve to illustrate the dynamics of institutional traditions and innovations surrounding medical training and certification.

Chapters 4 and 5 together analyze the transformation of medical education in London that took place in and around the metropolitan hospitals. In Chapter 4, I concentrate on the emergence of hospital ward-walking from the informal presence of surgeons' apprentices in 1700 to the hundreds of short-term pupils paying to follow staff men on their rounds in 1800. In Chapter 5, I examine the growth of private courses that medical men gave in a wide range of medical subjects, including physic, surgery, anatomy, midwifery, and chemistry, with particular attention to the ways that lecture courses entered some of London's hospitals. These chapters demonstrate how London's hospital men, their teaching colleagues, and their pupils expanded medical education by rearranging and revaluing existing institutions and practices over the course of the eighteenth century.

In Chapter 6, I develop the connections among medical knowledge, science, and hospital men during the first two-thirds of the eighteenth century. I argue that in this period hospital men, like their colleagues at the Royal College of Physicians or fellow serjeant–surgeons to the monarch, played out the concept of "doing science" as a gentlemanly pastime. Studying the natural world, including the human body and its health, placed them within the polite ranks of cultivated men and gave them intellectual respectability. Hospital work, especially for physicians, displayed their characters as charitable men as much as their dedication to teaching or absorbing clinical experience.

In Chapters 7 and 8, I show how a medical community developed in the second half of the eighteenth century and discuss the ways that doing science increasingly demarcated regular medical men from irregulars and, at the same time, shaped a new professional hierarchy. In Chapter 7, I concentrate on how a medical community based on medical societies and the medical press emerged after 1760. In it, I center on hospital physicians and surgeons as the core of a professional elite among a rank and file partly created by metropolitan associations and journals. During these decades, when London's hospital and teaching elite urged pupils to collect and describe useful case histories during their careers as private practitioners, they held out the promise that even modest medical men were men of science working in the fields. In Chapter 8, I return to the hospital elite as particular sorts of men of science and culture within the medical community between 1760 and 1820. They pursued both clinical investigations and research into chemistry, anatomy, physiology, and pathology that distinguished them from the rank and file, even as they supported the widespread use of case histories as contributions to knowledge. The physicians and surgeons who did research, moreover, concentrated on the medical sciences appropriate to their areas of clinical expertise. After consultations at the bedside, physicians returned to their libraries and chemical closets, surgeons to their books and bloody tables. And, equally important, I show how hospital men avoided discussions of the implications of their work, the hints that might suggest they held leanings toward materialism, irreligion, or democracy. They used science safely, participating in the construction of the "neutral" knowledge about nature that is so integral to modern medicine.

PART I

Institutions and education

A PLAN of the CITIES of LONDON, WESTMINSTER and Borough of SOUTHWARK, with the New Buildings to the Year 1786.

The London

St Thomas's

Guy's

St Bartholomew's

The Middlesex

The Westminster

St George's

Published Feb.y 1.st 1786 by I. Fielding, 23, Pater noster Row, Lond.n

2

The London hospitals: Virtue and value

In 1796, William Blizard, surgeon to the London Hospital and earnest Anglican, introduced one of his pamphlets with a revealing text. He chose a passage by William Blackstone, the eminent legal commentator, Member of Parliament, and judge.

The General Duties of all Bodies politic, considered in their corporate Capacity, may like those of Natural Bodies, be reduced to the single one, that of acting up to the End or Design, what ever it be, for which they were created by their Founder.[1]

Blizard went on to discuss the topic at hand – the importance of assistant surgeons in hospitals – as an application of this teleological principle. His essay resonated with the analogies he evoked with Blackstone's statement: hospitals were like "all Bodies politic," like "Natural Bodies," like God's creation. Inspired founders had shared God's vital spark, infusing their work with an all-encompassing Design. Blizard implicitly played out the rest of the analogy. Just as humans had to figure out God's Design to understand nature, hospital governors needed to grasp the founders' Design to carry out their "General Duties." Unfortunately, like corrupted churchmen, governors tended to forget "all the great objects they comprehend" and to fail to "appreciate their own true, high relation to the public." Blizard hastened to remind them that they were responsible "for their conduct to science, to humanity, to all mankind."[2]

---

1 William Blizard, "Reflections upon the Subject of Assistant Surgeons to Hospitals," in his *Suggestions for the Improvement of Hospitals and Other Charitable Institutions* (London: C. Dilly, 1796), 1. Blizard did not provide a citation for this quotation, but it came from William Blackstone, *Commentaries on the Laws of England*, 4 vols. (Dublin: J. Colles, 1766–7), 1: 467.

2 Blizard, "Reflections upon the Subject of Assistant Surgeons," 2–4. This was a published version of the memorial Blizard submitted to the hospital's governors in June 1795 urging that they create posts for three assistants, one for each full surgeon. London Hospital, Court of Governors Minutes, 3 June 1795, LH/A/2/5, London Hospital Archives. For Blizard's many reforming activities, see A. E. Clark-Kennedy, *The London: A Study in the Voluntary Hospital System*, 2 vols. (London: Pitman Medical, 1962), 1:182–8. Blizard had other reforming interests. See, for example, his *Desultory Reflections on Police: With an Essay on the Means of Preventing Crimes and Amending Criminals* (London: C. Dilly, 1785).

This was rather heavy-handed rhetoric for introducing an argument that the surgeons of the London Hospital needed help with their charitable duties, but Blizard was not one to resist a high moral tone when he held a pen. He was, moreover, quite serious. Upon his election in 1780, Blizard had thrown himself into making teaching appear to be as much a hospital's duty as care for the sick. In this pamphlet, Blizard asserted that relieving distress – the founders' explicit design – surely included the "cultivation, and advancement of medical knowledge." Better knowledge led to better practice, which improved care and lessened the misery of illness and trauma. But better knowledge was useless without better practitioners to apply it, and making better practitioners helped not only the poor in hospitals, but (once again) "all mankind," including the governors. Hospitals, which "may be considered as Nature's schools," should be "seminaries of medical science." In the meantime, assistant surgeons would not only train to become their seniors' skilled replacements, but would also instruct ward-walking pupils, "excit[ing] attention and diligence, in the rising student." Oh, and yes, assistant surgeons would help the patients, too. But Blizard could hardly make the relief of the immediate distress of the poor a major claim without implying that he and his peers shirked their duties. So, establishing new posts for assistant surgeons executed part of the founders' grand design – if seen from Blizard's cosmic viewpoint.

Faced with such radiant rewards "without incurring charge, or inconvenience," the governors tried Blizard's scheme.[3] They soon discovered, however, that it "is an impolitic measure, has not answered the expectations formed of it, and is not beneficial to the interests of the Hospital," doing away with the posts in 1797. They meant, of course, their interests, not Blizard's. It deprived "the Governors of their privilege of electing a Principal Surgeon, [which was] equally injurious to the Rights of the Governors & the Interests of the Charity."[4]

The surgeon's prose and the governors' responses illustrate several of the beliefs and relationships that defined hospitals in eighteenth-century London. On one hand, medical practitioners had to persuade hospital governors to change these institutions; in my book, at least, hospitals did not evolve through an unfolding of divine design. Appealing to the high ideals of charity to promote both moral and medical improvement was a constant theme in published reports and pamphlets. On the other hand, the governors at the London Hospital who actually decided to try having assistant surgeons, and then found the innovation "an impolitic measure," were not just vaguely defined readers of Blizard's eloquence. Not only were they the small minority of subscribers who bothered to attend meetings, but a look at the hospital's minute book also shows that different groups of men voted

3 Blizard, "Reflections upon the Subject of Assistant Surgeons," 4–11.
4 London Hospital, Governors Minutes, 6, 12 Sept., 6 Dec. 1797.

on these policies in 1795 and 1797. Two of those among the first group, by the way, were successful candidates for the assistant surgeons' posts they helped to create.[5] That is how the eighteenth-century hospitals worked. Staff men and active governors constantly balanced belief in public good with pragmatic choices on how best to run an inpatient medical charity.

In this chapter, I present the London hospitals both as symbols of virtue and authority, and as concrete institutions for medical care. The complex meanings of charity shaped the hospitals' foundation, funding, and roles as resources for the sick poor, emblems of civic humanitarianism, and places for the "cultivation, and advancement of medical knowledge." This is the view from a certain distance, one from which the detached observer can appreciate a nicely proportioned facade, as well as from the high moral planes of piety, good works, and rational improvement. For many Londoners, not to mention diverse audiences of eighteenth-century readers and travelers, these were the hospitals they knew.[6] Using this broad perspective, I introduce the seven general hospitals of eighteenth-century London, sketching out the similarities and differences among them. Their basic styles of funding and administration show how their founders and supporters translated broad charitable ideals – and less lofty interests – into self-perpetuating organizations.

In the abstract, the delegation of authority within the hospitals seems well defined. Governors had the ultimate power over everything, including medical affairs. Staff men had authority over patients' medical treatment, with physicians above the surgeons and both above the apothecary. Patients on the wards had control over nothing, except leaving if they could walk or get carried out. In practice, of course, the dynamics of authority among these people were a great deal more complicated. The mundane choices, compromises, and conflicts involved in hospital life reveal what authority actually meant in the boardrooms or on the wards. Hospital experience helped to construct the modern tensions between lay and medical authority, especially during struggles over who should have the final say in defining and performing "medicine" in these institutions. Yet, for

---

5 London Hospital, Governors Minutes, 3, 30 June 1795, 12 Sept. 1797. On 30 June, thirty-eight governors attended the Special General Court, which supported Blizard's proposal. Some disputes ensued, but the election for the three assistant surgeons was held on 30 Sept. Seven of the thirty-eight (18 percent) later appeared among the twenty (35 percent) on 12 Sept. 1797 at the Special General Court, which canceled the posts. At least one of these, the Rev. Thirlwall, disliked the measure, since he initiated the motion to end the appointments.

6 Browse through William Maitland, *The History of London from its Foundation to the Present Time*, 2 vols. (London: T. Osborne and J. Shipton, 1756), for an example of the way hospitals appear as part of civic life; Adrian Forty, "The Modern Hospital in England and France: The Social and Medical Uses of Architecture," in *Buildings and Society: Essays on the Social Development of the Built Society*, ed. Anthony D. King (London: Routledge and Kegan Paul, 1980), 61–93, esp. 62–74; John D. Thompson, *The Hospital: A Social and Architectural History* (New Haven, CT: Yale University Press, 1975).

the most part, apparent power plays between lay governors and hospital staff, such as the episode at the London in 1795–7 about assistant surgeons, were not about maintaining lay control over medical matters, but about different routes for, and degrees of, both lay and medical influence over the charity's responsibilities.

In the second part of this chapter, I turn to medical practitioners with staff positions in the hospitals, with an overview of how they got there, who they were, and what they did there. The hospitals' governors appointed or elected physicians, surgeons, and apothecaries to serve their charities. The medical qualifications that governors officially required from candidates for staff positions show where potential hospital men fit within the larger circles of urban practitioners. Yet the formation of a hospital elite among metropolitan medical men over the course of the eighteenth century depended very little upon the governors' scrutiny of professional expertise beyond some basic criteria. Using a few examples of elections and staff-men's status, I illustrate just how deeply embedded hospitals were in the cultural expectations of eighteenth-century English men and women.

CHARITY AND THE HOSPITALS

Giving time, care, goods, or money to needy strangers has long been a social virtue and religious duty. In the early modern West, people provided for the destitute sick and injured among the poor and abandoned in a variety of ways, from personal alms handed to individuals to parish-, city-, and state-based organizations, where publicly collected community funds replaced or subsidized private acts of guilt or kindness. Many historians have added new insights on the complex motives and meanings of charitable giving – and receiving – to the thoughtful efforts of generations of scholars who have traced the history of generosity and good works.[7] Not so long ago, simple religiosity, hopes for redemption, humanitarianism or the civilizing effects of material prosperity sufficed to explain charitable gifts, bequests, and foundations. The creation of medical charities throughout eighteenth-century England was, for historians such as Dorothy George and Mabel Buer, just one manifestation of a general snowballing of moral and medical improvement, especially among the middle

7 For the classics on charitable foundations in England, see M. G. Jones, *The Charity School Movement: A Study of Eighteenth-Century Puritanism in Action* (London: F. Cass, 1964 [reprint of 1938 edition]); W. K. Jordon, *The Charities of London, 1480–1660* (London: Allen & Unwin, 1960); David E. Owen, *English Philanthropy, 1660–1960* (Cambridge, MA: Belknap Press, 1964); B. Kirkman Gray, *A History of English Philanthropy: From the Dissolution of the Monasteries to the Taking of the First Census* (London: F. Cass, 1967 [reprint of 1905 edition]); Wilmarth Sheldon Lewis and Ralph M. Williams, *Private Charity in England, 1747–57* (New Haven, CT: Yale University Press, 1938).

classes.[8] More recently, however, scholars have probed, and sometimes exposed, the economic, political, and class interests underlying donors' ostensibly selfless motives to aid those less fortunate. Converting what givers once saw as acts of Christian virtue or Enlightenment humanitarianism into instruments of class oppression or cultural hegemony reveals the deep structures of eighteenth-century social order, the dark side of the Enlightenment.[9]

Hospitals' foundations and functions have started to attract their share of such historical reappraisal.[10] A few suggestive studies on those in London show the rewards of asking sharp questions about just whose interests they served at particular moments.[11] The governors' desire to bring religion and

8 Mabel C. Buer, *Health, Wealth and Population in the Early Days of the Industrial Revolution* (London: G. Routledge & Sons, 1926), 126; for Dorothy George, see Adrian Wilson, "The Politics of Medical Improvement in Early Hanoverian London," in *The Medical Enlightenment of the Eighteenth-Century*, eds. Andrew Cunningham and Roger French (Cambridge: Cambridge University Press, 1990), 5–10. Most historians of the individual London hospitals have taken this approach, too. See, for example, Hilary Aidan St. George Saunders, *The Middlesex Hospital, 1745–1948* (London: Parrish, 1949), 11; A. E. Clark-Kennedy, *The London*, 1: 18; Hector Charles Cameron, *Mr. Guy's Hospital, 1726–1948* (London and New York: Longmans, Green, 1954), 7–9.
9 See Sandra Cavallo, "The Motivations of Benefactors: An Overview of Approaches to the Study of Charity," in *Medicine and Charity Before the Welfare State*, eds. Jonathan Barry and Colin Jones (London and New York: Routledge, 1991), 46–62, for an especially insightful discussion of this issue. See also: Thomas L. Haskell, "Capitalism and the Origins of Humanitarian Sensibility," Parts 1 and 2, *American Historical Review* 90 (1985): 339–61, 547–66; T. J. Jackson Lears, "The Concept of Cultural Hegemony: Problems and Possibilities," *American Historical Review* 90 (1985): 567–93.
10 See, in particular, Mary E. Fissell, "Charity Universal? Institutions and Moral Reform in Eighteenth-Century Bristol," in *Still the Grumbling Hive: The Response to Social and Economic Problems in England, 1689–1750*, ed. Lee Davison, et al. (New York: St. Martin's Press, 1992), 121–44; Fissell, *Patients, Power and the Poor in Eighteenth-Century Bristol* (Cambridge: Cambridge University Press, 1991); Charles E. Rosenberg, *The Care of Strangers: The Rise of America's Hospital System* (New York: Basic Books, 1987); Arthur E. Imhof, "The Hospital in the 18th century: For Whom?" *Journal of Social History* 10 (1977): 448–70; Guenter B. Risse, *Hospital Life in Enlightenment Scotland: Care and Teaching at the Royal Infirmary of Edinburgh* (Cambridge: Cambridge University Press, 1986); Lindsay Granshaw and Roy Porter, eds., *The Hospital in History* (London and New York: Routledge, 1989); Peter Mandler, ed., *The Uses of Charity: The Poor on Relief in the Nineteenth-Century Metropolis* (Philadelphia: University of Pennsylvania Press, 1990); Jonathan Barry and Colin Jones, eds., *Medicine and Charity before the Welfare State* (London and New York: Routledge, 1991); Morris J. Vogel, *The Invention of the Modern Hospital, 1870–1930* (Chicago: University of Chicago Press, 1980); Charles Webster, "The Crisis of the Hospitals during the Industrial Revolution," in *Human Implications of Scientific Advance*, Proceedings of the International Congress for the History of Science, ed. Eric G. Forbes (Edinburgh: University of Edinburgh Press, 1977), 214–23. All of these offer perspectives that supplement those in the still-useful surveys: Brian Abel-Smith, *The Hospitals, 1800–1948: A Study in Social Administration in England and Wales* (London: Harvard University Press, 1964); John Woodward, *To Do the Sick No Harm: A Study of the British Voluntary Hospital System to 1875* (London, Boston: Routledge and Kegan Paul, 1974).
11 Donna T. Andrew, *Philanthropy and Police: London Charity in the Eighteenth Century* (Princeton, NJ: Princeton University Press, 1989); Wilson, "The Politics of Medical Im-

submission to the sick and to get laborers back to work, or staff practitioners' awareness that donating their medical services generated professional status and cash benefits from teaching, helps to explain why Londoners supported hospitals instead of (or in addition to) other charitable
enterprises. Yet finding economic, political, and social interests, no matter
how manipulative and mean-spirited they were, fails to wipe out the
sincerity and generosity with which eighteenth-century men and women
gave of their time and money. Nor does pointing out professional payoffs
negate hospital practitioners' honest attempts to give the best care they
could. Nor, in the end, did the undoubted demands of obedience, piety,
and deference on the wards cancel the relief patients got from rest, food,
warmth, and therapeutic attention. Charitable institutions that perpetuated
hierarchical relationships worked, it seems to me, precisely because they
often made everyone involved *feel* good at some level, even while using
one another. Acts of medical benevolence, in short, carried multiple coexisting motives and implications – some overt, some hidden, many ambiguous – all of which are needed to understand their power to embody both
social and medical knowledge.

Urban charity and the general hospitals

By 1750, seven general hospitals in London existed primarily to serve
"deserving" poor adults suffering from "curable" illnesses and injuries
(Table 2.1).[12] "General" applies to these institutions in two senses. First,
the Elizabethan Poor Law (1601–3), which managed assistance to those in
poverty through rates paid by local property holders, worked at the parish
level. According to an Act of Parliament in 1662, the poor could seek such

provement"; Craig Rose, "Politics and the London Royal Hospitals, 1683–92," in *The Hospital in History*, 123–48; Kathleen Wilson, "Urban Culture and Political Activism in Hanoverian England: The Example of the Voluntary Hospitals," in *The Transformation of Political Culture*, ed. Eckhart Hellmuth (London: Oxford University Press for the German Historical Institute, 1990), 165–84.

12 Unless cited otherwise, all the information on these seven hospitals I discuss later can be found in their individual histories. I cite other material, particularly various minute books on governors' meetings, found in hospital archives, the Greater London Record Office, the Guildhall Library, and the Corporation of London Record Office, only when I provide information that corrects errors in, or is absent from, these published sources. I also add notes when I believe it is important to supplement these sources with direct references to the archival material. These hospital histories vary in depth and several do not provide many citations.

St. Thomas's: Frederick G. Parsons, *The History of St. Thomas's,* 3 vols. (London: Methuen & Co., 1932–6); *St. Bartholomew's:* Sir Norman Moore, *The History of St. Bartholomew's Hospital,* 2 vols. (London: C. A. Pearson, 1918); Victor C. Medvei and John L. Thornton, eds., *The Royal Hospital of Saint Bartholomew, 1123–1973* (London: St. Bartholomew's Hospital, 1974); *Guy's:* Hector C. Cameron, *Guy's Hospital, 1726–1948* (London and New York: Longmans, Green, 1954); Samuel Wilks and G. T. Bettany, *A Biographical History of Guy's Hospital* (London: New, Ward, Lock, Bowden & Co., 1892);

Table 2.1. *The general hospitals of eighteenth-century London*

Hospital	Location	Foundation date	Size	Financial base
St. Bartholomew's	Smithfield	1123 Royal Charter - 1557 Enlarged - 1739	Inpatients - 428 (1788) Inpatients - 420 (1809)	Church lands/revenue; Endowed: plus further legacies and donations
St. Thomas's	The Borough, Southwark	c. 1173 Royal Charter - 1553 Enlarged - 1730s	Inpatients - 203 (1569) Inpatients - 440 (1788) Inpatients - 417 (1809)	Church lands/revenue; Endowed: plus further legacies and donations
Guy's	The Borough, Southwark	1726	Beds - 430 (1783) Inpatients -304 (1788), Beds - 411 (1809)	Endowed: plus further legacies and donations
Westminster	St. James	1719 - Infirmary 1777 - Hospital	Beds - 110 (1783) Inpatients - 85 (1788)	Voluntary: subscriptions, legacies, donations
St. George's	Hyde Park Corner	1734	Beds - 270 (1783) Inpatients - 185 (1788); 146 (1807)	Voluntary: subscriptions, legacies, donations
London	Whitechapel	1740 1758 - Incorporated	Beds - 160 (1783) Inpatients - 120 (1788) Beds - 400; inpatients - 180 (1814)	Voluntary: subscriptions, legacies, donations
Middlesex	Charles St. nr. Tottenham Ct.	1745	Beds - 150 (1783) Inpatients - 70 (1788), Beds - 179 (1814)	Voluntary: subscriptions, legacies, donations

Sources: John Howard, *An Account of the Principle Lazarettos*, 131-6. Anthony Highmore, *Pietas Londinensis: The History, Design, and Present State of the Various Public Charities in and Near London* (London: Cradock and Joy, 1814), 1-12, 71-5, 80-1, 124-8, 157-8, 223-7, 310-14; Samuel F. Simmons, ed. *The Medical Register* (London: 1783), 31-3; Parsons, *St. Thomas's*, 1: 206; Clark-Kennedy, *The London*, 1: 140-2; Wilson, *The Middlesex*, 15.

public aid only in their own parishes, where they had "settlement." In practice, this could be rather difficult for those who had migrated to London, ended up sick and destitute, and had to be returned to their place of settlement. The "general" hospitals, then, admitted those who found appropriate patrons to recommend them, without any restrictions on their origins. In this way, the hospitals, and other "general" charities, served the new mobility of labor and commerce in eighteenth-century society, especially in urban areas.[13]

Second, "general" contrasts these hospitals with the other types of hospital and residential charities that started to flourish from the mid-1740s. Donna Andrew has recently discussed many of the issues surrounding the establishment of more specialized hospitals. The Foundling Hospital (1739) and later lying-in hospitals, for example, relied upon strong appeals to the nation's need for healthy babies to increase its productive population, and upon the image of maternal care properly encouraged. The Smallpox Hospital (1745) aimed to attack the scourge of smallpox by providing inoculations and care during the course of the disease. The Lock Hospital tried to deal with the rampages of venereal disease among the poor. Magdalen House (1758) hoped to rescue prostitutes.[14] At the beginning of the nineteenth century, the London Fever Hospital, as W. F. Bynum has shown, similarly gained support because it spoke directly to a specific problem that its proponents wanted to ameliorate.[15] All of these hospitals

The Westminster: J. G. Humble and Peter Hansell, *Westminster Hospital, 1716–1766* (London: Pitman Medical, 1966); John Langdon-Davies, *Westminster Hospital: Two Centuries of Voluntary Service, 1719–1948* (London: John Murray, 1952); *St. George's:* Joseph Blomfield, *St. George's, 1733–1933* (London: Published for St. George's Hospital by the Medici Society, 1933); William E. Page, "Some Account of St. George's Hospital and School," *St. George's Hospital Reports* 1 (1866): 1–24; George C. Peachey, *The History of St. George's Hospital (1733–1753)* (London: J. Bale, Sons & Danielsson, 1910); *The London:* A. E. Clark-Kennedy, *The London: A Study in the Voluntary Hospital System,* 2 vols. (London: Pitman Medical, 1962); E. W. Morris, *A History of the London Hospital,* 3rd ed. (London: Arnold, 1926); *The Middlesex:* Hilary Aidan St. George Saunders, *The Middlesex Hospital, 1745–1948* (London: Parrish, 1949); Sir William J. Erasmus Wilson, *The History of Middlesex Hospital during the First Century of Its Existence, Compiled from the Hospital Records* (London: John Churchill, 1845).

13 Porter, "The Gift Relation," 160–1; Harold W. Hart, "Some Notes on the Sponsoring of Patients for Hospital Treatment under the Voluntary System," *Medical History* 24 (1980): 447–60; Woodward, *To Do the Sick No Harm,* 1–22. Hospital governors could waive the requirement that patients come with governors' letters, moreover, for emergencies or special circumstances. Clark-Kennedy, *The London,* 1: 32.

14 Andrew, *Philanthropy and Police,* 54–73, 115–27.

15 W. F. Bynum, "Hospital, Disease and Community: The London Fever Hospital, 1801–1850," in *Healing and History,* ed. Charles Rosenberg (New York: Science History Publications, 1979), 97–115; for the later development of specialist hospitals to serve professional interests, see Lindsay Granshaw, " 'Fame and Fortune by Means of Bricks and Mortar': the Medical Profession and Specialist Hospitals in Britain, 1800–1948," in *The Hospital in History,* 199–220.

had particular social and medical purposes that the general hospitals either refused to address, such as care of abandoned or sick infants, or did so tangentially. The Middlesex Hospital had a lying-in ward, for example, and all the general hospitals admitted some cases of smallpox, venereal disease, and fever, even when their policies excluded them. Yet they reserved most of their funds for adults beset by noncontroversial illnesses and injuries.[16]

Given the changing fashions of charitable giving, the general hospitals were fairly conservative projects. In this century of enthusiasm for collective improvement and moral reform, these institutions did not provoke the critics who worried that the Foundling Hospital and the Lock Hospital encouraged wantonness. They escaped the problems that plagued long-term residential charities, like the Magdalen, whose low turnover and doubtful "cures" kept it struggling for funds.[17] The hospitals faced the strongest attacks in the second half of the eighteenth century from the champions of dispensaries, who argued that providing medical advice and inexpensive medicines to outpatients, with some home visits, had decided advantages over inpatient care. Dispensaries assisted with the same sorts of illnesses, kept families together, fostered independence from excessive charity, prevented the spread of disease, and, above all, were cheaper. They could help more patients per pound than the hospitals. Donors and subscribers agreed, and dispensaries sprang up throughout the metropolis.[18] Most of the hospitals already had, or then established, outpatient services to compete. The Middlesex Hospital governors, feeling a definite pinch in 1788, resolved to do what they could "to encourage all Persons inclined to subscribe to such Charitable Institutions to pay their Money to a Regular established *Hospital* in preference to a Dispensary."[19] Some recent work on dispensaries has claimed that Dissenters' values and beliefs particularly inspired and shaped these efforts. While only applicable to part of the dispensary movement, a contemporary association of Dissent, dispen-

16 Woodward, *To Do the Sick No Harm*, 36–75; Cameron, *Guy's*, 71–72, for this hospital's lunatic house; Clark-Kennedy, *The London*, 1: 39, for the London's ward for venereal patients, which the staff sometimes used to isolate fever patients, as well.
17 Andrew, *Philanthropy and Police*, 127–34.
18 John Coakley Lettsom, "Hints designed to promote the Establishment of a Dispensary for extending Medical Relief to the Poor at their own habitations," in his *Hints Designed to Promote Beneficence, Temperance and Medical Science*, 3 vols. (London: J. Manman, 1801), 3: 185–208; John Herdman, *A Letter . . . Proposing a Plan for Improving Dispensaries and the Medical Treatment of the Diseased Poor* (London: Arch, Cornhill, 1809); Ulrich Tröhler, "Quantification in British Medicine and Surgery, 1750–1830, with Special Reference to Its Introduction into Therapeutics," Ph.D. dissertation, University of London, 1978; Irvine Loudon, "The Origins and Growth of the Dispensary Movement," *Bulletin of the History of Medicine* 55 (1981): 322–42; Andrew, *Philanthropy and Police*, 135–62.
19 Middlesex Hospital, Minutes of the Weekly Board, Court of Governors, 1 May 1788, original emphasis, Middlesex Hospital Archives; Wilson, *The Middlesex*, 45–52.

saries, and disparagement of residential charities could well have made the general hospitals seem socially safe places for a display of virtue among conservatives.[20]

Within London, the three endowed hospitals had the most financial stability during spells of doubting donors. Two of these, St. Thomas's and St. Bartholomew's, had medieval origins as Catholic foundations. After the upheavals of the early English Reformation, they were chartered as Royal Hospitals (along with Christ's, Bridewell, and Bethlem) and given to the City of London. St. Thomas's and St. Bartholomew's gradually became institutions specifically for the sick, distinct from the others, which educated children, took up vagabonds, and housed the aged and insane, respectively. At their chartering, the Crown endowed St. Thomas's and St. Bartholomew's with lands for revenue. Because of their relationship with the City, St. Thomas's and St. Bartholomew's admitted patients sent to them by the Corporation of London and by parish officers who had to promise to receive them back again when discharged or dead. St. Bartholomew's, in particular, submitted some hefty bills to the City for its work in caring for and clothing sick vagrants sent to them by the magistrates.[21] Guy's, the third endowed hospital, had no such formal obligations, but the governors did make arrangements to admit suitably recommended poor from local parish officers.[22] Thomas Guy founded his hospital between 1721 and his death in 1725, and it opened in 1726. Guy had risen from humble origins to become a respectable bookseller and publisher. During the early months of the South Sea Company, he made a huge fortune, much of which, after an Act of Parliament made his will's executors into a

20 Robert Kilpatrick, " 'Living in the light': Dispensaries, Philanthropy and Medical Reform in Late-Eighteenth-Century London," in *Medical Enlightenment,* ed. Cunningham and French, 254–80; I find Kilpatrick's argument that the dispensary movement as a whole was linked specifically to late-eighteenth-century Quakers too narrow. The reforming rhetoric he describes was ubiquitous among many social and religious groups, as Donna Andrew has shown.
21 Parsons, *St. Thomas's,* 2: 207; See City of London Record Office (CLRO) MISC MS 3.43, Orders to admit to St. Thomas's Hospital, 1783–4 and MS 331.8, St. Bartholomew's, Certificates for examinations of inpatients, for examples of the printed forms on which Aldermen or the Lord Mayor, sitting as Justices, filled in the blanks to recommend inpatients. Court of Aldermen, Repertory 182, 10 Feb. 1778; Repertory 186, 8 Oct. 1782; Chamberlains Office, Statements of Various Funds, c. 1780–1800, 17, 18, contains tallies of sums paid to St. Bartholomew's (1780–92) and St. Thomas's (1783–1792). St. Bartholomew's received £5,460 10s. 5p. in twelve years. This cost led to a committee of inquiry. See Common Council, Journal Book 73, 24 Oct. 1793, where the committee recommended that "the sitting Magistrate be requested to be very particular in his examination of the Objects claiming relief," and to try harder to get such poor back to their own parishes.
22 Guildhall Library, Broadside 32.51, is a printed form for parish "Churchwardens or Overseers" to use to send patients to Guy's. In this case, the patient, John Ridley, stayed in the hospital for twenty-one days; the hospital charged the parish 9s. 6p. for his admission (2s. 6p.) and "subsistence." Cameron, *Guy's,* 65–6.

self-perpetuating "body Politick and Corporate," endowed the hospital built next to St. Thomas's in Southwark.[23] Guy's was the last of the hospitals established with financial resources designed to make it independent of collection boxes, bequests, and donations.

The governors at St. Thomas's, St. Bartholomew's, and Guy's of course welcomed other funds, and regularly solicited additional money for special projects, especially for substantial renovations and new buildings. All three of these hospitals, moreover, required that all incoming patients have, or be supplied with, modest fees to cover their expenses for linen and possible burial. With good reason, their critics condemned this constraint upon the charitable objects needing help, who had to produce cash up front. The "taking-in" governors could waive this requirement if necessary, however, although how often they actually did so is an open question. These rules nevertheless ensured that the City and the parishes made appropriate payments for their poor, thus upholding the traditional responsibilities of local governments.[24]

The four voluntary hospitals had more precarious incomes. The Westminster, St. George's, the London, and the Middlesex depended upon subscriptions, gifts, and the proceeds of fund-raising events, such as concerts, for all of their operating and building costs. As they did *not* require payments or deposits from patients upon entry, much to the approval of those in favor of truly "general" charitable care, these hospitals shouldered greater expenses for food, linen, and burials.[25] Donna Andrew has explained in detail how voluntary charities appealed to donors anxious to avoid committing money posthumously. With donations during life, and perhaps token bequests at death, the charitably inclined watched over their good works and basked in public recognition, unless modesty or spiritual principles compelled anonymity. From the later seventeenth century on, charitable giving took an overtly pragmatic turn, both in its objects and in its disbursement. Charitable activists called for projects with demonstrable rewards in urban life: educating the poor, reforming vice-ridden manners, spreading religion, and curing the sick. Of course donors *"will be recompensed at the resurrection of the just,"* as Bishop Maddox proclaimed in 1743, for charity was, and remained, a virtue with sincere religious meaning.[26] In

23 Quoted from the Act (II George I, Cap. 12), in Cameron, *Guy's*, 49.

24 John Howard, *An Account of the Principal Lazarettos in Europe* (London, 1789), 132, 134–6; Parsons, *St. Thomas's*, 2: 207; In 1763, Guy's charged a parish 2s. 6p. for patient's admission, but charged "common" patients only 6p. The Steward received these fees, among others, as part of his prerequisites. Guy's Hospital, Minutes of the Court of Committees, 28 Oct., 16 Nov. 1763.

25 Howard, *An Account of the Principal Lazarettos*, 131, 133, 136–7. The London, however, like Guy's, charged 4s. a day for parish-supported patients and soldiers and sailors sent by the military.

26 Isaac Maddox, *The Duty and Advantages of Public Infirmaries* (London: H. Woodfall, 1743), 26. For more on Maddox, see Porter, "The Gift Relation."

the meantime, however, hospital organizers wanted their institutions run like businesses, accruing immediate and long-term social profits, with efficiency, effectiveness, and accountability. The voluntary charities allowed subscribers simply to stop giving if the enterprises' purposes or managements failed to please them, or when other projects promised more personal and public amelioration per guinea.

The seven general hospitals thus varied in their vulnerability to shifts in economic conditions, public opinions about worthy causes, and attacks on their reputations.[27] The endowed hospitals weathered such ups and downs better than the voluntary ones, yet had their own problems with lax administration and urban discord. As Sandra Cavallo has aptly put it, charitable enterprises were not just "an expression of policies towards the poor," but also the ongoing manifestations of "politics between elites."[28] Jockeying for the power to aid the poor, and to be seen doing it, rival groups shared beliefs about poverty and public responsibility, but differed over just who should control beneficence. Craig Rose has discussed how St. Thomas's and St. Bartholomew's faced internal and external disputes between 1683 and 1692, when their governors, supporters, and critics lined up with various political factions of the City, Parliament, and Crown. Ousting and reinstating Whig governors from St. Thomas's had little to do with the sick poor, for instance, but much to do with the patronage the governors held through the hospital's lands.[29] Similarly, Adrian Wilson has retold the story of the founding of the Westminster Infirmary, the first voluntary hospital, suggesting that its establishment gave high church Tories a way to maintain a public image of social seriousness and goodwill just before a general election in 1722.[30]

Throughout the century, all of London's medical charities responded and contributed to the complexities of urban experience. Much about their roles in particular neighborhoods, in parish, City, or county politics; in religious communities; and in local businesses awaits historians' efforts.[31] In broad terms, governors of the seven general hospitals shared a view of the multiple purposes of their charitable endeavors, even as they differed on who should implement these, and how. They assisted the sick, deserv-

---

27 Anne Borsay, " 'Persons of Honour and Reputation': The Voluntary Hospitals in an Age of Corruption," *Medical History* 35 (1991): 281–94.
28 Cavallo, "The Motivations of Benefactors," 53; Porter, "The Gift Relation," 153.
29 Rose, "Politics and the London Royal Hospitals, 1683–1692."
30 Wilson, "Politics of Medical Improvement," 18–24; in 1741, the Westminster governors ruled that the hospital would not admit Catholic patients, another sign of a conservative Church position; see Langdon-Davies, *The Westminster*, 49–50.
31 See, for example, Jeremy Boulton, *Neighbourhood and Society: A London Suburb in the Seventeenth Century* (Cambridge: Cambridge University Press, 1987), which has a few references to St. Thomas's Hospital in its detailed study of Southwark.

ing poor to recover from their illnesses and injuries and get back to work, hence the emphasis on curable conditions among adults, not on the disabled, the insane, or infants and children. These hospitals recovered future wealth potentially lost to the nation from those who had already produced it, the wealth embodied in laborers, mothers, sailors, servants, and down-on-their-luck artisans. To get admitted, possible patients had to pass governors' inspection as deserving relief. Many historians have explained how these decisions ensured the face-to-face acknowledgment of social order, paternalistic generosity, and individual discretion. And it extended such time-worn patronage among the middling sorts, especially at the voluntary hospitals, where subscribers of £3 to £5 annually could have one inpatient (and varying numbers of outpatients) on the books at a time.[32] "Deserving," then, was a category that nicely accommodated all sorts of notions of worthiness.

After admission, moreover, a period in the hospital could minister to the patient's soul as much as to his or her body. In 1761, governors at the Middlesex, for instance, wanted to start having regular prayers and services in the hospital. They were, they decided,

of the Opinion that the constant and regular instruction of the Patients in the Duties of Religion & Performance of Divine Worship will Probably Produce a reformation in the moralls [*sic*] of the Patients as their minds must be then more susceptible of instruction where their bodys are under Pain & Sickness.[33]

All the hospitals had strict rules against swearing, gambling, excessive drinking, and indecencies on the wards. Directions to see that a hospital's chaplain did his duty, to purchase spiritual readings for the wards, and to encourage visiting governors to instill submission to divine authority appear at intervals in the minutes of governors' meetings.[34] Attention to enforcing the rules, championing moral reform, and saving souls flowed and ebbed, however, with the governors' enthusiasm to do the work – or to pay someone else to do it.

Knowing who the governors, donors, and other benefactors actually were provides vital information about the general hospitals. Such details suggest the social range and geographical extent of those with interests in

32 Fissell, *Patients, Power and the Poor*, 112–17; Porter, "The Gift Relation."
33 Middlesex Hospital, Minutes of the Weekly Board, Court of Governors, 20 Jan. 1761; see also, William Blizard, "Cursory Observations Relative to Hospitals" in *Suggestions for the Improvement of Hospitals*, 34, 80–81.
34 For an overview, see Woodward, *To Do the Sick No Harm*; Parsons, *St. Thomas's*, 2: 207–13; Clark-Kennedy, *The London*, 1: 105–6; Cameron, *Guy's*, 74–7; Saunders, *The Middlesex*, 13; Langdon-Davies, *The Westminster*, 52. For an interesting discussion of the Johnsonian view on charity care at midcentury, see John Wiltshire, *Samuel Johnson in the Medical World: The Doctor and the Patient* (Cambridge: Cambridge University Press, 1991), 115–6.

46   *Institutions and education*

an institution's well-being.[35] At the endowed hospitals, current governors elected men to join them for life, and so operated as self-perpetuating oligarchies. Because St. Thomas's and St. Bartholomew's were technically under City governance, all governors were supposed to have the City's freedom and a certain number of Common Councilors were to sit as governors. In the eighteenth century, the governors pretty much ignored the former restriction and elected all sorts of prominent metropolitan figures, ending up with between two and three hundred names on their governors' lists at any one time.[36] (The latter rule, and indeed the whole relationship with the City's Common Council, sparked various disputes about who had final say in hospital matters, especially over financial decisions. But that is another story.)[37] Along with City politicians, St.

35 Andrew, *Philanthropy and Police*, discusses some of the major eighteenth-century philanthropists whom she identified through her study of subscribers' lists and wills. On the whole, identifying governors from the sources I have used (see nn 36, 38, and 39), is a difficult task. Printed lists, not to mention names noted in the minute books, often give no additional information with which to identify most of these people with any certainty. It is relatively easy, of course, to identify those with titles, or those whom other sources have detailed (such as well-known philanthropists). The work I have done to date is based on a combined list of names of governors elected, or subscribing to, the hospitals between 1700 and 1815. The data base contains 6,422 names, reduced to one entry per governor at each hospital (no matter how many times on different lists), where it was clearly the same person. I have used the following sources to make the conservative identifications I have presented as my impressionistic conclusions. It was soon apparent that most of the governors were *not* well-known metropolitan figures, and that any serious study of these men (and a few women) demands a well-planned sampling technique; considerable time with the hospitals' records, looking for addresses or occupations; and then sustained work with local records. I am grateful to David B. Morris for guiding me into this maze and helping me to stop. In addition to all the sources I refer to elsewhere to identify medical practitioners, then, I have consulted: Gerrit P. Judd, *Members of Parliament, 1734–1832* (New Haven, CT: Yale University Press, 1955); Sir Lewis Namier and John Brooke, *The House of Commons, 1754–1780*, 3 vols. (London: The History of Parliament Trust by Her Majesty's Stationery Office, 1964); Alfred B. Beaven, *The Aldermen of the City of London, Henry III–1908*, 2 vols. (London: The Corporation of the City of London, 1908, 1913); F. G. Hilton Price, *A Handbook of London Bankers* (London: Simpkin, Marshall, Hamilton, Kent & Co., 1890); among the various eighteenth-century directories for London (primarily the City), I have particularly used *Kent's Directory for the Year 1759* (London: Henry Kent, 1759) and *The London Directory for the Year 1772* (London: T. Lownes, 1772).

36 My observations on the hospitals' governors are based on partial study of the following sources: *St. Thomas's*, printed lists (British Library): *Governours* [sic] *of St. Thomas's*; manuscript registers of the governors' names, Greater London Record Office (GLRO) H1/ST/A64/1, 4, with names from c. 1679, 1770–1815. These provided a nearly complete data file of all the governors. *St. Bartholomew's*, printed lists (British Library): *A List of the Governors of St. Bartholomew's Hospital* [c. 1688–1702/3]; *The Names of the Governors . . .* [c. 1705–1712]; *The Names of the Governours* [sic]. . . [c. 1721–1723]; *A List of the Governors* . . . (1806); *A List of the Governors* . . . (1808). I have dated the earlier lists according to the periods in which the named President's and Treasurer's tenure overlapped.

37 The five Royal Hospitals and the City resolved their differences in 1782–3, both agreeing to an Act of Parliament that gave the hospitals' presidents, treasurers, and governors de facto power over the hospitals' lands and investments. In return, twelve common councilors (for each hospital) chosen by the City always served as full governors during their terms as councilors, and the City would act as the governors "whenever any legal process

Thomas's and St. Bartholomew's attracted bankers, merchants, and others with interests in London commerce, although they by no means restricted themselves to the money men. Nevertheless, anyone chosen for election had to have wealth enough to present the hospital with the customary £50 gesture of thanks for the honor bestowed upon him, a requirement that obviously limited the potential pool considerably. The governors at Guy's tended to elect men who moved in similar circles, and they understandably overlapped with those at St. Thomas's next door. Unlike the other hospitals, however, Guy's had been left by its founder with strict instructions that his institution could have no fewer than forty, but no more than sixty, governors. This kept the Guy's men a remarkably select group, and probably quite cautious about whom they chose to join them.[38]

Whereas the endowed hospitals were relatively closed corporations, the voluntary charities were extremely open ones. These charities depended upon large numbers of modest donations and constantly appealed for more public generosity. The four voluntary hospitals had between one and four hundred subscribers on each of their books at any one time in the eighteenth century. I tentatively estimate that one-fifth of these governors contributed to more than one hospital, while perhaps a third at each gave for more than ten years. Unlike some of the smaller, specialized charities that Donna Andrew has studied, the general hospitals seem to have had a high proportion of transient givers surrounding their cores of faithful philanthropists. Since these charities extended governors' privileges to anyone who paid the minimum annual subscription, they nicely point to the changing values of a commercializing society. Money, even small amounts of money, spoke louder than business, family, political, or religious connections for entrée into these groups. The lists of benefactors and subscribers that the governors at the Westminster, St. George's, the Middlesex, and the London chose to publish occasionally thus contain a wide range of people, with considerable variation in the names that appear in different neighborhoods at different times. Such lists both testified to the support

is threatened." [Quoted in Parsons, *St. Thomas's*, 2: 238, from the draft agreement of spring 1782]. For the details of these complex and underexplored events, see Nellie J. M. Kerling, "The Relations Between St. Bartholomew's Hospital and the City of London, 1546–1948," *Guildhall Miscellany* 4 (1971): 14–21; and, more importantly: Report of the Committee appointed 13 February 1756 to enquire into the Right of the Mayor and Commonality and Citizens of London to the Several Hospitals of this city. Presented 16 Dec. 1766. CLRO PD 114.26; Minute Papers of the Committee appointed to enquire into the right of members of the Common Council to be Governors of the Royal Hospitals, 1775–1782, CLRO MS 62.5 (see also CLRO MS 62.7, 2 vols., for the other committee work, the printed report, and miscellaneous letters); Papers re Governors, 1782–3, CLRO MISC MS 331.13; Journals of the Common Council, Jor. 68.

38 Guy's, printed lists (British Library): *A List of the President and Governors*. These were annual flyers apparently sent to all the governors each year. This collection includes the years 1735, 1738, 1777–1815; Cameron, *Guy's*, 97, remarks that Guy's shared St. Thomas's reputation as a center for Whigs and Dissenters.

the hospital attracted and displayed individuals' participation in its worthy efforts.[39]

For the voluntary hospitals, a parade of royals, nobles, and bishops as hospital benefactors, particularly when dukes, earls, and viscounts served as presidents and vice-presidents, gave these enterprises the cachet crucial for fund-raising among the better sort, whom others then followed. The splendid names, the glittering turnout at benefit services, concerts, and other celebrations, gave these charities public faces, the ones that beamed with civic pride and urban humanitarianism. The far larger display of less-splendid names contributed substantially to this public face, for they united the middling sort with their social superiors, demonstrating that good works transcended the distinctions of birth, wealth, or royal promotion. Historians have regularly observed that voluntary charities let ordinary folk mingle with the great as "equal" contributors to public good. Tradesmen, minor clerics, medical men, social climbers, and hangers-on clearly hoped to promote private good, too, their own in particular, through useful introductions and connections.[40] Even if they never met members of the elite, their names shared the same printed lists, which might be casually left in strategic places or offhandedly mentioned in the right conversations.

From this perspective, the voluntary hospitals revealed and maintained the traditional social hierarchy, in which eighteenth-century people defined themselves through appropriate expressions of deference to those above and polite, but carefully distanced gestures of recognition to those below. But, as Kathleen Wilson has argued, voluntary hospitals also embraced a

39 The governors' names used for my general observations here came from the following printed sources, supplemented by names from hospital minutes. *The London:* Isaac Maddox, *The Duty and Advantages of Public Infirmaries* (London: H. Woodfall, 1743), 34–40; *Account of the Rise, Progress and State of the London Hospital . . . 1740 to . . . 1765* (London, 1765); *Account of the Rise, Progress and State of the London Hospital . . . 1740 to . . . 1785* (London, 1785), 13–28; *General State of the London Hospital . . .* (London, 1787); *Middlesex: A List of the Governors and Contributors to the Middlesex Hospital* (London, 1750); *A List of the Governors . . .* (London, 1753); *A List of the Governors . . .* appended to Thomas Church, *A Sermon preached . . . before the Governors of the Middlesex Hospital* (London, 1754); *St. George's: A List of the Governors and Contributors to St. George's Hospital* (London, 1734); *An Account of the Proceedings . . . 1734 . . . to 1744 at St. George's Hospital* (London, 1744); supplemented by transcriptions of the governors present at sampled weekly boards, plus full lists of those attending General Courts for staff elections, in St. George's Hospital, Board of Governors Minutes, 11 May 1792, 27 May 1796, 21 Mar., 27 Apr. 1800, 18 Mar. 1808. *The Westminster:* attendance samples from weekly board meetings, in Westminster Hospital, Proceedings of the Trustees, 1782–1815. Many more names of governors at all of these hospitals could be gleaned from surviving financial records, where the names of subscribers are given with their payments. See, for example, London Hospital, Cash Book, 1757, LH/F/2/4, and Cash Book, 1777, LH/F/2/5, District Archives, Tower Hamlets Health Authority.

40 Wiltshire, *Samuel Johnson in the Medical World*, 115–7; Andrew, *Philanthropy and Police*; Porter, "The Gift Relation"; Cavallo, "The Motivations of Benefactors."

set of values at odds with "the imperatives of patrician society" in the way that they were organized and managed.[41] They were, as I noted, open to a wide range of people, and every subscriber had the same privileges, including an identical vote at the governors' meetings and the right to inspect the hospitals' minute books, account books, and contracts. Wilson stresses that these procedures allowed men in the middle ranks, who had quite circumscribed political influence within the kingdom, to deploy power and to participate in social authority. Through charitable organizations, then, the middling sort identified with the elite not only by hoping to better themselves by contact with the right circles, but, more important, by having yet another way to distance themselves from the poor, the marginal, and the disreputable.[42] Hospital subscribers were on the other side of a widening cultural divide and could demonstrate this with their own public acts of generosity and efficient management.

Active governors and medical men

Understanding the hospitals' public faces – the images they projected with their buildings, their newspaper announcements for benefit concerts, and their printed reports and lists of governors – shows how important hospitals were as cultural symbols of charitable activity. These images, however, did not run the hospitals. The governors who actually showed up at board meetings did.[43]

At all of the hospitals, a group of governors met weekly to take care of the routine chores, including deciding upon patients' admissions and seeing to complaints or new proposals. Governors attending the annual general meeting usually elected or appointed members of these groups, called "weekly boards" or the "House Committee" (except at Guy's, where it was the "Court of Committees," each governor serving on it being a "committee"), although any governor could attend any weekly meeting if he chose. These committees passed on their resolutions, decisions, and motions to the Quarterly General Courts for discussion and confirmation, rejection or tabling, with one of the quarterly courts usually overlapping with the annual meeting. At any time, the weekly boards or the president could call for Special (or Extraordinary) General Courts, for which notices

41 Wilson, "Urban Culture and Political Activism," 173.
42 Wilson, "Urban Culture and Political Activism."
43 Identifying the men who attended board meetings entails the same, if not more, problems as identifying those on the full lists, since many of their names simply do not appear in published sources. Wilson, in his "The Politics of Medical Improvement," and Rose, in his "Politics and the London Royal Hospitals," have made the most detailed attempts to identify specific governors acting at specific times. Their work shows the difficulties, and hazards, of "identifying" well-known men, especially to give them solid enough party affiliations and religious orientations on which to generalize about the governors' motives.

were sent to all the governors noting the topic to be addressed. The president was supposed to chair the General Courts but could delegate that honor to one of the vice-presidents or to another governor. The hospital secretary and treasurer, both elected officials, shared the day-to-day administrative power with the weekly board. Governors also regularly visited the wards and inspected the hospital, reporting irregularities to the weekly boards. Sometimes appointed from members of the weekly boards, sometimes from the governors at large, these Visiting Governors were the ones who interacted most with the patients and hospital servants. Any governor could visit and raise complaints if he wished, so it appears that hospital boards created Visiting Governors because few patrons spontaneously took this duty seriously.[44]

Many of the men and women who subscribed to the voluntary hospitals, and a good proportion of the men elected to the endowed ones, could well have agreed with Lord Bute. When solicited for a subscription in 1763, he replied to the Middlesex governors that he would give "if it did not require any Attendance, or put him to any Trouble."[45] And a far smaller number of governors bothered to take "any Trouble" with these charities than the number who subscribed, except at exciting moments such as the contested staff elections that I discuss later. Thus, to establish that any of the hospitals' particular administrative decisions and acts arose directly from broader political, religious, economic, and social positions demands considerably more work in London's archives. From the attempts that I have made to identify active governors, I believe that most were the lesser lights on the governors' lists. At the voluntary hospitals especially, the faithful seem to have been local clergy, shopkeepers, tradesmen, retired military officers, and middling gentlemen, with a sprinkling of sirs, honorables, and right-reverends. Even those regularly attending meetings at the endowed hospitals tended not to be current Directors of the Bank of England, or the Honorable East India Company, much less the Lord Mayor. How involvement for these men varied over their careers and life cycles (did retired bankers and merchants spend more time at meetings? or the newly elected sons of prominent men go to mingle?) remains an interesting question for social historians.

44 W. B. Howrie, "Complaints and Complaint Procedures in the Eighteenth- and Early-Nineteenth-Century Provincial Hospitals," *Medical History* 25 (1981): 354–62, gives close descriptions of what visiting governors did and his characterizations apply equally well to the London hospitals in this period. See, for example, London Hospital, Visitors Book, 1781–94, LH/A/16/3, District Archives, Tower Hamlets Health Authority.
45 Middlesex Hospital, Minutes of the Governors, 4 May 1763. The London, the Middlesex, St. George's, and the Westminster all had "lady" governors, who could vote by proxy in staff elections. For discussion of women subscribers and charity, see Andrew, *Philanthropy and Police,* and idem, "Two Medical Charities in Eighteenth-Century London: The Lock Hospital and the Lying-In Charity for Married Women," in *Medicine and Charity Before the Welfare State,* ed. Barry and Jones, 82–97.

The active governors usually had plenty to do at their meetings. Dealing with patients occupied a relatively small proportion of their time, particularly at General Courts, where the records hardly ever mention specific patients' names or problems. The minute books of governors' meetings are full of business: cash flow, orders for repairs, inspections of accounts, hiring and dismissing of nurses, and all the other tasks for keeping these large enterprises going. On the local level, hospital governors wielded patronage over the contracts for the charities' groceries, meat, cheese, bread, beer, drugs, and fuel. Suspicion of undue influence made most of the hospitals proclaim that tradesmen providing these goods could not serve as governors, meaning that it was up to their brothers, uncles, cousins, and friends on the boards to help their bids get approved.[46] At the Middlesex, however, to note the inevitable contrary example, the governors formally decided that preference should be "given to Tradesmen who are subscribers."[47]

The minute books also reveal the chains of influence that governors used to further hospital interests, from individuals' connections not only to the grand and mighty, but also to more modest areas of power. The active governors at the endowed hospitals handled some complex financial affairs, for their corporations held numerous investments, including land that they leased to scores of tenants. Some of the properties included rights to fill the local clerical livings, thus giving the governors the patronage roles enjoyed by landed elites and other corporate bodies, such as Oxford and Cambridge.[48] As I have mentioned, Craig Rose has shown how control over property had significant political meaning for St. Thomas's and St. Bartholomew's in the later seventeenth century. Property and patronage clearly continued to shape the endowed hospitals' relationships with the City and the Crown, especially the induction of governors throughout the eighteenth century, although the precise influences remain to be explored. For all of the hospitals, the active governors' connections with various groups in London were a staple of regular business. In 1796, for instance, the governors at the London Hospital thanked John Liptrap, Sheriff and life governor, "for his help on the Court of Common Council." Liptrap and the chair of the weekly board, Christopher B. Metcalf, both fairly middling

46 Borsay, "'Persons of Honour and Reputation'"; Clark-Kennedy, *The London,* 1: 142; London Hospital, Court of Governors Minutes, 19 Dec. 1750, LH/A/2/2.
47 Middlesex Hospital, *Laws, Orders and Regulations,* 13; John Howard strongly disapproved of this practice at the Middlesex. Howard, *An Account of the Principal Lazarettos,* 133.
48 See, for example, Guy's Hospital, Minutes of the Court of Governors, 10 May, 2 Aug. 1737, 8 Nov. 1765, 10 Feb. 1767; H9/GY/A1/1/1. At the August 1737 meeting, the governors had a living to grant, with two petitioners. They "called in & heard as to what they had to further offer" before deciding on William Willim. In 1765, the governors reminded the candidates for rector of Peterstow in Hereford that the rector had to reside in the living and was "personally to discharge the duties of the rector." Cameron, *Guy's,* 58–61, discusses the Guy's governors' management of Thomas Guy's endowment.

men, had worked hard to persuade the City of London to give the hospital an immediate donation of £500, a generous sum for a charity outside the City's jurisdiction.[49]

Medical practitioners, too, sat as governors at all the general hospitals along with their friends and relatives, mixing with possible patrons and patients. Getting elected or choosing to subscribe was as just as available to them as to anyone else in metropolitan society, under the conditions I have just described. The governors at St. Bartholomew's, St. Thomas's, and Guy's very rarely elected medical men, however. Dr. Edward Hulse, for example, joined the St. Thomas's governors in 1723. He was physician in ordinary to King George I, after serving Queen Anne in the same post. But many other royal physicians and surgeons never were elected, so it is perhaps equally telling that his brother-in-law, Richard Levett, was a governor at the time.[50] Most of the medical practitioners elected at these endowed hospitals were the select few among the staff physicians and surgeons whom the governors decided to honor with an appointment when they retired from duty. John Belchier, for instance, was surgeon to St. Thomas's for thirty-two years (1736–68). When he stepped down, the governors at both St. Thomas's and at Guy's invited him to join them. Similarly, William Saunders, physician to Guy's from 1770 to 1802, became a governor at both hospitals in 1804 and attended Court meetings at Guy's fairly regularly thereafter.[51] Medical governors at the endowed hospitals, in short, were men well established in society and in their careers, if not already quite finished with practicing medicine.

In contrast to the endowed hospitals, the voluntary ones split over the question of whether or not current staff physicians and surgeons could have governor's privileges, even if they subscribed. They all started off with the staff as full governors, many of whom regularly attended weekly board meetings and General Courts. At the Westminster and St. George's,

49 London Hospital, Governors Minutes, 26 July 1796. For the details of this request to the City, and the hospital's fulsome thanks, see Common Council, Journal, v. 76, 23 June, 4 Aug. 1796. The request reminded the Common Council that "Many of the Objects relieved are Artificers, Labourers or Journeymen employed in the City and its Suburbs," especially accident victims, who were admitted immediately, "without any recommendation or any expense to the Patient."

50 William Munk, *The Roll of the Royal College of Physicians of London, comprising biographical sketches of all the eminent physicians whose names are recorded in the Annals*, 2nd ed., 4 vols. (London: Royal College of Physicians, 1878), 2: 65–6; for Richard Levett, son of Sir Richard Levett, Hulse's father-in-law, who died in 1711, see Beaven, *Aldermen*, 2: 124. The St. Thomas's governors elected Dr. David Orme, a noted but not especially famous man-midwife and lecturer, in 1776, for reasons I cannot even guess. For practitioners and royal appointments, see W. F. Bynum, "Medicine at the English Court, 1688–1837," in *Medicine at the Courts of Europe, 1500–1837*, ed. Vivian Nutton (London and New York: Routledge, 1990), 262–89.

51 Cameron, *Guy's*, 98.

the medical staff had all the governor's rights throughout the century, as long as they kept up their subscriptions. The active physicians and surgeons at these hospitals sometimes comprised most of the governors who showed up for the weekly boards, even, on occasion, for an Annual General Court.[52] At the London and the Middlesex in the 1750s, however, the governors decided to exclude staff from acting as governors during their service to the charity, to take effect with the next elections for physicians and surgeons. The London governors stuck to the policy they passed on 19 December 1750 and it became part of the provisions of the hospital's charter in 1758.[53] The staff at the Middlesex clearly disliked the 1752 regulation, for it obviously distinguished them from their governor-colleagues in the other nonchartered, West End institutions. In 1760, an attempt to revoke the rule failed when, after much debate, the staff "withdrew their Motion." Ten years later, a new set of bylaws omitted the exclusion, and staff governors immediately became regulars again at the weekly board meetings and at the General Courts.[54] While most hospital physicians and surgeons could not act as governors at their own hospitals, moreover, technically nothing prevented them from paying to do so elsewhere. William Saunders, for example, while a physician at Guy's, subscribed as a life governor (with a single payment of £30) to the London.

52 See, for example, St. George's Hospital, Board of Governors Minutes, v. 12, 3 Jan. 1776, v. 14, 8 Feb. 1788, which I chose at random for samples of meetings. Eight governors attended the weekly board meeting on 3 Jan. 1776: the chair, Mr. Rennald, Reverend Clarke, and six current staff: the four surgeons, John Hunter, Charles Hawkins, John Gunning and William Bromfield, and two of the four physicians, Drs. Richard Wright and John Burgess. At the Yearly General Court held 8 Feb. 1788, only twelve governors were present: three of the four full surgeons (Hunter, Gunning, and William Walker); two assistant surgeons, Thomas Keate (to Gunning) and Everard Home (to Hunter); and three physicians, Drs. John B. Robertson, Matthew Baillie, and George Pearson. The remaining, and clearly outnumbered, nonstaff governors were D. Gib (*possibly* the surgeon Daniel Gibs listed in the *Medical Register* of 1783), George Medley, Mr. Setlow, and Rev. James Clarke.
53 London Hospital, Governors Minutes, 19 Dec. 1750; Clark-Kennedy, *The London*, 1: 30, 141. Staff men could still pay subscriptions, of course, even if they did not get the privileges. William Blizard, for example, was listed as a life governor in the hospital's report, *General State of the London Hospital . . .* (London, 1787).
54 The decision on 2 Apr. 1752 stated: "No Physician, man-Midwife or Surgeon, or other Officer or Servant of this Charity who shall hereafter be elected shall act as a Governor of this charity during his Continuance in office." The wording was important, as several staff men elected before this date continued to act as full governors, including the surgeons Henry Watson (to 1762), Pennell Hawkins (to 1756), and William Young (to 1758), and the physicians Charles Morton (to 1754) and Henry Hinkley (to 1756). Henry Watson raised the motion to reinstate staff as governors in 1760 on behalf of his colleagues. Since he was the only one left by then, he probably had good reason to insist. Watson resigned from the Middlesex to serve the Westminster – as surgeon and governor – a year and a half after his motion had to be withdrawn. Middlesex Hospital, Minutes of the . . . Governors, 2 Apr. 1752, 19 Feb., 18 Mar., 1 May 1760, 3 May 1770. Middlesex Hospital, *Laws, Orders and Regulations*, 1770, n.p.; Wilson, *The Middlesex*, 16, 222.

Few staff men did this, however, perhaps from loyalty and good manners, or lack of time, or a surfeit of charitable goodness expressed through their hospital duties.[55]

Whether or not allowed to act as independent governors, some staff men had considerable involvement in managing their hospital's medical affairs along with active lay governors. Three of the voluntary hospitals, for instance, St. George's, the London, and the Middlesex, established "medical committees" responsible for inspecting the apothecary's laboratory, surgery room, and medical supplies; approving candidates for the apothecary's post; and generally seeing to medical matters.[56] The one created at the Middlesex in 1763 was the most elaborate, with twenty governors and staff men appointed by a Quarterly General Court. Only hospital physicians and surgeons, however, tended to show up for its monthly meetings, where they primarily discussed drug orders, inventories, and medical costs.[57] Lay governors at the voluntary hospitals also appointed staff physicians and surgeons to special committees formed to address specific problems, such as revisions to the bylaws or regulations for hospital pupils. When faced with major complaints against one of the medical staff about poor medical care, nevertheless, the governors carefully excluded their medical officers from committees of inquiry.[58]

Throughout the eighteenth century, as my sketch has emphasized, the general hospitals in London served many individuals' purposes. Assigning specific motives for charitable giving, for the effort some governors put into the hospitals or for its absence among others, remains tricky at best. "Medical" versus "lay" concerns and interests might seem easy to identify from a distance but become closely intertwined in the hospitals' board-

55 Among the other staff men who were governors at one hospital while staff at another were Dr. Charles Cotes and Ambrose Dickins. Cotes was physician to the Westminster from 1733 to 1739. During that time he was elected MP (1734) and elected a governor of St. Thomas's (1736). Munk, *Roll*, 2: 137; Ambrose Dickins had a distinguished career as serjeant-surgeon to Queen Anne, George I, and George II. He was elected a governor of St. Bartholomew's in 1721. In that year he became surgeon to the Westminster Infirmary and, when St. George's split off, surgeon to St. George's from 1733 to 1738. Bromfield, *St. George's*, 8, 10. These examples suggest political connections as much as possible hospital alliances.

56 St. George's Hospital, Laws and Regulations . . . extracted from the Minute Books (manuscript compiled in 1805), 281–2; London Hospital, Governors Minutes, 28 Dec. 1748; *By-laws of the Governors of the London Hospital* (London: H. S. Woodfall, 1769), 3; Middlesex Hospital, *Laws, Orders and Regulations*, 28; Langdon-Davies, *The Westminster*, 148; Westminster Hospital, Proceedings of the Trustees, 15 Feb. 1792. In 1792 the hospital physicians proposed a medical committee, but nothing seems to have come of it until 1826.

57 Middlesex Hospital, Minutes of the . . . Governors, 3 Nov. 1763; Middlesex Hospital, Minutes of the Medical Committee 1773–8, Middlesex Hospital Archives. This volume includes notes to 1783; it is the only surviving manuscript minute book for this committee in the archives.

58 For details on a report about complaints against staff men, see Clark-Kennedy, *The London*, 89–95; Middlesex Hospital, Minutes of the . . . Governors, 3 May 1770.

rooms. The men who were governors to more than one hospital, or who moved in the same business, religious, or social circles with other governors and subscribers, moreover, connected these charities to one another, through both public displays of metropolitan-wide munificence and private discussions among boardroom associates.[59] As much as the London hospitals were distinct institutions, with one or another offering an exception to almost any generalization, they shared clusters of people who took their charitable beliefs, social values, medical practices, rivalries, prestige, patrons, and problems along with them. The governors reached decisions about hospital policies and procedures, such as the regulations for staff hours or privileges to pupils, knowing what other hospitals did.[60] The medical men who served them, too, knew a great deal about what went on in their colleagues' charities – before, when, and after these practitioners had direct authority to change patients' lives.

HOSPITAL PRACTITIONERS

In the episode I discussed at the beginning of this chapter, the governors at the London Hospital objected to appointing assistant surgeons because these new posts interfered with "their privilege of electing a Principal Surgeon."[61] They discovered this in the late spring of 1797, for two of the new assistants promptly stepped into positions opened when one full surgeon died in April and another died in June. The governors held elections for the full surgeons' posts as usual, but only the senior assistant surgeon at the time appeared as a candidate, making the choice pro forma. Whether or not a clever behind-the-scenes contrivance among the surgical staff and would-be candidates, this succession of appointments annoyed enough governors to have the positions simply abolished, not reformed.

The governors' power to elect all of a hospital's medical officers further underscores the social webs entangling lay and medical interests and expectations. While most elections proceeded calmly, especially when just one candidate was left because all the others judiciously withdrew beforehand, others rivaled the exciting hustings at Parliamentary polls.[62] At contested staff elections, hundreds of governors showed up to ballot for candidates

59 When the Middlesex governors were concerned about the rise in dispensaries, for example, they wanted to work with St. George's and the Westminster on the problem. They formed a committee to formulate proposals and directed "that the governors of this Hospital, being governors of one or both of those hospitals, be requested to procure a meeting of some of the governors from each of these hospitals" to discuss them. Middlesex Hospital, Minutes of the . . . Governors, 9 May 1788. Also quoted in Wilson, *The Middlesex*, 51.
60 See, for instance, Middlesex Hospital, Minutes of the Governors, 21 June 1757. I draw further connections in Chapter 4.
61 London Hospital, Governors Minutes, 12 Sept. 1797.
62 Clark-Kennedy, *The London*, 1: 80–4.

who had lobbied hard, some even going into debt to line voters' pockets with subscription fees. Hospital elections publicly bestowed lay approval upon certain practitioners, granting them respect for their medical knowledge and responsibilities for patient care in places where their work and ideas could be watched and commented upon. When the governors chose a hospital physician or surgeon, they picked a man who represented the charity's major purpose, the cure of the deserving poor, through his orders about care and medications or his performance of operations. Yet they also selected a man who displayed their social values and public loyalties, quite apart from considerations of his medical skill.[63] And they guarded their rights to make these judgments through trial by democratic fire, affirming that *they* knew a good man, and a good practitioner, when they, or friends, business partners, patrons, or relatives, saw one.[64]

Having a hospital post defines the group who emerged as an elite among London practitioners in the eighteenth century, for reasons I explore later, but the process of *getting* a hospital post exposes why its members had very diverse intellectual, social, educational, and medical concerns. At all of the hospitals, staff men had certain minimal duties to fulfill for their charitable service. Some put in their required visits and immediately went off to paying patients; others spent extra hours on the wards, instructing paying pupils; still others devoted themselves to hospital attendance. As these men varied in their commitment to hospital work among themselves and over their careers, they also differed in their attitudes toward the sick and injured men and women whom they admitted into the hospitals, saw on the wards, and watched depart, either living or dead. Whether superficially rhetorical or deeply felt, beliefs that practitioners must treat hospital patients with as much Christian kindness, compassion and conservatism as they had for their private patients were expressed by several staff men. With this stance, physicians and surgeons used hospital cases for "experiments," as I discuss in Part II, under the same personal constraints they had when trying out a new remedy or operation on a nonhospital case. No set of ward rules or governors' dicta, however, presumed to direct those practitioners who lacked compassion or experimental restraint in their private work to behave differently when they walked

63 Astley Cooper, for example, who initially favored the French Revolution, had a reputation as a "political partisan" that endangered his election to the surgeon's post at Guy's. I discuss his decision to give up political opinions in Chapter 8. Bransby B. Cooper, *Life of Sir Astley Cooper*, 2 vols. (London: J. Parker, 1843), 1: 293–7; M. Jeanne Peterson, *The Medical Profession in Mid-Victorian London* (Berkeley: University of California Press, 1978), has an excellent discussion of nineteenth-century hospital elections (see pp. 140–57).

64 For a pointed contemporary criticism of governors' power to elect practitioners, see Medicinae Studiosus, *A Letter to Thomas Keate, Esq. . . . with some general remarks on the medical profession occasion'd by the approaching election of a Surgeon to St. George's Hospital* (London: T. Hurst, 1800).

into the hospital, exuding comfortable self-confidence and issuing commands.[65]

Getting in

Hospital governors elected three sorts of practitioners – physicians, surgeons, and apothecaries – as well as other hospital officers, such as the chaplain, treasurer, resident steward, and, in some institutions, matron. Those in elected positions had greater medical, financial, or moral responsibility than those simply hired for wages, such as nurses and day laborers. By 1745 all of the hospitals had three full physicians and three full surgeons serving at a time (except for St. George's, which had four of each). The number and status of assistant physicians and assistant surgeons, however, varied by hospital.[66] Both full and assistant hospital physicians and surgeons donated their time, an expression of their own charitable virtues and financial independence, and so a mark of their presumed gentlemanly status. None of the physicians or surgeons lived *in* the hospital, either, as most of the other officers did.[67] Each hospital had only one apothecary, who sometimes had official assistants or help from his apprentices. Unlike his fellow practitioners, the hospital apothecary was required to be single, to live in the hospital, and to forgo private practice. For this service, the apothecary received a salary, living quarters, board, and coals and, for all intents and purposes, had the status of an upper servant, rather like the resident steward and matron. Over the course of the 1700s, as independent apothecaries and surgeon–apothecaries became the de facto general practitioners of eighteenth-century society, the hospital apothecary remained in a circumscribed and subordinate position within an institutional hierarchy. Although responsible for patient care when staff physicians and surgeons were not in the hospital, the apothecary took orders from the other staff about treatment.[68] By the late eighteenth century, resident apothecaries,

---

65 See, for instance, Moore, *St. Bartholomew's*, 2: 531, on Dr. Pierce Dod's pompous manner, and his place in Hogarth's caricature, "The Consultation of Physicians."

66 See Appendix I.B. For examples of regulations covering assistant physicians and surgeons, see: London Hospital, Governors Minutes, 16 July 1746, 6 Feb. 1750/1; Westminster Hospital, Proceedings of the Trustees, 21 Mar. 1787; St. Thomas's Hospital, Court of Governors, 28 July 1790.

67 At the endowed hospitals, St. Bartholomew's, St. Thomas's, and Guy's, the staff received a token fee of £30 to £40 per year. For references to this salary, see Guy's Hospital, Minute Book of the Court of Governors, 5 Mar. 1744, where the candidates for an additional physician's and surgeon's post had to have "offered to serve with:t Salaries." St. Thomas's, Court of Governors, 12 Dec. 1679, 9 Oct. 1702; Cameron, *Guy's*, remarks that staff physicians received their honorary £40 until 1948, such was the persistence of tradition. Cameron, *Guy's*, 55.

68 At St. George's, for example, from the 1780s the hospital apothecary had plenty of reminders of his lower status. The governors named "Visiting Apothecaries" from among their ranks, who inspected the House Apothecary's work and were available for medical

then, had neither the prestige nor the authority of the other medical staff and so stayed on the margins of the hospital elite emerging among London practitioners.

I have listed the names, posts, and dates of service for all of the physicians and surgeons elected to the seven general hospitals from 1700 through 1815 in Appendix I. A total of 310 men filled 331 posts (including assistants); 21 staff men moved from one hospital to another during their careers.[69] All told, 132 positions for full surgeons and 182 positions for full physicians came open (314) in this period, since 16 surgeons and 2 physicians resigned or died without moving up to full status. When each of the five London hospitals founded in the eighteenth century started, six or so practitioners immediately became hospital men, usually by appointment, not election. After midcentury the size of this metropolitan group stabilized at 45 men, with 22 physicians and 23 surgeons holding full positions at the general hospitals at any one time.[70] The small number of places was another reason why practitioner-inspired medical charities, especially dispensaries, proliferated in the later eighteenth century, when institutional affiliations increasingly marked medical status and visibility, but so few men could become physicians or surgeons at the general hospitals.

The number of chances for ambitious physicians and surgeons to obtain one of these hospital posts depended, of course, on the turnover among those who had them. Staff men were elected for life, and many served until they died or retired from practice. In general, hospital surgeons stayed at their posts longer than hospital physicians, especially after the number of ward-walking pupils increased and the surgeons took home a nice income from their fees.[71] William Blizard, for example, resigned from the London in 1833. He was ninety years old and had been staff surgeon for fifty-four years. His was an extreme case, no doubt inspiring much muttering among his juniors, yet other hospital men served for decades. Other staff, of course, resigned after only a few years of attendance, as the pressures of private practice, lack of interest in ward care, or other avocations made

consultations. St. George's Hospital, Board of Governors' Minutes, 12 Apr. 1799; Clark-Kennedy, *The London*, 1: 41; Middlesex Hospital, *Laws, Orders and Regulations*, 36–7. On the status of apothecaries in the eighteenth century, see Juanita G. L. Burnby, *A Study of the English Apothecary from 1660 to 1760*, Medical History, Supplement No. 3, 1983; Irvine Loudon, *Medical Care and the General Practitioner, 1750–1850* (Oxford: Clarendon Press, 1985).

69 William F. Bynum has explored the career patterns and choices of staff men to the general hospitals, specialized hospitals, and dispensaries, as well. See his "Physicians, Hospitals and Career Structures in Eighteenth-Century London," in *William Hunter and the Eighteenth-Century Medical World*, ed. William F. Bynum and Roy Porter (Cambridge: Cambridge University Press, 1985), 105–28; and Bynum, "Medicine at the English Court, 1688–1837."

70 See Appendix I.B. I have excluded the physician–accoucheurs to the Middlesex from this analysis.

71 See Chapter 4.

them choose to move on. On rare occasions, internal disputes led the active governors to encourage their medical officers to depart voluntarily. In 1765, for instance, Samuel Howard and Isaac Minors, staff surgeons at the Middlesex, and Dr. William Baylies, staff physician, stopped consulting with James Moffat, the other staff surgeon. At a Special General Court, which attracted seventy-three governors, an apparently intense discussion ended with the Court's voting "to request Mr. Moffat to withdraw his attendance on the Hospital," and Moffat did, although he never formally resigned.[72]

When a surgeon or physician died or resigned, the governors officially announced a vacancy at a weekly board meeting or general court, sometimes ordering that an advertisement be sent to the newspapers.[73] Notices for an election, usually called as a Special General Court, went out in due course, with a least a month or two between the acknowledged vacancy and the election. In this period, a practitioner declared himself as a candidate at a weekly board meeting and the governors examined his credentials – if, that is, they required any. During the eighteenth century, as I discuss in detail in Chapter 3, formal licensing carried little weight as a check on those who could or could not practice in London. Many medical men simply did not bother with the expense of joining the Corporation of Surgeons or the Royal College of Physicians (RCP), whose powers to prosecute nonmembers in the City of London and seven miles around were not only quite weak, but rarely tested. Membership had social rewards, however, for ambitious practitioners. While not necessarily a mark of competence, corporate connection signified occupational status, a self-identification with the expectations about background, training, and

---

72 Middlesex Hospital, Governors Minutes, 31 Oct. 1765. See also 22, 29 Oct., 5 Nov. 1765. Moffat simply stopped going to the hospital. The weekly board governors waited five days before declaring a vacancy. Wilson, *The Middlesex,* 224–5. During a dispute at St. Thomas's in 1768, the governors forced one of the surgeons, Benjamin Cowell, to resign, and Thomas Baker, Cowell's surgical colleague, resigned soon after. St. Thomas's, Minutes of the Grand Committee, 27 July, 19 Aug. 1768, GLRO H1/ST/A1/7; Parsons, *St. Thomas's,* 2: 223–5, 265. In neither case did the governors record specific complaints against these men. Baker, however, in 1767 had lost a legal case, in which a private patient, Mr. Slater, complained that Baker had incorrectly treated his fractured leg. Not only had Baker not informed Slater of his plan to rebreak the leg, but the testimony also pointed the judge to the decision that "Mr. Baker wanted to try an experiment with [his] new instrument." George Wilson, *Reports of the Cases Argued and Adjudged in the King's Courts at Westminster,* 4th ed., 3 parts (Dublin: Luke White, 1792), 2: 362. (In the case description Baker is incorrectly given as surgeon to St. Bartholomew's Hospital.) I am extremely grateful to Dr. Catherine Crawford for this reference. The story of Baker's defeat was well known to contemporaries: see Sylas Neville, *The Diary of Sylas Neville, 1767–1788,* ed. Basil Cozens-Harely (Oxford and London: Oxford University Press, 1980), 141.

73 See, for instance, Westminster Hospital, Proceedings of the Trustees, 29 Mar. 1786. Hospital governors became annoyed when candidates began to canvass for votes before a vacancy was announced. See, for example, Middlesex Hospital, Minutes of the . . . Governors, 8 Mar. 1814.

knowledge that defined these traditional groups. Among physicians, the distinction between Fellows (FRCP) and Licentiates (LRCP) especially marked a gulf between the College's elite, the Fellows who ruled it, and the Licentiates, whom the Fellows examined, licensed, and excluded from power. Fellows had MDs from Oxford or Cambridge, and so had to belong to the Church of England; Licentiates took their MDs elsewhere, at Leiden, Edinburgh, or any number of Continental universities, and so had no single religious hoop to jump through. I focus on hospital physicians in the following discussion of staff positions, in large part because of the accessibility of sources to identify them individually and collectively.[74] With physicians at the top of the medical hierarchy, debates and evidence about whom to elect reveal the issues at stake, yet unfortunately do leave the surgeons still in the shaded background. Here it must suffice to stress that when the hospitals' governors acknowledged candidates for their medical posts, they usually faced Corporation surgeons and Collegiate physicians, partly because these were the men who thought themselves appropriately placed for hospital service.

Before the last third of the eighteenth century, however, the evidence is not at all clear about how much hospital governors actually cared that their candidates conformed to corporate or Collegiate requirements. In many cases, the hospitals' clerks and secretaries simply did not record in the minutes just what contenders did to verify their suitability to stand for election.[75] The lack of routine procedures for documenting professional status has significant implications for the formation of London's hospital elite from the 1740s to the 1780s. On one hand, it is quite probable that evidence of membership in the Surgeons' Company or holding of an LRCP or FRCP was simply so obvious that the governors may not have bothered to have it recorded, especially if the candidate were personally known to them. On the other hand, a few telling examples show that the governors at some of the voluntary hospitals felt no obligation to pay attention to the Royal College of Physicians' paper power over London practice. Approximately one-sixth of the physicians elected either never bothered to sit at the Royal College of Physicians for examination, or did so after they

74 Complete lists of the names of members of the Barber–Surgeons' Company, the Surgeons' Company, and the Royal College of Surgeons (before the 1830s) are available only from the manuscript records of these bodies. Unfortunately for my study, these have not been accessible enough to me to pursue systematic identification of the hospital surgeons. Since retired military surgeons did not need membership in the surgeons' corporations to practice legally in London, moreover, another large potential pool of surgeons existed outside corporate jurisdiction.

75 The secretary sometimes noted that candidates had "testimonials" in support of their petitions, but then gave no clues about the contents of such papers. See, for example, Westminster Hospital, Proceedings of the Trustees, 5 Apr. 1786, 12 Mar. 1788, 8 June 1791.

obtained their hospital posts.[76] Dr. W. H. Muckleston, for instance, served as physician to St. George's for five years (1783–7) without ever seeking the benefit of Licentiate or Fellowship letters to follow his name. John Brisbane, who received his MD from Edinburgh in 1750, became physician to the Middlesex in 1758, but did not obtain a College Licentiate until 1766.[77] A similar analysis of hospital surgeons' memberships in the Surgeons' Company remains to be done, but I suspect that governors were sometimes equally flexible when accepting surgical candidates for election.[78]

Concern about formal professional qualifications so rarely became an explicit issue for the governors that when it did, sparks flew. Among those incidents that provide glimpses of personalities and patronage at work in the boardrooms, a revealing episode at the Middlesex in the mid-1750s nicely illustrates the interplay of medical and lay interests over staff positions. In 1751, the active governors decided that henceforth "no Physician who shall have practiced as a Surgeon or Apothecary be admitted a Candidate for, or be appointed a Physician to this Hospital."[79] This interesting

76 See Appendix I.C.
77 Thirteen (7 percent) of the physicians elected to hospital posts never received the blessings of the Royal College of Physicians. Since physicians who did not enter the Royal College of Physicians are absent from Munk's *Roll,* finding biographical details on them has been difficult, especially as I could not find evidence for MDs for them from the standard sources. At least three of these are cases where the elected physician had an MB degree from Oxford or Cambridge, which allowed him to practice in England. Gowin Knight (Westminster) and Richard Bathhurst (Middlesex) went this route. Francis Biddulph, elected physician at St. Bartholomew's in 1793 with an MB from Cambridge, promptly died in January 1794. See J. A. Venn, *Alumni Cantabrigiensis,* part II, 6 vols. (Cambridge: At the University Press, 1940), 1: 259; Edward Richardson, physician to the London in 1764, similarly died within a year (Morris, *The London,* 241), as did John Watkinson, physician to St. Thomas's in 1783, but I have not traced any medical degrees they held. A further twenty-two (12 percent) physicians did not possess a College Licentiate on their elections, and half of them then waited several years before applying for College recognition. I have *not* included physicians elected with an Oxford or Cambridge MB, or Oxbridge license to practice, while waiting the number of years necessary to get the MD, for such men were clearly in line for eventual Fellowship status from the College, and all of them (except the ones who remained nonmembers, counted previously) obtained it. Those later getting the Licentiate, in contrast, had MDs from other universities. For Brisbane, see Munk, *Roll,* 2: 275.
78 St. Thomas's required memberships in the Surgeons' Company at least from 1691; St. Thomas's Hospital, Court of Governors, 26 May 1691; Parsons, *St. Thomas's,* 2: 124. In the 1795 discussion about assistant surgeons at the London, the governors decided that candidates had to be members (Clark-Kennedy, *The London,* 1: 188), but I found no mention of this requirement in the discussion about assistant surgeons in 1751. See London Hospital, Governors Minutes, 6 Feb. 1750/1. Since active governors did not always follow their hospitals' regulations, moreover, the names of obscure staff men and candidates simply must be checked in the appropriate records.
79 Middlesex Hospital, Minutes of the . . . Governors, 1 Nov. 1753. This entry refers to a minute of 22 Oct. 1751. This volume of the Minutes was missing at the time I consulted the archives.

measure excluded quite a number of eighteenth-century physicians, men who started out as apprentices to, or simply spent time practicing as, surgeons and apothecaries, before taking an MD degree. Considering that two of the serving physician–governors at the Middlesex had been elected without membership in the RCP, this resolution neatly omitted any requirement for collegiate status. Yet it laid down an unmistakable qualification for background and status dear to elite physicians' hearts for the next century.[80] It did not last. Two years later (with only one of the physician–governors, Charles Morton, left over from 1751, but now possessing the LRCP), the active governors added the clause "*except* that He be a Fellow or Licentiate of the College of Physicians of London."[81] Apparently collegiate membership wiped out the taint of more menial practice from the past. In a remarkable series of Quarterly General Courts in 1754, however, the governors overturned this new clause, overturned the whole requirement, then reinstated the entire resolution, and then overturned it again.

By September the episode had an obvious focus. Dr. Richard Bathhurst, MB (not MD) from Cambridge and one of Samuel Johnson's dear cronies, had offered himself as a candidate. He was neither a member of the RCP, nor, apparently, a physician with an undivided following. At the Special General Court called to attend to this problem, the vote split over the legality of a previous Court that had admitted Bathhurst as a candidate but in the end elected him physician. In the minute book, the secretary recorded a letter from Sir Kenrick Clayton, Vice-President of the hospital and long-time Member of Parliament, which probably helped the governors along. "Permit me," Sir Kenrick told them, "to recommend your unanimous choice of Dr. Bathhurst." His presence, the knight concluded, "will be a Credit to the Hospital." And Sir Kenrick's servant waited for the Court's answer, suggesting that more would be heard from him if they rejected Dr. Bathhurst.[82] Not until 1770 did the Middlesex governors lay down qualification rules again, and this time they lasted. Physicians, finally, had to be members of the RCP *or* graduates of Oxford, Cambridge, or Dublin. Surgeons had to belong to the Surgeons' Company, and could not have been "bred" to practice as an apothecary or man-midwife. Appropriate conformity established, the Middlesex proceeded to attract Fellows as candidates, and a flurry of FRCPs graced their wards.[83]

80 Loudon, *Medical Care and the General Practitioner*, 19–20; Peterson, *Medical Profession*, 6, 225, 255.
81 Middlesex Hospital, Minutes of the . . . Governors, 1 Nov. 1753. Wilson, *The Middlesex*, 188–9.
82 Middlesex Hospital, Minutes of the . . . Governors, 17, 24, 26 Sept. 1753. Wilson, *The Middlesex*, 188–9. For Bathhurst, see Wiltshire, *Samuel Johnson in the Medical World*, 94–6.
83 Middlesex Hospital, *Laws, Orders and Regulations*, 33–4; Anthony Highmore, *Pietas Londinense: The History, Design and Present State of the Various Public Charities in and Near London* (London: Cradock & Joy, 1815), 233.

The shifting fate of the resolution specifying the physicians' qualifications, and Bathhurst's candidacy, not only shows traces of governors working behind scenes to manipulate meetings, but also underscores the impossibility of demarcating a "medical" interest different from a "lay" one. Stories of other candidacies and contested elections repeat the same messages, some involving religious issues, others overtly political ones. In a much publicized episode at the London Hospital, for instance, Samuel Leeds was elected physician in 1768 with a strong Quaker backing, winning over four other contenders, three with LRCPs in hand.[84] In this case, Leeds's lack of an RCP qualification became a way for his opponents to make his life miserable. His critics included the well-respected Quaker physician Dr. John Fothergill, and the animosity between them went before the Society of Friends (who fined Fothergill £5,000 for a damning remark about Leeds) and then to civil court (where Lord Mansfield ruled for Fothergill). In the midst of this dispute, a group of active governors passed a resolution that hospital physicians had to belong to the RCP. Leeds proceeded to examination – and failed, twice. He resigned, humiliated, on 6 June 1770. At the next election, immediately held on 20 June, both candidates had their Licentiate papers with them to show the 401 governors who attended.[85] Every hospital election, in short, tells a tale of influence, factions, and patronage that boosted one man into a post giving him prestige and medical authority, whatever his knowledge or skill.

From the perspective of aspiring candidates, trying to get a hospital position could be a long, tedious, expensive, and potentially embarrassing process.[86] Apprentices to hospital surgeons had a decided entrée into hospital life and connections, and at least by the early nineteenth century this expensive training and patronage had become an understood requirement

84 Five hundred thirty-three governors showed up to vote for one of five candidates. James Brickenden was already physician to the Westminster. William Saunders, who already gave lectures in London, was soon elected to Guy's. They both had the LRCP, as did William Vaughan, while Thomas Cogan and Samuel Leeds did not. These qualifications were not noted in the minutes. London Hospital, Governors Minutes, 25 May 1768; for Brickenden, Saunders, and Vaughan, see Munk, *Roll*, 2: 242, 274, 399–401.

85 Clark-Kennedy, *The London*, 1: 163–4; London Hospital, Governors Minutes, 7 Mar., 6 June, 20 June 1770; John Fothergill, *An Appeal . . . on the late differences between J. Fothergill and S[amuel] L[eeds]* (London, 1773). Other elections at the London occasioned disputes over the next forty years, but all of the candidates at least were members of the Royal College of Physicians. See London Hospital, Governors Minutes, 28 July, 18 Aug., 1 Dec. 1784; 9 June, 2 Sept., 15 Sept., 1807; James J. Abraham, *Lettsom: His Life, Times, Friends and Descendents* (London: Heinemann, 1930), 104, 222–8.

86 For examples of some of the especially nasty pamphlets that elections and hospital service could inspire, see Caesar Hawkins and John Ranby, *The True Account of all the Transactions before the Right Honourable Lords, and others of the Commissioners for the Affairs of Chelsea Hospital; as far as relates to the admission and dismission of Samuel Lee, Surgeon* (London: J. and P. Knapton, 1754); Thomas Skeete, *An Exact Representation of the Very Uncandid and Extraordinary conduct of Dr. John Coakley Lettsom, as well previous to, as on, the day of election for Physician to the Finsbury Dispensary* (London: J. Fielding, 1786).

for advancement.[87] Physicians developed similar ties by walking the wards as physicians' pupils. Six out of the eighteen physicians elected to St. Thomas's between 1750 and 1815, for instance, registered as hospital pupils, some with medical degrees in hand.[88] Hopeful hospital candidates worked to develop other links, too, in order to maintain or to create a presence in the charities. At the voluntary hospitals, future candidates for physicians' and surgeons' posts signed up as governors months or years before a position became open, and some attended meetings assiduously.[89] At the endowed hospitals, since becoming a governor was not an easy option, aspirants joined the hospitals' medical societies, when these appeared in the later eighteenth century, and evinced great interest in hospital practice.[90] As sincere as such efforts to gain hospital experience probably were, they nevertheless served to enhance a practitioner's visibility to the governors and staff men they needed to support them, come time for an election.[91] Such experiences, moreover, may well have helped those with secret goals for eminence realize the extent of the competition long before risking a public declaration of their hopes to serve.

A few personal recollections from hospital men underscore how much the formation of a hospital elite was a story of anxiety and failure as often as ambition and arrogance, even for those who made it in. Ludford Harvey, for instance, confided his electioneering frustrations to his diary. Apprenticed in 1777 to Percival Pott, a St. Bartholomew's surgeon, and considered Pott's personal assistant, Harvey had bright prospects of succeeding to Pott's private practice. With Pott's support, he fully expected to be elected an assistant surgeon, the post that all full surgeons began in at St. Bartholomew's. Suddenly, however, James Earle, already an assistant

87 Peterson, *Medical Profession*, 141–6.
88 St. Thomas's, Register of Physicians' Pupils. George Fordyce, for example, went to London with an Edinburgh degree in 1758 and walked the wards that year. George Gilbert Currey signed up as a physicians' pupil in 1800. He was elected assistant physician in 1802, received his Oxford MD in 1804, and became a Fellow of the Royal College of Physicians in 1805. Munk, *Roll*, 2: 373, 3: 26.
89 At the Westminster, for example, Drs. Alexander Buchan (elected 1813), George Maton (elected 1800), and George Leman Tuthill (elected 1812) all appeared at governors' meetings before their elections; Dr. Donald Mackinnon, an unsuccessful candidate, did so as well. At the Middlesex, John Obadiah Justamond, surgeon (in 1770) and governor at the Westminster, attended meetings at the Middlesex between 1763 and 1770, standing for election at the Middlesex in 1765. For William Blizard's active role as a hospital governor before his election, see Clark-Kennedy, *The London*, 1: 149–51.
90 Susan C. Lawrence, " 'Desirous of Improvements in Medicine': Pupils and Practitioners in the Medical Societies at Guy's and St. Bartholomew's Hospitals, 1795–1815," *Bulletin of the History of Medicine* 59 (1985): 94–5.
91 Closer to election time, candidates did even more to become known. See, in particular, the detailed newspaper notices published during the contest among George Neale, Richard Hamilton, Gabriel Risoliere, and Henry Thompson for places as assistant surgeons to the London in 1753, in the *Public Advertiser*, 6, 14 Feb., 17 Mar. 1753. See also: *The Gazetteer and New Daily Advertiser*, 11 Jan. 1759, 26 Dec. 1768; *Times*, 30 Sept. 1795.

surgeon to the hospital, married Pott's daughter after a two-week court-ship. He became Pott's heir apparent and Harvey "never afterwards re-ceived the slightest notice or favour from Mr. Pott." At an election for assistant surgeon in 1784, five years after the last opening, Harvey found himself on his own, and wrote bitterly that

the contest was very severe; as the Event was long Expected. . . above 15 friends of Mr. Long in one day having made themselves Governors in his behalf gave him on that day a decided majority ———— this Event I had endevour'd to parry by also *making* Governors & 4 Gentlemen were nominated who were so *generous* as to permit *me* to pay their fines of £50 each – which I veryly believe exhausted the last penny I was master of.[92]

Luckily for Harvey, another full surgeon soon died. James Earle, his re-placement in Pott's affections, stepped into the full position, leaving his assistant surgeon's post open, and Harvey was elected.[93]

Even for apparently well placed physicians, the competition for enough favor to win was intense. Thomas Young, the young natural philosopher and classicist who was elected to the Royal Society at age twenty-one for his work on optics, stood for election at St. George's in 1811. By this time, at thirty-eight, he had inherited a tidy estate from his uncle, Dr. Brocklesby, and had taken an MD degree at Göttingen and another at Cambridge. He canvassed hard among his connections to challenge the other candidates, one of whom had substantial "local interest," the other of whom could draw upon "parliamentary influence." "It is remarkable," Young noted, "what a variety of interests I have been obliged to bring into play." He won, and "Mrs. Young has emerged from death to life by the event of this contest."[94] Dr. Young's wife, at least, had obviously suffered the effects of her physician–husband's ambitions.

In his search for support, Thomas Young had an advantage over the other candidates, one that returns my discussion to the significance of professional status in elections. He was a Fellow of the Royal College of Physicians. As I have stressed, governors at the voluntary hospitals had mixed feelings about requiring collegiate membership of their candidates. But they were well aware of the status of those who held it when casting votes. In every election for a physician for which I have the names of the rival candidates, if Fellows stood against Licentiates at the ballot, a Fellow

92 Ludford Harvey, Private Diary and Memorandums, St. Bartholomew's Hospital Archives [no reference number], Section 2, pp. 52, 55. Emphasis in the original. Long won with seventy-two votes, Harvey received sixty-two votes, and John Heaviside only twenty-four. The fourth candidate, Valentine Jones, withdrew before the election. Moore, *St. Bartholomew's*, 2: 647.

93 Harvey was the only candidate, likely because he had come so close to Long in the previous election and still had "his" governors' support. Moore, *St. Bartholomew's*, 2: 647.

94 Quoted in Alexander Wood and Frank Oldham, *Thomas Young, Natural Philosopher, 1773–1829* (Cambridge: At the University Press, 1954), 74.

won – with one exception.[95] In 1811, William Babington, a dearly beloved physician at Guy's, stepped down from a full physician's spot because of the pressures of his private practice among the metropolitan privileged. Upon receiving his letter of resignation, the governors resolved that the hospital should try "to avail itself of the services of Dr. Babington if they can be afforded in any situation consistent with his professional engagements." With that remarkable display of enthusiasm, Babington decided to serve again as an assistant physician, and was unanimously reelected to this lower post a week later. The governors ignored James Tattersall, a rival candidate who had a brand-new MD from Oxford and a sure future as a Fellow.[96] Thomas Young's experience was more typical of governors' decisions, in the sense that his reputation as a physical scientist, classical linguist, and medical scholar gave a cultural luster to St. George's, along with the prestige of another FRCP physician. His election displayed the governors' good taste and appreciation of rank, as much as their possible attention to his medical merits compared with those of his lesser rivals.

While being a Fellow or Licentiate hardly determined an individual physician's character, his friends, his politics, or his medical skills, of course, these ranks nevertheless stood for definite differences in education, training, collegiate prerogatives, formal relationships with other practitioners, and attitudes toward medical reform. As the hospital elite gained new prestige within the broad community of London practitioners at the end of the eighteenth century, the character of the physicians within it shifted. At midcentury the number of Licentiates equaled the number of Fellows who obtained hospital posts. By the early nineteenth century, Fellows had started to renew the majority they had had among hospital physicians sixty years before, when St. Bartholomew's, St. Thomas's, Guy's, the Westminster, and St. George's nearly always had Fellows who wished to serve these charities.[97] Fellows brought the shadow of the col-

95 This conclusion is based on the following samples. *St. Bartholomew's:* all physicians' elections, from Moore, *St. Bartholomew's*, 2: 516–52 (spot checked for accuracy against St. Bartholomew's, Journal of the Board of Governors, HA1/12, 14, 16); *Middlesex:* all elections, from Wilson, *The Middlesex*, 182–204, and detailed notes from Middlesex Hospital, Minutes of the . . . Governors; *London:* Clark-Kennedy, *The London*, vol. 1, passim, but more names of candidates from the London Hospital, Governors Minutes; *Westminster:* Proceedings of the Board of Trustees, for elections between 1780 and 1815; *St. Thomas's:* St. Thomas's, Court of Governors, for elections between 1780 and 1815; *Guy's:* Guy's Hospital, Minute Book of the Court of Governors, 1725–1815, for elections between 1779 and 1815 (I am extremely grateful to Sue Palmer, who, when Guy's archivist at the GLRO, extracted this information for me from a volume unfit for consultation); *St. George's:* St. George's Hospital, Board of Governors, for elections between 1790 and 1815.
96 Guy's Hospital, Court of Governors, 6, 13 Nov. 1811.
97 See Appendix I.C and I.D. These figures include physicians elected without the RCP but who later obtained the Licentiate, since the later LRCPs still represent "lower"-ranking MDs.

lege's conservatism and respect for classical learnedness with them, in increasing contrast to the Licentiates' enthusiasms for newfangled ideas, methods, and medical power that already undermined the traditional elite's claims for authority over medical knowledge. And Licentiates, for whatever mix of social and professional reasons, won hospital posts only when they competed with other Licentiates, or were such clearly favored choices that other candidates withdrew before election day arrived. When Fellows wanted hospital posts, they usually won them.[98]

Getting into a hospital post called all of a practitioner's social and occupational circumstances into play with those of the governors who elected him. Once in, staff men interacted with governors, in ways that religion, politics, status, and learning continued to shape, but now they all had patient care and hospital management to talk about, as well as where they learned medicine, whom they knew, how they stood on current events, and what church or chapel occupied their Sundays. New staff men took on duties and privileges that gave them access to different conditions for clinical experience, to contact with students, and to expressions of charitable care for the poor. And, barring discord and scandal, physicians and surgeons could stick with these opportunities for a few months, a few years, or the rest of their lives. Although members of the emerging hospital elite ended up overlapping with the inner circles of the Corporation (or, after 1800, the College) of Surgeons and the Royal College of Physicians, moreover, neither corporate body had any formal role in determining specific candidates, much less winners. Where the ruling groups of these bodies passed their authority on to their worthy juniors more or less by seniority, in the hospitals the governors handed it over by ballot – a

98 The London, for instance, off east in Whitechapel and supported by Dissenters, had only four Fellows serve of the hospital's nineteen physicians (21 percent) elected between 1740 and 1815. The relative status of physicians at the Middlesex rather suddenly reversed its proportions around 1770, as I have mentioned. Before the hospital settled into respectability, the governors elected twenty physicians: four non-RCP practitioners, four Fellows (20 percent), and twelve Licentiates (60 percent). During the next forty-five years, 80 percent (twelve of fifteen) of the new physicians were Fellows, who served from time to time with one of the three Licentiates who made it in. St. Bartholomew's, in contrast, close to St. Paul's in the City and with a history of affiliation with high church interests in the Church of England, had only one Licentiate succeed among the roll of Fellows elected physicians. Moore, *St. Bartholomew's*, 2: 516–52. At Bart's, Dr. Robert Pate, physician from 1752 to 1762, was the exception, and he held an MD from Aberdeen. Moore found this episode peculiar. "Some circumstances which I have failed to discover must have affected this election," Moore confessed, since Pate faced Dr. Anthony Askew, a candidate with Fellowship credentials (p. 534). Bart's had a close connection with the Royal College of Physicians. In his will, Dr. Balwin Hanney directed that £40 a year be given as a salary for a physician at the hospital. His bequest required that the physician have the FRCP and be one of two candidates recommended by the College (see St. Bartholomew's, Journal of the Board of Governors, 1 Feb. 1749, HA1/12). In election proceedings, the minutes record the RCP's "candidates," but they regularly declined actually standing for election (cf. 17 Mar. 1774, 14 Aug. 1801), a detail that Moore omitted.

process that subtly shifted the pathways to the power over who made and disseminated acceptable medical knowledge.

Duties and deference

Relationships between hospital practitioners and poor patients were always configured by rank, by the disparities in dress and deportment, knowledge, and background, that marked interactions up and down the deference scale of eighteenth-century British society. Medical authority was inextricably intertwined with social authority, as historians and sociologists have frequently emphasized for early modern (and modern) clinical encounters.[99] Yet, while some staff physicians and surgeons disdained the poor, others evidenced respect for individuals they found on the wards. Similarly, while most patients seem to have passively obeyed and done what they were told, others rebelled and walked out of a hospital when it suited them.[100] Some, indeed, simply got their own way on the wards. Dr. Thomas Young, FRCP, for instance, mentioned the case of one of his patients in St. George's in his learned book on consumption. Dr. Young strongly advised against excessive bloodletting in such conditions, but this patient insisted on them, and not only received them, but (of course) soon died of debility. Perhaps Dr. Young decided to let the patient have what he wanted, rather than force him to endure treatment that he distrusted in order to prolong the inevitable. In such small ways, as well as in large ones, medical men displayed their social and medical power on a spectrum between cruelty and kindness, all the while in institutions where the rituals of rank and deference underlay their contact with the sick.

Upon election, physicians and surgeons agreed to attend to hospital patients during times that the governors established for medical visits and rounds. The details of hours and duties varied from hospital to hospital, but all included a basic set of responsibilities. At least one hospital physician and surgeon attended when the governors' weekly boards saw to the taking-in of new patients and reviewed the number discharged during the previous week. The staff men determined whether the petitioner had an admissible condition for inpatient or outpatient treatment, once the governors had decided upon his or her worthiness as a deserving object of charity. If a bed was available, the sick person needing in-house care was admitted as either the physician's or the surgeon's patient, on the basis of an initial brief diagnosis. With staff rotating in turn, each physician and surgeon had new inpatients every three weeks. The entering sick were

99 Foucault, *Birth of the Clinic*, 83–4; Ivan Waddington, "The Role of the Hospital in the Development of Modern Medicine," *Sociology* 7 (1973): 211–25; Nicholas Jewson, "The Disappearance of the Sick-Man from Medical Cosmology, 1770–1870," *Sociology* 10 (1976): 225–44; Fissell, *Patients, Power and the Poor*.
100 Clark-Kennedy, *The London*, 1: 88, 106.

placed in the vacant beds throughout the hospital's male and female wards, without any organization by condition, unless the charity had reserved space for venereal patients, lying-in women, or, as at Guy's, a few luna-tics.[101] Whatever the rules about admissions, moreover, at taking-in staff men managed to manipulate the committee when they had good reason. Henry Earle, for example, surgeon at St. Bartholomew's, reported in an article that he convinced a young mother to take her baby to the hospital in 1812. He "promised," Earle stated, "to procure his admission, as [he] was very anxious to watch the progress of the case," and he did.[102]

During the rest of the week, the physicians and surgeons had regular hours set for visiting their patients. At the London, the governors expected a physician and at least one surgeon to visit patients on the wards daily from eleven to one o'clock, excluding Sundays, consulting among them-selves as necessary.[103] Compared with that of the other hospitals, this was an extremely onerous schedule for the physicians, and another probable reason why Fellows avoided positions there. Elsewhere physicians had regular hours, but the regulations specified only their taking-in and con-sulting duties. With such flexibility, physicians set their own hospital days, seeing their patients about two or three times a week. Hospital surgeons tended to make regular rounds every other day. At St. Thomas's, for example, the surgeons visited on Tuesdays, Thursdays, and Saturdays from eleven to one; at Guy's, they visited on Mondays, Wednesdays, and Fridays at the same time and appeared at midday on Saturdays for further consultations.[104] All in all, hospital physicians might get by spending just six to eight hours a week in charitable service. Surgeons routinely devoted more time to hospital work, especially when they performed major opera-tions. After consulting each other about the necessity for the knife, they had notices posted about scheduled operations so that other staff and pupils could watch, probably performing surgery at midday as often as possible, when the light was best. In addition to regular visits, moreover, physicians and surgeons were supposed to respond to messages seeking their help in emergencies. In practice, the resident apothecary and designated pupils did most of this work, with assistant physicians and assistant surgeons those next in line to be called.[105]

101 Parsons, *St. Thomas's*, 2: 208, 212; Cameron, *Guy's*, 59, 93; Clark-Kennedy, *The London*, 1: 32, 61.
102 Henry Earle, "A Case of Diseased Testicle, Accompanied with Disease of the Lungs and Brain, and Terminating Fatally," *Transactions of the Medical and Chirurgical Society* 3 (1812): 64.
103 Clark-Kennedy, *The London*, 89–94.
104 Cameron, *Guy's*, 79, 91–3; Clark-Kennedy, *The London*, 1: 48.
105 Parsons, *St. Thomas's*, 2: 209; Clark-Kennedy, *The London*, 1: 89–94. In 1749–50, the governors decided that if staff surgeons were unavailable in emergencies, the apothecary could send for "any other surgeon–governor of this charity," a custom that seems to have soon disappeared (p. 90); see also Chapter 4.

The interactions of physicians, surgeons, and patients on the wards constantly demonstrated the relationships among these men and their knowledge to both lay and medical audiences. Governors, patients, and hospital pupils saw these medical men at work. At taking-in, most cases were easily assigned to either a physician or a surgeon, and so maintained the distinctions that physic and surgery had long imposed upon different sorts of diseases, knowledge, and therapeutic skills. Since the causes and consequences of illnesses and injuries crossed over the neat boundaries between physic and surgery, however, all of the hospitals established certain hours each week for the physicians and surgeons to consult with one another on patients with mixed conditions.[106] Such collaborations between physicians and surgeons brought considerable learned expertise to the bedsides of the poor, who when on their own in the community saw practitioners using drugs and potions alongside lancets, bandages, and limb-splints without regard for the niceties separating the practices of physic and surgery among their betters. When cases blurred, moreover, hospital students, the majority of whom went on to practice both physic and surgery, learned about the manners appropriate for consultations and the nuances of dominance, debate, and approval, exchanged from physician to surgeon and surgeon to physician. The demarcations between hospital physicians and surgeons, and, of course, between them and the obedient hospital apothecary, thus displayed the rituals and courtesies of their professional elites to young men preparing themselves even for the fringes of polite practice.[107]

Meeting formally for joint consultations meant that at least once a week hospital staff men explicitly negotiated the boundaries of their respective professional territories. And they did so through questions centered on specific cases, not in the abstract, as they could in books or lectures or corporate charters. They acted out the traditional hierarchy between the ranks when surgeons deferred to physicians in decisions about patient care. At the same time, however, these men had continuing opportunities to transform old distinctions between learned physicians and craft-trained surgeons through mutual interests and collegial respect. Whether they did so or not depended, of course, upon each individual's desire to preserve time-worn dignity and decorum, his willingness to expose possible ignorance, or his eagerness to seek enlightenment from practitioners with lower status, less experience – or a more recent education. These ostensibly personal variations mattered for hospital medicine in London. Later I dis-

---

106 At Guy's and St. Thomas's, all staff gathered on Saturdays from eleven to one o'clock, going "in pairs to visit their patients." Cameron, *Guy's*, 91; at the Middlesex, physicians and surgeons met together on Mondays at 11:00 a.m. Middlesex Hospital, *Laws, Orders and Regulations*, 34; at the London, they consulted on Wednesdays. Clark-Kennedy, *The London*, 1: 48.

107 Relationships between hospital physicians and surgeons gave rise to disputes, as well. See, for example, Clark-Kennedy, *The London*, 1: 84–6.

cuss the fact that hospital physicians with RCP Licentiates tended to work much more closely with their surgical colleagues on problems in research and practice than did many of the Fellows with hospital posts. Chance interactions on the wards, formal conversations at weekly consultations, and interchanges elsewhere in the hospitals thus shaped much more than the care that the sick poor received.

What the sick poor in London thought about that care, much less about the smiles and snubs exchanged by the gentlemen walking busily around the wards, remains obscure. As much as historians have tried to glimpse patients' experiences of hospital treatment in the eighteenth century, nearly all of the scant written evidence touching on patients' feelings was reported by others – and usually those with complaints, not praise.[108] Most observers, such as John Howard, an earnest reformer who toured hospitals throughout Europe and Britain in the 1780s, remarked on hospitals' general standards of cleanliness, ventilation, and diet, not on patients' opinions or staff attitudes toward the objects of their care.[109] William Nolan, whose connections to any of the London hospitals have eluded me, was one of the few authors who took these charities to task for the "wanton abuse" that he claimed went on in them. In an acidic pamphlet published in 1786, Nolan criticized both nasty nurses and humming pupils for their lack of "compassionate attention" and "sensibility." As for the physicians and surgeons, he "earnestly recommend[ed] to these gentlemen a more humane regard to the feelings of their unhappy patients." At the very least they should cease using "harsh language" unsuitable to their dignity, remembering that some of the poor were just like infants in their need for "affability."[110] Nolan's comments display the anxieties marking the eighteenth-century "man of feeling," a popular hero in middle-class novels, not the day-to-day concerns of the active governors dealing with ward discipline or of staff men annoyed with patients' noncompliance.[111] Yet his opinion returns me to the point that belief in Enlightenment humanitarianism, of

---

108 Risse, *Hospital Life*, 15, 86, 89, and Porter, "The Gift Relation," 168–72, describe the only known example of a patient's rhapsodies over his hospital care, a poem by Joseph Wilde; Fissell, *Patients, Power and the Poor*, 148–70; Clark-Kennedy, *The London*, 1: 89–94; Westminster Hospital, Proceedings of the Trustees, 4, 11 Sept. 1811.
109 John Howard, *An Account of the Principal Lazarettos*. See Clark-Kennedy, *The London*, 1: 177–80, and Cameron, *Guy's*, 73–4, for examples of Howard's visit and the governors' responses to his criticisms. Howard was a subscriber to the London, by the way, and gave it a fairly favorable report; John Aikin, *Thoughts on Hospitals* (London: Joseph Jackson, 1771).
110 William Nolan, *An Essay on Humanity: or, a view of abuses in Hospitals with a Plan for correcting them* (London: J. Murray, 1786), 19, 24–5, 37–8; I have been unable to find any clues on when and where Nolan might have observed London practice. He has not appeared on any list of governors' names, or among the active governors I have noted from hospital minute books. Nor does he appear as a hospital pupil on the lists of register names I have available.
111 G. J. Barker-Benfield, *The Culture of Sensibility: Sex and Society in Eighteenth-Century Britain* (Chicago: University of Chicago Press, 1992), e.g., 257–60.

good works designed to tend and to ease both bodies and souls, had a potent power to sway eighteenth-century readers' understanding of appropriate behavior to the unfortunate. Hospital men, too, could have wished to be men of feeling, dispensing compassion along with their compounds and bleedings.

In the early nineteenth century, a few hospital physicians and surgeons began to speak up about the ways that their charitable work put virtue before mere medical value. Alexander Marcet, physician to Guy's, reminded the students attending his introductory clinical lecture at the hospital that "we shall take every opportunity of trying new and promising remedies, but we shall carry on our inquiries with the same caution as if we were experimenting upon our friends or upon ourselves."[112] He offered a tender analogy, not a moral argument, to guide the pupils' care. After 1815, moreover, hospital men contended with the formidable lure of the Paris schools, finally accessible again to English students after the Napoleonic wars. The Paris schools, having been restructured during a godless revolution, had a considerable reputation for their harshness to the poor and their cavalier use of hospital patients' corpses for dissection. Of course London men tried to use the Paris evil in order to keep students at home (and paying their "schools" instead), but they did so in ways that capitalized on the long history of the London hospitals as the voluntary expressions of civic virtue and individual values. "In England," John Abernethy, surgeon to St. Bartholomew's, exclaimed to a crowd at the Royal College of Surgeons in 1819,

the indigent who suffer from illness and injury are supported and relieved chiefly by the liberality of that benevolence which is so creditable to our national character; and as much as I wish for the promotion of medical knowledge, I should be sorry if the bodies of the poor were to be considered as public property . . . in our country. Far better would it seem to me, that medical science should cease, and our bodily sufferings continue, than that the natural rights and best feelings of humanity could not be equally respected in all classes of society.[113]

Perhaps Abernethy exaggerated his feelings a bit; perhaps not. Certainly not all hospital men, much less many other practitioners, agreed with him. The significance of his passion rests neither with his sincerity, nor with his behavior toward his hospital patients, but with the figure of a senior hospital surgeon publicly expressing this view to other surgeons at a College celebration without, I presume, expecting laughter at his earnestness or incredulity at his priorities.

112 Alexander Marcet, *Some Remarks on Clinical Lectures* (London: G. Woodfall, 1818), 19.
113 John Abernethy, "Hunterian Oration (1819)," in his *Surgical and Physiological Works*, 2 vols. (London: Longman, Hurst, Rees, Orme and Brown, 1825).

The meaning of charity, the way that governors ran these institutions, and the qualifications, elections, and duties of hospital physicians and surgeons laid out in this chapter are inextricably connected to the metamorphosis of each hospital as a site for teaching, learning, doing research, and acquiring collective professional identity. The very diversity among the seven hospitals I have studied, as much as or more than their similarities, highlights how little specific religious orientations, political affiliations, or economic conditions at these institutions at particular times directly shaped the century-long transformation of hospital medicine in London. Anglicanism at St. Bartholomew's, Dissent at the London, Whiggery at St. Thomas's, and Toryism at the Westminster; boom years; trade slumps; peace and war: all mattered dearly to their governors, and probably to their physicians and surgeons. Such factors constantly influenced specific decisions and policies, just as many individual patients fashioned practitioners' and pupils' experiences of diseases, injuries, cures, and death. But despite the hospitals' differences, ward teaching emerged at all of them at about the same time.

In case notes, lectures, and published articles, moreover, hospital governors and patients take on a sense of being nearly interchangeable parts in the changing educational and intellectual systems of eighteenth-century medical knowledge, no matter what their personal circumstances or peculiar conditions were. These people sometimes appear as abstract concepts in the rest of my story, then, in part because practitioners and pupils wrote of them as "the governors" and "the patients," as though each group comprised a self-evident, unitary category. Indeed, such labels for lay administrators and the institutionalized sick were essential elements in the construction of hospital medicine. They helped to distance those other people from the men who medical practitioners seemed to think mattered most – themselves.

3

The corporations, licensing, and reform, 1700–1815

No degree of discipline, nor any kind of examination, can ensure the public against having a certain number of persons who are indifferently qualified included in the list of well-qualified practitioners. Young men may be compelled to have opportunities of study, but they cannot be compelled to learn.

Quarterly Review, 1840[1]

The history of medical education in London seen through official records, from the minute books of the Surgeons' Company to Acts of Parliament, is a patchwork of regulations and traditions that hides as much as it reveals about medical organization and practice. From the bureaucratic perspective that such documents offer, London medical men were separated into the familiar tripartite division of physicians, surgeons, and apothecaries, each with its own corporate body, public voice, and standards of appropriate medical training.[2] Entry into the Royal College of Physicians, the Surgeons' Company, or the Worshipful Society of Apothecaries certainly marked professional status and acceptance into the mainstream of metropolitan practice. Yet, as much recent work has shown, defining the medical profession(s) according to these corporations' claims flies in the face of contemporary understanding of who could and should practice medicine. The lines between "quacks" and "regulars," so bitterly drawn by medical men threatened for their livelihoods and so frequently ignored by their potential patients, are more realistically cast as the shades of gray between regular and irregular practitioners. Community acceptance and length of

---

1 Review of the "Report from the Select Committee on Medical Education, 1834," *Quarterly Review* 67 (1840): 54. The review has been attributed to Benjamin Brodie, surgeon to St. George's Hospital.
2 Bernice Hamilton, "The Medical Professions in the Eighteenth Century," *Economic History Review*, 2nd ser., 4 (1951): 141–69; Charles Newman, *The Evolution of Medical Education in the Nineteenth Century* (London: Oxford University Press, 1957), 1–24; Ivan Waddington, *The Medical Profession in the Industrial Revolution* (Dublin: Gill and MacMillan Humanities Press, 1984), 1–8.

experience could matter as much as − or more than − formal licensing, university degrees, or corporate membership in establishing a full-time medical career in much of eighteenth-century Britain.[3]

Given such fluidity, the London corporations' licensing regulations and forays into medical education have limited value for assessing how a large number of practitioners either identified themselves within the tripartite structure or trained for their occupations. The corporations' regulations reveal, instead, their own concerns to perpetuate elite definitions of medical practice. In this chapter, I focus on the corporations' licensing regulations and their minimal roles in educating their members. The corporations' lack of interest in medical education encouraged the laissez-faire conditions that allowed private lectures, hospital ward-walking, and open medical societies to flourish in eighteenth-century London. I summarize the medical reform movements of the 1790s to 1810s, which other historians have amply detailed, in order to clarify the relationships between the public debate about standards for medical education and the transformation that had already occured in metropolitan training and licensing. London's ad hoc system of ward-walking and lecturing, the subjects of Chapters 4 and 5, respectively, literally created the rank and file whom activists tried to organize and inspire at the beginning of the nineteenth century.

The reformers' rhetoric, which encapsulated ordinary practitioners' anxieties about competition and their anger at the corporations' closed elites, is wonderful for telling colorful stories about professional identity during this period. From the perspective of medical education, however, reformers (not surprisingly) had little criticism of their own medical training. Indeed, I show that the reformers' suggestions for licensing standards raised what many of them had done voluntarily − going to lectures and attending hospitals − to formal requirements. Activists' ringing denunciations of corporate lethargy and elitism, moreover, ignored changes in institutional practices that I believe were quite significant for shaping the ultimate provisions of the Apothecaries' Act of 1815. This Act established the first nationwide licensing certification (the Licentiate of the Society of Apothecaries, or LSA) for all those who compounded medicines.

The power the Act gave to the Apothecaries' examiners mirrored that

3 Irvine Loudon, *Medical Care and the General Practitioner, 1750–1850* (Oxford: Clarendon Press, 1986), 11–28; Roy Porter, *Health for Sale: Quackery in England 1660–1850* (Manchester and New York: Manchester University Press, 1989), 1–15; Mary E. Fissell, *Patients, Power and the Poor in Eighteenth-Century Bristol* (Cambridge: Cambridge University Press, 1991); William Bynum and Roy Porter, eds., *Medical Fringe and Medical Orthodoxy, 1750–1850* (London: Croom Helm, 1987). Contemporaries, not just historians, referred to the professional elite as acknowledged "regulars"; see, for example, *The Ill State of Physic in Great Britain: Truly Represented to all Lovers of Health and of their Country and an Apology for the Regular Physicians* (London: J. Roberts, 1727); and the anonymous review of Edward Harrison's "Address to the Lincolnshire Benevolent Society" and Jeremiah Jenkin's, *Observations on the Profession*, in *Critical Review, or Annals of Literature*, 3rd. ser., 21 (1810): 187.

already held by the examiners at the Royal College of Surgeons. I argue that military demand for qualified practitioners, along with the public horror at decimation of soldiers by epidemic diseases during the wars with France and Napoleonic Europe, spurred changes to licensing requirements at the Royal College of Surgeons much more than reformers' vigorous complaints about unqualified civilian competitors. And these seemingly minor modifications – the power to demand and to accept or reject an applicant's certificates of course and hospital attendance – established the subsequent authority of London's licensing bodies over medical teaching in the nineteenth century. Until then, however, as this chapter demonstrates, the corporations' concern for medical training in London wavered between providing a few lectures for their members' apprentices and steering clear of any activities that could infringe on their members' rights to teach, or on universities' traditional claims to educate learned physicians.

THE LONDON CORPORATIONS: MEMBERSHIP AND LICENSING

In bald terms, nearly anyone could practice physic, surgery, or midwifery at any time and anywhere in England and Wales in the eighteenth century. Even where licensing bodies existed, as in London, their powers to restrict practice to their own members were severely limited, either by lack of legal backing for their claims (as for the Company of Surgeons) or by disinclination for the expensive, time-consuming, and potentially embarrassing process of taking nonlicensed practitioners to court (as for the Royal College of Physicians).[4] Provincial regulars relied upon registered apprenticeships, medical degrees, the remnants of city guilds, and, to a much lesser extent in the eighteenth century, Bishops' licenses, for formal recognition of their occupations. Whether such distinguishing marks mattered either to local magistrates or, more important, to many patients is doubtful.[5]

---

4 Juanita G. L. Burnby, *A Study of the English Apothecary from 1660 to 1760* (*Medical History*, Supplement No. 3, 1983), 2–3; Cecil Wall, *History of the Surgeons' Company, 1745–1800* (London: Hutchinsons, 1937), 42–7, 145–7; George Clark, *A History of the Royal College of Physicians of London*, 3 vols. (Oxford: Clarendon Press, 1964–6), 2: 463, 507–16; for examples and discussion of the Company's ability to restrict surgical practice in London, see Company of Surgeons, Minute Book of the Court of Assistants, 3 May 1753, 7 July 1768, 1 July 1773, 2 Feb. 1775, 5 Mar. 1778, 4 Apr. 1782, 6 Oct. 1785, 2 Feb., 5 Oct. 1786, Royal College of Surgeons Library.
5 John R. Guy, "The Episcopal Licensing of Physicians, Surgeons and Midwives," *Bulletin of the History of Medicine* 56 (1982): 541–2; Burnby, *English Apothecary*, 94–5; Fissell, *Patients, Power and the Poor*. For the most comprehensive, yet still incomplete, list of eighteenth-century medical men, see P. J. Wallis and R. V. Wallis, *Eighteenth Century Medics (Subscriptions, Licenses, Apprenticeships)*, 2nd ed. (Newcastle-upon-Tyne, UK: Project for Historical Biobibliography, 1988).

The three London organizations that in principle controlled medical practice in the City and for seven miles around thus served to demarcate hierarchies of status rather than to police the care of the sick. These corporations varied considerably in their relationship to the Crown, the City, and metropolitan society in the eighteenth century, and all warrant far more study of their economic, cultural, and political roles.[6] They unquestionably promoted their own interests, especially those of the ruling members, who represented a minority of the practitioners accepted within their halls, and repeatedly battled each other over the demarcations among physic, surgery, and pharmacy. As corporate groups, all three bodies had essentially self-perpetuating, closed leaderships.[7] Any debates about entry qualifications, licensing regulations, or teaching thus fell to men who had already made it to the top, through means that defined, in part, their own claims to knowledge and legitimacy. Most references, in short, to the Royal College of Physicians, to the Company/Royal College of Surgeons, or to the Society of Apothecaries refer to their guiding oligarchies, not to all members or licentiates, and certainly not to all those practicing as physicians, surgeons, or apothecaries.

The Royal College of Physicians (RCP) obtained its first charter in 1518. It weathered the interruption of royal patronage during the Civil War and Interregnum and found renewed if lackadaisical support from the Crown under the Restoration.[8] In line with its foundation by humanist physicians, the RCP insisted that its members belonged to a learned profession. According to the statutes in force in the 1700s, they required a university MD degree for London practice, plus an oral examination conducted in Latin and based upon reading and explaining classical texts.[9] Full members, the Fellows (FRCP), had Oxford or Cambridge MDs (or degrees incorporated there), could serve as Elects (the ruling members), and were forbidden to practice a trade; those seeking the Fellowship spent a year or more as Candidates. These provisions effectively defined an educated, genteel elite who could not dispense drugs, perform surgical operations, or practice midwifery. A physician with an MD degree from another university obtained only the status of Licentiate (LRCP). He could not vote on College

6 Harold J. Cook's work on the RCP offers a model for such studies. See his "Policing the Health of London: The College of Physicians and the Early Stuart Monarchy," *Social History of Medicine* 2 (1989): 1–34; and *Decline of the Old Medical Regime in Stuart London* (Ithaca, NY: Cornell University Press, 1986); George Unwin, *The Gilds and Companys of London,* 2nd ed. (London: Methuen, 1925).
7 Clark, *Royal College of Physicians,* 1: 77, 90–2, 175, 304, 356; 2: 537.
8 Clark, *Royal College of Physicians,* vol. 1.; Cook, *Decline of the Old Medical Regime,* 192–253.
9 Clark, *Royal College of Physicians,* 2: 518–19; Andrew R. Cunningham, "Aspects of Medical Education in Britain in the Seventeenth and Early Eighteenth Centuries," Ph.D. dissertation, University of London, 1974, 113, 130–9, 242–8.

matters and was allowed to dabble in "trade" or midwifery. The license clearly carried the stigma of a second-class qualification and LRCPs fiercely and frequently criticized the College Fellows for their exclusivity during the eighteenth century.[10] From the 1770s, the Fellows raised a handful of distinguished Licentiates to the FRCP on an ad hoc basis, an action that worked to divide and diffuse Licentiates' reforming zeal.

The College also offered an "extra-Licentiate" (ERCP) for provincial practitioners, although this was not required for practice outside London. The RCP did not require a medical degree for the ERCP, relying instead on recommendations and an oral examination (sometimes in English, if the candidate had no verbal skill with Latin) of the applicant until 1807. That very few medical men bothered to take the ERCP suggests that the marginal status associated with hanging on the fringes of the London college was hardly worth the application, unless the licentiate served to enhance local status. Finally, the RCP instituted a midwifery license in 1783 (MRCP), designed to recognize successful and high-ranking practitioners in London, rather than in any way to control men–midwives. As in the process for the FRCP and LRCP, the College demanded an oral examination, first in English and then in Latin, in order to exclude run-of-the-mill surgeons and apothecaries from aspiring to the MRCP. When it was discontinued in 1804, only ten accoucheurs had obtained midwifery licenses.[11]

London surgeons had had a guild at least from the fourteenth century, but joined with the Company of Barbers in 1540 to form a new City Livery company of Barber–Surgeons. In 1745, the surgeons again separated from the Barbers, creating the Company of Surgeons. The new company had an ambiguous relationship with the City. Since they were not a Livery company, new members were no longer entitled to gain entry by patrimony or redemption, nor were they Parliamentary voters in the City, as liverymen were. Yet the company did claim traditional rights to oversee practice in London and seven miles around[12] and to disfranchisement, whereby they could fine members who entered another corporation, particularly the Royal College of Physicians. According to the new 1745 bylaws, the Court of Assistants comprised twenty-one members who limited their practice to "pure" surgery, thus excluding those who also prepared medications and attended normal childbirth. The ten most senior Assistants comprised the Court of Examiners and, like the rest of the Assistants, served for life. The Company of Surgeons, as a result of various upheavals and irregularities, was dissolved with the creation by royal charter of the Royal College of Surgeons of London in 1800. The new Royal College differed very little

10 Clark, *Royal College of Physicians*, 2: 552–72; see Chapter 7.
11 Clark, *Royal College of Physicians*, 2: 588–9, 637.
12 Hamilton, "Medical Professions," 150.

from the prior Company, however, especially in membership of the ruling Court of Assistants, except that it formalized its separation from the City of London.[13]

In contrast to practitioners of the learned profession of physic, Barber–Surgeons relied on the traditional training for craft and trade to determine membership. In addition to formal apprenticeship to a member, registered at the Hall, they required an examination or certification of the apprentice's general education, including a knowledge of Latin, upon indenture.[14] After the 1745 separation, the company's examiners no longer required apprenticeship, although many entrants continued to train under a master. Instead, the examiners at the Surgeons' Company relied on oral interrogation of the applicant, who had to be at least twenty-two years old.[15] Finally, the charter for the Royal College of Surgeons simply confirmed the company's habits. Again, no apprenticeship was demanded for membership (the post-1800 "MRCS"), only "satisfactory evidence of anatomical and chirurgical education." This wide-open clause left the surgeons' Court of Examiners with sole control over what they would require of their applicants, from oral examination to later certificates demonstrating attendance at lectures and hospital practice.[16]

Both the Barber–Surgeons' Company and the later Surgeons' Company supervised entry, by examination, into naval and, after 1745, into army service, but full membership in the company was not required for military practice.[17] Thus military applicants did not have to produce evidence of apprenticeship or other training, although they usually needed some expertise to qualify for a commission.[18] In 1749 and again in 1763, the Crown confirmed a privilege granted to all discharged military officers, including

---

13 Hamilton, "Medical Professions," 149–59; Zachary Cope, *The Royal College of Surgeons of England: A History* (London: A. Blond, 1959), 1–21; John Flint South, *Memorials of the Craft of Surgery in England,* ed. D'Arcy Power (London: Cassell, 1886); Wall, *Surgeons' Company,* 78, 183–208. I cite documents printed in South's collection, instead of archival references, where the information is equivalent.

14 South, *Memorials,* 112–8; Wall, *Surgeons' Company,* 49, 55.

15 Wall, *Surgeons' Company,* 55–7; Hamilton, "Medical Professions," 149–50; Company of Surgeons, Examination Book, 1745–1800, Royal College of Surgeons (RCS) Library. This manuscript register records the indentures of apprentices to members, but few references were made to proof of apprenticeship when candidates appeared for their examinations.

16 W. Willcock, *The Laws Relating to the Medical Profession, With an Account of the Rise and Progress of its Various Orders* (London: J. and W. T. Clarke, 1830), cxcviii, 65–6.

17 W. N. Boog Watson, "Four Monopolies and the Surgeons of London and Edinburgh," *Journal of the History of Medicine* 25 (1970): 311–22; Barber-Surgeons Company, "Lists of Surgeons & Mates Examined, 1734–1745," Guildhall MS 5263; Barber-Surgeons Company, "Lists of Certificates to Navy Surgeons, 1709–1744," Guildhall MS 5264; James Wallace, Bond, 3 June 1740, and Augustine Gradwell, Bond, 2 October 1744, in Guildhall MS 9833, illustrate the formal acceptance of membership into the Company of Barber-Surgeons.

18 South, *Memorials,* 264–8, 270.

surgeons, that allowed them to practice their trades without apprenticeship or the freedom of City companies. This law further weakened the Surgeons' claims to a monopoly over metropolitan practice. Military service thus became a valid route to a London (or provincial) career, although it is impossible to estimate how frequently medical men deliberately chose this path, with its low pay and even lower status.[19]

The third medical corporation, the Worshipful Society of Apothecaries, obtained a royal charter as a City Livery company in 1617, when the apothecaries separated from the grocers. It had two major economic and public functions from the early seventeenth century. First, all those practicing as apothecaries in London and seven miles around technically fell under the Society's control. The Court of Assistants, or the executive subgroup called the Private Court, determined entry into membership, by registering indentures, certifying completion of a seven-year apprenticeship, and giving oral examinations. Illegal and unqualified apothecaries could be called to the Society and fined £5 per month for their unlicensed work. Second, and more important in their marketplace role, was their supervision over trade. Senior members inspected shops, examined the materials used to prepare medications, and oversaw the business at the Hall; from the late 1600s, their enterprises included two limited joint-stock groups, in chemical manufacturing and navy procurements.[20]

As both apothecaries and physicians dealt with prescribing medications, friction between the Society and the College frequently erupted in the seventeenth century and continued well into the 1700s. The most famous example of overt conflict is the Rose case, which began with the successful RCP prosecution of William Rose, a Liveryman of the Society, for illegally practicing medicine. In 1704, however, the House of Lords overturned the previous decision, acknowledging the apothecary's right to give medical advice as well as to fill physicians' prescriptions, which confirmed the status quo of such practice. The Lords' conclusion supported public recognition that the College's claim to a learned monopoly over physic rested on shaky grounds.[21] A growing proportion of apothecaries thus practiced as regular medical men, and the Society of Apothecaries had to juggle its dual functions as a City company concerned with business and a "professional" corporation speaking for medical practitioners.

The three London corporations thus attempted to demarcate their claims

19 Lloyd G. Stevenson, "A Note on the Relation of Military Service to Licensing in the History of British Surgery," *Bulletin of the History of Medicine* 27 (1953): 420–7; Hamilton, "Medical Professions," 151–2.

20 Hamilton, "Medical Professions," 159–69; Cecil Wall, *A History of the Worshipful Society of Apothecaries of London, 1617–1815*, ed. E. Ashworth Underwood and H. C. Cameron, [1 volume only] (London: Oxford University Press, 1963), 1: 8–22, 79–82, 148–61.

21 Harold J. Cook, "The Rose Case Reconsidered: Physicians, Apothecaries and the Law in Augustan England," *Journal of the History of Medicine* 45 (1990): 527–55; and Cook, *Decline of the Old Medical Regime*, 246–53.

to knowledge and practice. Their official boundaries, however, obscure movement among the three divisions. Throughout the 1700s apothecaries' apprentices joined the Company of Surgeons, while surgeons left their Company and acquired Licentiates from the Royal College of Physicians.[22] Practitioners' choices underscore the search for upward mobility, but they also suggest the mutability of educational standards that ignored formal curricula and concentrated instead upon educational labels (like the MD and apprenticeship indentures) or claims from experience, for licensing.

EDUCATION AT THE HALLS AND COLLEGE

By the early eighteenth century, the three London corporations each had a few activities designed to instruct their members or, for the Society of Apothecaries and the Barber–Surgeons' Company, their members' apprentices. These exercises followed their officially separate spheres, reflecting learned profession, trade, and craft. As they developed during the eighteenth century, the lectures and other educational opportunities provided at Apothecaries' Hall, Surgeons' Hall, and the College of Physicians remained clearly delimited; while fulfilling the responsibilities laid down in charters and endowed lectureships, the corporations steadfastly avoided expanding their teaching.

Since several Court members taught privately, simple lack of interest in lecturing hardly accounts for apparent corporate apathy. Instead, as the debates at the Company/Royal College of Surgeons make abundantly clear, the issue centered on public responsibility. None of the original charters (or their revisions) enjoined the London bodies to educate all aspirants for practice, only to certify their qualifications. For the physicians, of course, such a teaching expectation was socially absurd, as only a university could prepare a man for the intellectual challenges of medicine. For the surgeons and apothecaries, equal weight fell upon apprenticeship, which had no rivals at the beginning of the eighteenth century. By the time that alternate routes could challenge apprenticeship and, indeed, allow it to be criticized, the corporate leaderships refused to compete with their own colleagues. They could then effectively deny direct responsibility for comprehensive instruction, while championing a public duty to control qualifications indirectly, through their assessment of a candidate's account of his education.

Royal College of Physicians

Expecting that aspiring physicians arrived in London with their MD degrees at least close to completion, the Royal College of Physicians upheld

22 Burnby, *English Apothecary*, 82.

the universities' claims to produce qualified medical men. The only area where academic training might be weak, the RCP acknowledged, was in anatomy, as access to corpses was limited in provincial towns. From the midsixteenth century, the College had permission to obtain the corpses of executed criminals for dissections at their premises. Until at least the early seventeenth century, the College required that candidates for the Fellowship, Licentiates, and first-year Fellows attend the College's dissections or be fined. This rule, however, either disappeared or was not enforced in the eighteenth century. Throughout the 1700s, the rest of the College's teaching centered on their endowed lectures: the Lumleian (established in 1581/2), the Gulstonian (1639), and, from 1749, the Croonian. The Gulstonian lectures, given for three days over a dissected corpse, rotated among the Fellows; the Lumleian lectures, originally founded to teach surgery, had a more varied schedule and until the mid-eighteenth century the lecturer held the post as long as he chose. The Croonian fund, in contrast, supported an annually chosen member of the College to give a single lecture on an anatomical topic.[23]

While little is known about the audiences for the College's lectures in the eighteenth century, they certainly were not advertised as public talks or designed for beginning medical pupils. Rather, they provided a forum for discourses on contemporary ideas, their originality depending upon the skills, resources, and ambitions of the Fellows chosen. Such lectures served primarily as demonstrations of elite knowledge, suitably given – and occasionally published – in Latin. Similarly, when the RCP began its first museum in 1809, a collection of materia medica specimens, access to it was limited to the Fellows and, with permission, to others who could inspect the material in the curators' presence.[24] Like the College's dinners and library, the lectures and museum symbolized the Fellows' authority within the College and, presumably to their satisfaction, within metropolitan practice.[25]

Society of Apothecaries

During the 1700s, the Society of Apothecaries sponsored herbalizing field trips, arranged to acquaint young men with practical botany. (Complaints

23 Clark, *Royal College of Physicians*, 1: 122, 151–2, 178–9, 251, 345; 2: 456, 505–6, 526–7; William Munk, *The Roll of the Royal College of Physicians of London*, 3 vols. (London: Royal College of Physicians, 1878), 3: 350–60.
24 The museum expanded in the 1820s, especially when Matthew Baillie gave the College his anatomical preparations, but still remained more of a research than a training facility. Clark, *Royal College of Physicians*, 2: 635, 658. The RCP library holds several manuscripts relating to the collections of materia medica and pathological preparations, especially letters from various London medical men which accompanied specimens given to Baillie or the Royal College of Physicians.
25 Clark, *Royal College of Physicians*, 2: 526, 529–30, 577–8, 635.

about the apprentices' unruly behavior suggest that the students took them as a chance to picnic and have fun with their London peers.) The Society's Physic Garden at Chelsea, revived in the early eighteenth century, also served to teach apprentices about medicinal simples, as well as providing a growing ground for diverse botanical specimens.[26] Since most apothecaries with apprentices, especially in London, could not afford much time to wander in country fields or to keep their own gardens, both the herbalizings and the Physic Garden show where the Society took public responsibility to supplement apprenticeship.

Members of the Society repeatedly proposed that the gardener or demonstrator of plants give lectures to the apprentices at the Physic Garden, but most of these attendants appeared not to have the time or desire to do so on their meager salaries.[27] At the Apothecaries' Hall in the City, members also tried to institute lectures on the materia medica and chemistry at midcentury. The materia medica course seems to have been given, at least in 1753, but the committee in charge of the Laboratory vetoed the chemistry lectures, since they "would interfere with the business of the Laboratory," which centered on the commercial assessment and sale of simples and chemical compounds. In the same year the Society also refused Dr. James Greive's request to use their Hall for an introduction to his chemistry lectures.[28] Thomas Wheeler, appointed demonstrator of plants at Chelsea in 1778, then began a series of botanical lectures at the garden, with moderate success in drawing members' apprentices. Wheeler, himself a product of apprenticeship to a London firm and ward-walking at St. Thomas's Hospital, also offered lectures on botany at Apothecaries' Hall in 1784, but gave them up in 1786 as they were poorly attended.[29] Not until 1803 did the Society sponsor an entire series of lectures on materia medica in their Hall, fulfilling the terms of a bequest by William Prouting.[30]

Company of Barber–Surgeons to Royal College of Surgeons of London

The surgeons' corporations have a similar history of demonstrations, formal lectures, and resisted suggestions for innovation. Compared with the Royal College of Physicians and the Society of Apothecaries, however, the surgeons' companies had much more responsibility to instruct their members' apprentices. Their Courts' eighteenth-century debates display ambivalence about balancing their members' public functions, namely teaching anatomy and preparing public dissections, and their private inter-

---

26 Wall, *Society of Apothecaries*, 88–90.
27 Wall, *Society of Apothecaries*, 167–70, 177–81.
28 Charles R. B. Barrett, *The History of the Society of Apothecaries of London* (London: Elliot Stock, 1905), 140. The quotation is from an unspecified Society document.
29 "Thomas Wheeler," in *Dictionary of National Biography* [hereafter *DNB*]; Wall, *Society of Apothecaries*, 177–9.
30 Barrett, *Society of Apothecaries*, 166, 170.

ests, especially offering lucrative independent courses and attracting ward-walking pupils to the hospitals. For some, comprehensive anatomical instruction could enhance the Surgeons' Company's prestige, promote their claims to professional competence, and, perhaps, provide free publicity for their private lectures and hospital posts. For others, when the specter of Company competition loomed large, they exorcised it with the passive resistance of tradition. Increasingly dominated by hospital men, the Court of Assistants created a company that implicitly supported the proliferation of unregulated medical teaching across the metropolis.

According to the terms of their charter, the Company of Barber–Surgeons and, after 1745, the Company of Surgeons held public dissections and presented anatomy lectures on the bodies of executed criminals. These lectures, based on the traditional process of dissecting a single corpse, usually took place over a few consecutive days. Until the 1730s, moreover, physicians gave the Arris and Gale lectures, endowed for anatomical topics.[31] In 1734, new Company regulations specified that the Court of Assistants would henceforth choose "one or more examined Surgeons . . . to be Demonstrators or Teachers of Anatomy." The earlier posts of masters and stewards of anatomy, who were responsible for obtaining the executed criminals and preparing them for public demonstrations, continued.[32]

The 1734 guidelines for anatomy teaching at Surgeons' Hall outlined the topics to be covered in demonstrations and lectures, from "the System of the Arteries and Veins" to extra summer sessions on osteology. Half the corpse, if possible, moreover, should be spared to demonstrate "Chirurgical Operations." The Company offered both public demonstrations and "private Anatomys," depending upon the supply of bodies. The surgeons restricted such displays, except for the "publick Lectures" where the criminal's body was opened for public humiliation, to their members and

all [such] Apprentices as have served 3 compleat years and have been bound at the Hall, they bringing a note signed by their respective Masters and date[d] with the day of the month and year that he gives them leave to come: the notes are to be filed and left open for the Inspection of any Members of the Company that desire it.[33]

By the 1740s, therefore, the Barber–Surgeons' Company had reiterated its public and professional obligations to teach anatomy using bodies provided

31 South, *Memorials*, 224–8, 239–40, 367–73; George C. Peachey, *A Memoir of William and John Hunter* (Plymouth: William Brendon and Son, 1924), 1–5. Clark, *Royal College of Physicians*, 1: 150–1; 2: 500. The last reference so far discovered to a physician's giving anatomical lectures at Surgeons' Hall is in 1746–7, when "Dr. Goddard" received £16 for the task. South, *Memorials*, 228; see also, Andrew Cunningham, "The Kinds of Anatomy," *Medical History* 19 (1975): 11–13, for the seventeenth century.
32 "Order for the New Regulation of the Demonstration [1734]," in South, *Memorials*, 242.
33 "Order for the New Regulation of the Demonstration [1734]," in South, *Memorials*, 242–4.

by the state. They also made explicit their expected audience, keeping the privilege of learning anatomy (not just watching a public lecture) to members and their bonded apprentices. Whether enforced or not, the regulations upheld the idea that knowledge of craft secrets distinguished its members from other practitioners.

Official permission to dissect executed criminals hardly spared the Company from popular revulsion and reaction.[34] The records of the Company show that the Barber–Surgeons spent much of their energy trying to enforce their rights to claim dead bodies from sheriffs at public executions. Popular feeling against dissection ran so high during the first half of the eighteenth century that even the soldiers sent to keep order during the executions helped to prevent the bodies from being turned over to the surgeons.[35] In 1734, the Company still required that notices of the public dissections be sent to various daily papers, but, in 1742, it ordered that the advertisements cease.[36]

Both protecting craft secrets and coping with popular resentment engaged the Barber–Surgeons' Company during the decades before 1745. Its Court of Assistants attempted to control the proliferation of "private anatomys," at the Hall and elsewhere, primarily to preserve the Company's rights to executed criminals. Too much has been made, however, of the Company's single act to censure a surgeon for holding a private anatomy course outside the Hall. In 1715 the Barber–Surgeons called William Cheselden (1688–1752) to account because he

did frequently procure the Dead bodies of Malefactors from the place of execution and dissect the same at his own house, as well during the Company's Publick Lectures as at other times without the leave of the Governors. . . . By which means it became more difficult for the Beadles to bring away the Companies Bodies and likewise drew away the members of this Company and others from the Public Dissections and Lectures at the Hall.[37]

Cheselden appeased the Company's Court by promising "never to dissect at the same times as the Company had their Lecture at the Hall, nor without leave of the Governors for the time being," and likely found other sources of human material.[38] This episode, often taken to show the stultifying restrictions that the Company placed on the study of anatomy,

---

34 Ruth Richardson, *Death, Dissection and the Destitute* (London and New York: Routledge and Kegan Paul, 1987), esp. 32–40; Thomas Forbes, " 'To Be Dissected and Anatomized'," *Journal of the History of Medicine* 36 (1981): 490–2.
35 South, *Memorials*, 234–9; Peter Linebaugh, "The Tyburn Riot against the Surgeons" in *Albion's Fatal Tree: Crime and Society in Eighteenth Century England,* ed. Douglas Hay, et al. (New York: Pantheon, 1975), 65–117.
36 South, *Memorials*, 245–6.
37 South, *Memorials*, 233, n. 2, quoted from the minutes of the Court of Assistants, 25 Mar. 1714 [OS].
38 Peachey, *Memoir*, 97; South, *Memorials*, 233–4, n. 2.

instead reveals that the Barber–Surgeons acted to maintain their public access to corpses.[39] Indeed they tolerated dozens of private lecture courses, including Cheselden's, apparently as long as such offerings did not conflict with the Company's public functions. Such private courses (see Chapter 5) arose as supplements as much as alternatives to the work at Surgeons' Hall and many of them, despite the Company's concern over illicit dissections, offered demonstrations on human material and, by the early 1740s, student practice on corpses.[40]

When the Surgeons separated from the Barbers in 1745, the new Company dispensed with the seventeenth-century bylaw that forbade private dissections without prior permission. This decision technically freed anatomists from the Company's supervision and hence is usually cited as the reason for a surge in private courses, especially William Hunter's notable success.[41] Probably much more significant, however, was the absence of the Company's lectures and dissections from 1745 to 1752, while the surgeons built a new hall and theater. Private courses then emerged as necessary alternatives, not supplements, to the Company's lectures. With more topics covered in greater detail than those at the Barber–Surgeons' Hall, illustrated by preparations, models, and drawings, and, increasingly after 1746, with opportunities advertised for students to dissect, private lectures captured the market.

When the new Surgeons' Hall was finally ready in 1753, including "iron spikes in the Theatre to prevent the Mob getting over the outer rail," teaching resumed.[42] The traditional pattern of giving a short set of public lectures over the dissected corpse continued. Filling one of the offices devoted to anatomy proved to be difficult, as it required considerable effort for apparently meager honor and payment.[43] Between 1753 and 1766–7, thirty-nine men served as stewards (two), wardens (two) and anatomy master (one), a series of rotating offices filled by seniority among the

39 Cope, *Royal College of Surgeons*, 5; Peachey, *Memoir*, 17.
40 Among the earlier courses for which Peachey gives details, those by George Rolfe (1701), James Douglas (1706), William Cheselden (1711), Peter Macculloch and Nathaniel St. André (1719), and Frank Nicholls (1727) referred to demonstrations on human bodies or the making of preparations. William Hewitt and James Vitrack both offered courses in 1740 and 1741, respectively, specifying that pupils would be able to dissect with their own hands. George Peachey claimed that the interference of the Company probably prevented these courses from being given or, at least, continued. Since he assumed that other courses, which did use bodies for demonstrations, were allowed to go on, perhaps with the permission of the Company, his argument is not convincing. Peachey, *Memoir*, 12, 14, 20, 28, 38, 45, 97.
41 Peachey, *Memoir*, 2, 38, 94–8; Cope, *Royal College of Surgeons*, 12; Toby Gelfand, "The 'Paris Manner' of Dissection: Student Anatomical Dissection in Early Eighteenth-Century Paris," *Bulletin of the History of Medicine* 46 (1972): 99–101.
42 "Regulations as to the Anatomy Lectures at Surgeons' Hall [1753]," in South, *Memorials*, 381.
43 In 1746–47, for example, the surgeons who dissected a body received only £4 each. South, *Memorials*, 228.

London members; but forty-three preferred to pay the £21 fine to be excused from office when their names came up.[44] Isaac Minors, who rotated from Anatomy Steward to Master between 1753 and 1755, was well aware of the inconveniences and dissatisfaction with the system. On 19 August 1755, he proposed an elaborate plan for "a school of anatomy at Surgeons' Hall, in order to raise both profit & reputation to the Surgeons' Company." The details, which included a salaried professor to lecture three days a week at the cost of five guineas per pupil, were circulated to all members of the Court.[45] The Court of Assistants, all of whom were too senior to fill the anatomical offices, rejected the plan on 2 September. They noted only that the current system of the new Company, with rotating lectures on specific topics, had not yet had "a proper Tryal."[46]

When the matter was raised again in July 1766, the Court referred the question of "improving the Lectures and rendering them more credible to the Company and easy to the Members thereof" to a Court committee. Significantly, five of the six committee men were surgeons to one of the general hospitals: John Belchier and Joseph Warner, of Guy's; Percival Pott, of St. Bartholomew's; William Bromfield, of St. George's; and Richard Grindall, of the London. This group not only proposed that the Master be replaced with a "Professor," who would give "a complete course of lectures" each year, but also that part of his privileges should include use of the theater, dissecting room, and library for his private lectures.[47] The Court rejected this ambitious and radical suggestion. The new professor, elected for a three-year term, was, as usual, only required to give six lectures in the fall on the muscles, six in the winter on the viscera, and three in the summer on osteology, all for a gold medal. The Court gave no reasons for overturning the suggestion that the professor use the Hall for private lectures, which some hospital men so clearly endorsed.[48] Already the possibility of corporate monopoly, of unfair competition, perhaps even of the work that would be involved in turning the Company into a

44 Wall, "Anatomical Officers," in *Surgeons' Company*, 228–30; Company of Surgeons, Minutes of the Court of Assistants, 11 Oct. 1753; the Master was to lecture on a topic decided by the Court, Wardens demonstrated the material in lecture for the Master, and Stewards prepared and dissected the bodies for the lectures.
45 Company of Surgeons, Minutes of the Court of Assistants, 19 Aug. 1755; the proposal is reprinted in South, *Memorials*, 378–80. Isaac Minors was surgeon to the Middlesex hospital from 1753 to 1779, a member of the Court of Assistants from 1773 to 1797, and Examiner from 1784 to 1797.
46 Company of Surgeons, Minutes of the Court of Assistants, 2 Sept. 1755.
47 Company of Surgeons, Minutes of the Court of Assistants, 9, 23 July 1766. Christopher Fullanger was the last member of the committee; he had been on the Council since 1745.
48 Company of Surgeons, Minutes of the Court of Assistants, 23 July 1766. South in his *Memorials*, 278, conflates the proposal with what was actually passed. The last, and minor, innovation occurred in 1779, when the Court decided to add six lectures on surgery in the fall and winter, bringing the professor's total to twenty-one for a year's course. Company of Surgeons, Minutes of the Court of Assistants, 1 July 1779.

"school," likely discouraged the Court from opening its doors to free enterprise.

Supported by annually rotating anatomy stewards and wardens, thirteen "professors" declaimed at the Hall between 1767 and 1799, more than half of whom had hospital posts and their own lecture courses in anatomy: Joseph Else, Henry Watson, Henry Cline, William Blizard, John Abernethy, Astley Cooper and Thomas Blizard. Ninety-three surgeons served as stewards and/or wardens to the professors; yet, again, a further 102 decided to pay the fine, including John Hunter (in 1776–7), then surgeon to St. George's and with his own private courses, Lewis Way (in 1768–9), surgeon to Guy's, and James Chafy (in 1775–6), surgeon to the Middlesex.[49]

During the 1770s and 1780s, the company appeared especially marked by complacency and conservatism, with the required lectures given perfunctorily. The Company's torpor finally provoked John Gunning to lash out at the Court on 1 July 1790, the day he stepped down from his year as Master of the Company. Gunning, surgeon to St. George's, member of the Court of Assistants since 1784, and Examiner since 1789, took them to task for numerous irregularities, neglect, and apathy in all of their duties. Their only excesses, he complained, were in "the number & expense of your Dinners."[50] Among his criticisms, Gunning pointed to the poor quality of anatomical teaching and the lack of instruction in surgery, coupled with the remarkable expense of the few lectures regularly given. By 1790, the reason to limit the Company's function was patently obvious: "I know it will be said that our Hall can never be a School of Anatomy. The situation of the different Hospitals, the extent of the Town, together with its interference with private courses prohibit it."[51] Recognizing the flourishing trade in private lectures and their close connections to the hospitals, where students walked the wards and whose surgeons dominated the Court, however, did not deter Gunning from arguing that the Company still had avoided its duty. He recommended that a series of fifteen lectures on surgery be given "in May & June, when the Anatomical Lectures should be over, & before the Students have left the Town." These, offered free to all London students and presented by "Men of Experience in the profession . . . could not fail of being highly useful to the Students as well as being

49 Wall, "Anatomical Officers," in *Surgeons' Company*, 230–5; Cope, *Royal College of Surgeons*, 12; South, *Memorials*, 276–7.
50 "Speech Delivered by Mr. Gunning," in South, *Memorials*, 382–401, quotation p. 387; this well-known speech is also discussed in Cope, *Royal College of Surgeons*, 13–15; Wall, *Surgeons' Company*, 107. Gunning had begun reforms of the Company the previous January, including limiting the amount spent on the dinners. Company of Surgeons, Minutes of the Court of Assistants, 1 Jan., 1 Apr. 1790.
51 "Speech Delivered by Mr. Gunning," in South, *Memorials*, 395. Also quoted by Cope, *Royal College of Surgeons*, 14.

honourable to ourselves." The "Men of Experience," moreover, were "such Members from your Court of Assistants as are in practice, and are Surgeons to Hospitals, and for which they should be liberally paid."[52] In other words, Gunning saw an opportunity for the Company to supplement private teaching in a way that would demonstrate its authority over surgical knowledge, consolidate the hospital surgeons' position as surgical elites and, by offering a short course, not compete with its members' livelihoods.

The Court acquiesced to Gunning's appeal to their vanity, deciding on 7 October 1790 to appoint a professor of surgery the following July to give fifteen lectures for £80. To John Gunning's evident dismay, the Court then elected him for this honor, which he refused. None of the Company's luminaries seemed to want this position and a motion was put forward to cancel the professorship. In January 1792 Gunning responded with an irate letter, changing the tactics of his argument. Now he reminded the Company that it had long condemned various laws that exempted discharged military surgeons from taking any further licensing examinations. Since the Assistants believed that military men were ill-trained, Gunning insisted that they had both the responsibility and the resources to provide needed additional instruction. Furthermore, if the lectures were free, then the poorest students – who, he implied, were most likely to join the military – would benefit.[53] Gunning pleaded in 1792 that a member of the Company who was not on the Court of Assistants be appointed.

I am at loss to assign sufficient reasons for your objections. The gentlemen may not think these lectures of so much Importance if read by a younger Man as they would if read by members of this Court. Possibly not, it is admitted, but Gentlemen regularly bred to the profession of Surgery alone, who have the care of Hospitals and who read lectures at these Hospitals both Chirurgical and Anatomical, are capable surely of giving them Here for the instruction of Young Men destined for the service of the Army and Navy.[54]

This change of approach, from distinguished senior lecturers to younger hospital surgeons, however, still threatened their pocketbooks, as Gunning knew well.

But it may interfere in some degree with the Profits of the different Hospitals and encourage the pupils to discontinue their attendance there. – The little Anatomical Shops for Demonstrations as they are called and the custom of admitting pupils on false pretenses [without paying], to see the Chirurgical operations [at the hospitals] will greatly interfere with this, if not totally prevented, as it is.[55]

52 "Speech Delivered by Mr. Gunning," in South, *Memorials*, 395–6.
53 Company of Surgeons, Minutes of the Court of Assistants, 7 Oct., 4 Nov. 1790, 1 July, 6 Oct. 1791, 5 Jan. 1792; see also Wall, *Surgeons' Company*, 107–9.
54 Company of Surgeons, Minutes of the Court of Assistants, 5 Jan. 1792.
55 Company of Surgeons, Minutes of the Court of Assistants, 5 Jan. 1792.

Although few on the Court of Assistants lectured in the early 1790s, its hospital members shared in the ward-walking fees of all the surgeons' pupils who signed up at their institutions.[56] As lectures likely attracted students to the hospitals, the Assistants still feared the potential competition. The vexed question of the surgery professor was repeatedly postponed for future discussion until the Company dissolved in 1800.[57]

For the new Royal College of Surgeons, turning their Hall into any kind of school with complete courses on anatomy and surgery was effectively a dead issue. The only change in the new College's public duty occurred when it became a repository for John Hunter's vast collection of anatomical and pathological specimens. The College recognized that the museum was "of great national benefit [for] promoting and extending the knowledge of anatomy and surgery." To ensure that the collection fulfilled these goals, the museum was to be available to "properly introduced" individuals. The surgeons also planned to deliver an annual course of lectures on comparative anatomy, "illustrated by the preparations."[58] The museum finally opened in 1813 and Everard Home, surgeon to St. George's and John Hunter's protégé, gave the first course in comparative anatomy.[59] There is little evidence to suggest, however, that the College saw this work as part of the professional knowledge *required* for pupils and apprentices, although it could be a useful accomplishment for them as well-educated gentlemen.

The disparity between many London surgeons' efforts to offer private courses, provide instruction at their hospitals, and create medical societies, while serving (or not) the Company that gave them formal status and defined them as regular practitioners, epitomizes the corporations' ambiguous positions in the eighteenth century. Wanting both free enterprise in teaching and control over licensing in practice led the Surgeons' Company to endorse the status quo. Yet their decisions are contradictory – or self-defeating – only from narrow twentieth-century definitions of professionalization, which emphasize uniform standards and closure. In the hallowed

56 In 1790, sixteen of the twenty-one members of the Court of Assistants were, or had recently served as, hospital surgeons to one of the seven general hospitals; in 1792, seventeen of twenty-one were hospital men. Wall, *Surgeons' Company*, 219–23, lists the members. Only two members of the Court, John Hunter of St. George's and James Earle of St. Bartholomew's, were actively lecturing in 1790, although Henry Watson, of the Westminster, had previously had a private anatomy theater. See Appendix I.E for the number of hospital men on the Court of Assistants for sampled years from 1745 to 1820.
57 Company of Surgeons, Minutes of the Court of Assistants, 2 Feb. 1792, 10 Jan. 1799, 2 Jan. 1800.
58 Company of Surgeons, Minutes of the Court of Assistants, 26 Apr. 1799; Cope, *Royal College of Surgeons*, 22–26; see also Jessie Dobson, "John Hunter's Museum," in Cope, *Royal College of Surgeons*, 274–306.
59 In 1810, Everard Home and William Blizard gave a few lectures on anatomy and surgery, and Home had presented a short course on comparative anatomy, but the annual series only began in 1813. Cope, *Royal College of Surgeons*, 31–2; Dobson, "John Hunter's Museum," 273–7.

traditions of City livery companies, the corporate surgeons first looked to their Council's interests, then to their members', and, when useful, to those of the "public." Even though only one or two Court members actually offered independent lecture courses on anatomy or surgery in 1755, 1766, or 1790–2, the hospital majority acted for their self-proclaimed elite: those who practiced "pure" surgery, untainted by the apothecary's trade. Only when the rank-and-file members, the ubiquitous surgeon–apothecaries, found their college and company unresponsive to calls to assume a public duty to license all practitioners in England and Wales did the hospital surgeons' power in the College and the apparent conflict between their private and public interests become scandalous.[60]

EDUCATION, WAR, AND THE COLLEGES: REFORM AND RESPONSES, 1780–1815

The movements for medical reform in the late eighteenth and early nineteenth centuries demonstrate the political and economic concerns of the rank and file. But it is a mistake to credit the vocal critics of the medical elite with the policy changes that took place in the corporations at the turn of the century. The wars with France, beginning in 1793 and lasting with a few lulls through the summer of 1815, had a much more pervasive impact on certification at the Royal College of Surgeons. Unlike previous military entanglements, especially the Seven Years' War and the War of American Independence, the early-nineteenth-century continental offensive drew heavily on British resources. Medical men fell in large numbers alongside soldiers and sailors, who died not only of wounds but of ravaging epidemics. However much civilian concerns for irregular practice exercised reformers, the RCS responded instead to the military's pragmatic needs, first codifying educational requirements in 1809.

Over the past decades, historians and sociologists of medicine have probed and reprobed the history of the medical reform movements.[61]

60 Adrian Desmond, *The Politics of Evolution: Morphology, Medicine and Reform in Radical London* (Chicago: University of Chicago Press, 1989), 101–92. Desmond offers an excellent account of later reforming agendas and the role of the rank and file within radical politics; Waddington, *The Medical Profession*, 54–69, provides another overview of criticisms of the RCS in the 1820s to 1840s.
61 Loudon, *Medical Care and the General Practitioner*, 129–301; Hamilton, "Medical Professions"; Wall, *Society of Apothecaries*, 192–209; Clarke, *Royal College of Physicians*, 2: 614–50; Newman, *Medical Education*, 56–81, 135–93; Waddington, *The Medical Profession*; Noel Parry and José Parry, *The Rise of the Medical Profession* (London: Croom Helm 1976), ch. 6, esp. 104–17; S. W. F. Holloway, "The Apothecaries' Act, 1815: A Reinterpretation," *Medical History* 10 (1966): 107–29, 221–36; idem, "Medical Education in England, 1830–1958: A Sociological Analysis," *History* 49 (1964): 299–324; D. L. Cowen, "Liberty, Laissez-faire and Licensure in Nineteenth-Century Britain," *Bulletin of the History of Medicine* 43 (1969): 30–40; M. Jeanne Peterson, *The Medical Profession in Mid-Victorian London* (Berkeley: University of California Press, 1978), 16–39; Ivan Waddington, "General Prac-

Irvine Loudon recently pointed out that much of the debate about the significance of this apparent crusade has hinged on when medicine became "professional," a focus which quickly becomes a circular, dead-end approach. Instead, as both Loudon and Roy Porter stress, eighteenth-century medical men struggled to capture their share of a buoyant, diverse, and quixotic market for medical services. The regulars' reforming rhetoric of the early 1800s repeated refrains heard throughout the century against quacks, disreputable practice, and exploitation of an ignorant populace. With often little difference between the regulars' and irregulars' therapies, concepts of disease, and techniques of self-promotion, the regulars claimed authority by virtue of class and education, as much as through knowledge and therapeutic efficacy.[62]

During the mid-eighteenth century, many surgeon–apothecaries had found their occupations reasonably lucrative and moderately respectable. They coexisted, if not happily at least patiently, with both irregulars and the corporate elites. At the end of the century, however, competition sharpened. Particularly worrisome for these general practitioners was their perception that druggists and chemists were encroaching on their territory, dispensing (cheaper) prescriptions, even offering medical advice, instead of simply selling toiletries and patent therapies in the shops that sprang up throughout Britain. Surgeon–apothecaries could hardly raise a public outcry over unfair competition in laissez-faire England, but they could harness their antiquack calls. Pointing once again to differences in education and training, general practitioners sought to undermine the druggists' claims to competence.[63] Medical activists increasingly declared that truly regular general practitioners (like them) had training beyond apprenticeship to shop-bound druggists, particularly emphasizing the lecture courses and hospital experience available in London. Although medical men by no means universally concurred with the challenge to training by apprenticeship alone, courses and ward-walking became a useful standard against which druggists' training would inevitably be found lacking. In 1815, the Society of Apothecaries agreed.

Reforming rhetoric, mass meetings, failed Parliamentary Bills, and supercilious corporate snubs all highlight the most visible battles waged against the elite for public recognition of surgeon–apothecaries. The effects of the early reform movements on medical practice and patients' choices

titioners and Consultants in Early Nineteenth-Century England: The Sociology of an Intra-Professional Conflict," and Ian Inkster, "Marginal Men: Aspects of the Social Role of the Medical Community in Sheffield, 1790–1850," in *Health Care and Popular Medicine in Nineteenth Century England*, ed. John Woodward and David Richards (New York: Holmes & Meier, 1977), 164–88, 128–63; Joseph F. Kett, "Provincial Medical Practice in England, 1730–1815," *Journal of the History of Medicine* 19 (1964): 17–24.

62 Loudon, *Medical Care and the General Practitioner*, 13–18; Porter, *Health for Sale*, 15–17, 21–59.

63 Loudon, *Medical Care and the General Practitioner*, 129–138; Holloway, "Apothecaries' Act," 109.

are difficult to gauge, however, considering the general resistance to limiting the public's freedom to decide on their own medical care. Yet the publicity given to debates over certification probably influenced some aspiring practitioners in the early nineteenth century to obtain corporate sanction. The number of "diplomas," which the Company, then the Royal College, of Surgeons granted to recognize full membership (MRCS), for example, rose dramatically from 47 in 1780 to 348 in 1815.[64] During the eighteenth century, provincial medical men had routinely ignored the London corporations. Surgeon–apothecaries like Matthew Flinders and Thomas Bayley, who walked the wards in London hospitals, both settled in reasonably prosperous practices in the 1770s and neither secured any licenses. Bayley told his apprentice, John Green Crosse, that membership in the Company of Surgeons simply had not been necessary for him. Crosse, in contrast, sat for the MRCS examination as a matter of course in 1813, after hearing lectures and walking hospital wards in London for two years. Both more ambitious and mobile than his master, Crosse nevertheless typifies those who saw official affiliation as both socially and professionally critical, whether or not Parliament would respond to demands for provincial licensing.[65]

Societies and associations

The shift from the perennial pamphlet squabbles about irregulars and quacks to mass meetings, petitions, and bills to Parliament rested upon very basic changes in how, where, and when medical men associated with each other. The emergence and shape of this community are covered in Chapter 7, so I merely stress here that reforming associations surfaced within a much broader context of interactions among practitioners of all

64 Sampled years from the Examination Books show the following increases in the number of full diplomas (membership) compared with the number of military certificates. Where applicants received both a "diploma" and a military certificate, they were counted under "diploma."

	Diploma	Military certificates	Total
1780	47 (12%)	331 (88%)	378
1790	109 (29%)	262 (71%)	371
1800	142 (35%)	265 (65%)	407
1810	164 (33%)	335 (67%)	499
1815	348 (79%)	90 (21%)	438

The 1815 diploma figure may include a high proportion of military men retiring from service and wishing to upgrade their professional qualification. The Court of Examiners in the early nineteenth century charged £22.10s. for a diploma to practice in the provinces, £32.10s. for a London diploma, £3.3s. for examination of military and East India surgeons and £1.1s. for examining mates. Company of Surgeons, Examination Book, 1745–1800; RCS, Court of Examiners, Examination Book, 1800–1820.

65 For Flinders, see Loudon, *Medical Care and the General Practitioner*, 103–9; Flinders registered as a pupil at the London Hospital on 11 July 1769, Pupil Register, London Hospital LX/X/13/9. For Bayley and Crosse, see the letters from Bayley to Crosse, 4 Apr. 1812, 18 Dec. 1813, Norwich Record Office, MS 4306 T 138A.

sorts in the metropolis and provinces. By the end of the eighteenth century, medical men had far more extensive networks of connections, both within London and, through corresponding members of medical societies, with the provinces, than they had ever had previously. Such connections materialized with the gradual formation of medical societies and a medical press, which became such obvious engines of early-nineteenth-century activism.[66] At least from the early decades of the eighteenth century, the increasing metropolitan fascination with coffeehouses, dining groups, semiformal coteries, and formal organizations celebrating occupational, intellectual, or political brotherhood created a thriving social basis for associational politics. The techniques that medical reformers employed to energize the rank and file and solicit support from those more powerful had familiar precedents in contemporary culture. In the 1790s, moreover, when the events of the French Revolution inspired many with either exhilaration or terror, some of these suddenly seemed more radical – or possibly more efficacious – than they had in the 1760s or 1780s.[67]

When the first group of reforming apothecaries got together in the early 1790s, they hardly sought to overthrow the corporations and institute a new regime of medical democracy. They were all for hierarchy – just against their place in it. The commercial prosperity of druggists, who kindly offered advice on medicines in their shops, threatened both their status and their security as "general" practitioners, and the initial impulse for their political action was to outlaw such untrained practitioners. To organize such a project, however, demanded far more work than simply requesting the Society of Apothecaries to act, since that body was not particularly responsive to problems outside its immediate City purview and company business. Hence London men began the General Pharmaceutical Association of Great Britain (GPA) in 1794, using the same methods to mobilize mass support as that politically dangerous group, the London Corresponding Society (started in 1792) did for their cause, the recognition of the politically disenfranchised. The GPA, while not sympathetic to the

---

66 Susan C. Lawrence, " 'Desirous of Improvements in Medicine': Pupils and Practitioners in the Medical Societies at Guy's and St. Bartholomew's Hospitals, 1795–1815," *Bulletin of the History of Medicine* 59 (1985): 89–104; see Loudon, *Medical Care and the General Practitioner*, 279–82, for nineteenth-century medical societies and reform. Dr. Edward Harrison, for example, who championed reform between 1805 and 1809, found strong support from, among other London physicians, Sir John Hayes and William Blackburne. All three were members of the London Medical Society in 1789. "List of the Members . . . 1789," *Memoirs of the Medical Society of London* 1 (1787), n.p.
67 E. P. Thompson, "The Moral Economy of the English Crowd in the Eighteenth Century," *Past and Present* no. 50 (1971): 76–136; P. Corfield, "Class by Name and Number in Eighteenth Century Britain," *History* 72 (1987): 38–61; John Brewer, "English Radicalism in the Age of George III," in *Three British Revolutions*, ed. J. G. A. Pocock (1980), 323–67; Nicholas Rogers, "Crowds and People in the Gordon Riot," in *The Transformation of Political Culture*, ed. Eckhart Hellmuth (London: Oxford University Press for the German Historical Institute, 1990), 57–118; E. P. Thompson, *The Making of the English Working Class* (London: Pantheon Books, 1963).

London Corresponding Society's radical goals, shared its vision of harnessing the discontents of fellow sufferers throughout the kingdom. Initiated with a mass meeting at a tavern in the Strand, the GPA charged its elected committee to write to all "regular" apothecaries in England, asking them to join the association and to fill in a questionnaire about local practitioners.[68] Such tactics – whether used to undermine the state or to undermine druggists – sought to lift dissatisfaction from individual to collective perception, and hence to inspire action. In this sense, just as E. P. Thompson observed that the London Corresponding Society helped to "create" the working class, so did the GPA help to "create" the general practitioner.[69]

After reporting on the extent of irregular practice that the GPA compiled from the responses of its correspondents, the association organized a few meetings with the London corporations and, as a final measure, presented a petition to Parliament. The GPA disappeared in 1795, however, unable to sustain its members' allegiance in the face of corporate obstinacy.[70] Increasing government repression in 1794–5, moreover, may well have discouraged practitioners from any activity that hinted of radical criticism. Then, in 1797, a "Surgeons' Committee" was formed at the Crown and Anchor Tavern; it was organized to protest the Company of Surgeons' plans for a Parliamentary Bill that would absolve the Court of Assistants of their recent peccadillos, such as holding elections without quora and buying property valued beyond their legal limits. This committee of non-Court members argued for numerous reforms, especially to open the Court to surgeon–apothecaries elected from the membership at large and to press for the power to license practitioners throughout England and Wales. The Company's Court circumvented the popular uprising in their midst by successfully applying for a royal charter, instead of an Act of Parliament, to become the Royal College of Surgeons.[71]

Calls to protect the public from unscrupulous druggists and other irregu-

---

68 Quoted from John Mason Good, *The History of Medicine, so far as it relates to the Profession of the Apothecary* (London, 1795), in Holloway, "Apothecaries' Act," 109–10.

69 E. P. Thompson, *The Making of the English Working Class*; George Rudé, *Hanoverian London, 1714–1808* (Berkeley: University of California Press, 1971), 248–9; Loudon, *Medical Care and the General Practitioner*, 130–1. Loudon discounts any connection between medical reform and the aims of "political radicals and religious dissenters" (p. 130). Certainly the major figures in each of these groups did not overlap, but the similarity of methods and challenge to elite oligarchies suggest that the apothecaries gained indirect inspiration from their more dangerous and disruptive contemporaries. See also Parry and Parry, *The Rise of the Medical Profession*, 106–7; Waddington, "General Practitioners and Consultants," 181–3; Holloway, "Apothecaries' Act," 111.

70 Loudon, *Medical Care and the General Practitioner*, 138.

71 Company of Surgeons, Minutes of the Court of Assistants, vol. 2 (1790–1800); Hamilton, "Medical Professions," 157–9; Cope, *Royal College of Surgeons*, 17–21; Wall, *Surgeons' Company*, 78, 183–208. The composition of the Surgeons' Committee is unknown, but the spokesmen included John Mason Good, who brought reforming experience from the General Pharmaceutical Association to help mobilize the surgeons against a Bill which did nothing to help the lower-ranking practitioners.

lars through comprehensive licensing lay dormant until 1806, when Dr. Edward Harrison, a provincial practitioner, nearly singlehandedly formed the Associated Faculty (1806–11). When Harrison gave up, the Association of Apothecaries and Surgeon–Apothecaries was formed in 1812, starting off with a London meeting to protest a recent tax on glass. Harrison, like the members of the GPA, solicited practitioners throughout the kingdom to report, in quantitative terms this time, about their local practice. The Association of Apothecaries and Surgeon–Apothecaries similarly drew on subscribers from all over England and Wales to lend weight to its proposals. Throughout this later period, the corporations, generally in response to the platforms of these organizations, formed committees of their ruling members to consider the ideas for reform and occasionally to introduce their own suggestions.[72] The licensing bodies primarily reacted, however, with blanket objections to any bill which would infringe upon their own powers, control, or sense of dignity.

Medical reform and London medical education

For all of the reform organizations and reforming authors, discussion of medical education was subsumed under the larger, and more significant, problem of licensing "qualified" men and excluding usurpers and quacks. From the General Pharmaceutical Association's program to the final resolutions of the Apothecaries' Act, the key points were apprenticeship and the criteria required for taking the licensing examinations. Apprenticeship remained a central plank in medical training, despite criticisms of its narrowness and associations with "trade," primarily because it was the traditional and accepted route to acquire sound knowledge and one which many reformers had followed.[73] In the early nineteenth century, only a very few would even think of denouncing it totally. It took a radical physician, Dr. Thomas Beddoes, to sneer, "I allow little or nothing for apprenticeship; during which the mind is too apt to be choked up with moral and medical rubbish."[74] For the rank and file, taking apprentices gave them both status

72 Loudon, *Medical Care and the General Practitioner*, 138–66; and Holloway, "Apothecaries' Act," 109–26, give the details of these organizations and the corporations' responses.
73 William Chamberlaine, *Tirocinium Medicum, or a Dissertation on the Duties of Youth Apprenticed to the Medical Profession* (London, 1812), chapter VI; James Lucas, *Candid Inquiry into the Education, Qualifications and Offices of a Surgeon Apothecary* (London: S. Hazard, 1800), 16–33; Fissell, *Patients, Power and the Poor*; Joan Lane, "The Role of Apprenticeship in Eighteenth Century Medical Education in England," in *William Hunter and the Eighteenth Century Medical World*, ed. William Bynum and Roy Porter (Cambridge: Cambridge University Press, 1985), 61–3, 99–100.
74 Thomas Beddoes, *A Letter to the Right Honorable Sir Joseph Banks, Bart., On the Causes and Removal of the Prevailing Discontent, Imperfection and Abuses in Medicine* (London: Phillips, 1808), 81; for Thomas Beddoes in context, see Roy Porter, *Doctor of Society: Thomas Beddoes and the Sick Trade in Late-Enlightenment England* (London: Routledge, 1992).

as masters and a modest source of income. To threaten regular apprenticeship would undercut such practitioners' claims to expertise and open the floodgates to those unwilling to devote at least five years to learning their craft. Thus for the reforming apothecaries in the General Pharmaceutical Association of 1794 proper control over competence rested entirely on the hope that "none be at liberty to settle until examined; nor any person [be] entitled to an examination until he shall have faithfully served an apprenticeship of five years at the least."[75]

While apprenticeship remained the bedrock for educating all but physicians, it was nevertheless not enough to distinguish regular practitioners from others with more dubious backgrounds. The focus shifted to additional licensing requirements, necessary in order to be examined by one of the corporations. In 1806, both Dr. John Latham, FRCP and retired physician to St. Bartholomew's, writing for the Royal College of Physicians, and Dr. Harrison and his Associated Faculty circulated proposals that urged more extensive qualifications. In the draft Bill he wrote for the RCP to endorse, Latham suggested that surgeons and apothecaries serve five-year apprenticeships preceding a required period of hospital attendance: "Two Years in a Provincial Hospital, or One Year at least in any of the Hospitals in London, Dublin, or Edinburgh."[76] The Associated Faculty recommended that, first, physicians had to be graduates of a university in the United Kingdom (a charming statement of British loyalty); second, both surgeons and apothecaries had to have served five-year apprenticeships; and third, surgeons had to have studied "anatomy and surgery for two years," while apothecaries had to study physic for a year beyond apprenticeship.[77] Plans for Parliamentary bills promoted by the Association of Apothecaries and Surgeon–Apothecaries in 1812–13 displayed a similar range of standards for preliminary education, from coursework and hospital experience to apprenticeship or military practice.[78] Clauses in their early drafts dispensed with mandatory apprenticeship, substituting certificates of attendance at lectures on anatomy, chemistry, midwifery, and medicine, plus six months' work at a London hospital or a year at a provincial institution. This alternative route did not last long in their proposed bills, however, and apprenticeship plus some additional training became the preferred requirements for examination.[79]

During the middle wave of reforming zeal between 1804 and 1808, the only institutional change occurred at the RCP. While rejecting Harrison's

75 Quoted from John Mason Good, *The History of Medicine, so far as it relates to the Profession of the Apothecary* (London, 1795), in Holloway, "Apothecaries' Act," 111.
76 Clark, *Royal College of Physicians*, 2: 624–7, 772–5; Holloway, "Apothecaries' Act," 115.
77 Holloway, "Apothecaries' Act," 116; Newman, *Medical Education*, 61–2.
78 Loudon, *Medical Care and the General Practitioner*, 154–9.
79 Holloway, "Apothecaries' Act," 119–20; Loudon, *Medical Care and the General Practitioner*, 157–8.

proposals and finding Latham's plan impossible to promote, as it centered on having the physicians regulate practice throughout the country, the RCP made a telling internal regulation. Probably picking up the Associated Faculty's concern for the quality of provincial practitioners, the RCP altered its regulations for the entry of extra-Licentiates in 1807. Candidates for this provincial qualification thenceforth had to "produce certificates of one year's residence at a university or of one year's attendance on the practice of a hospital in London or two years' at a provincial hospital, with certificates of having attended lectures on anatomy and physic."[80] Since extra-Licentiates were long regarded as inferior physicians, the College's elite apparently did not object to the obvious blurring of the extra-Licentiate category with the training thought appropriate for surgeons and apothecaries. Extra-Licentiates were not supposed to dispense medicines, so the most important distinction between them and apothecaries was maintained. It is not surprising, however, that very few chose to obtain the extra-Licentiate, since it cost £17. 3s. and was neither mandatory for provincial practice nor at all prestigious.[81]

While various associations and the corporations held their committee meetings and jockeyed for compromises that might result in Parliamentary action, pamphleteers and reviewers contributed their thoughts to fan public awareness and professional reactions. In this diverse literature, two significant points about medical education stand out. First, despite a range of opinions on the efficiency and efficacy of apprenticeship, no one criticized the system of lectures and hospital practice already in place in London, except to claim that too few practitioners took advantage of such opportunities. Second, requiring post- or extra-apprenticeship courses and hospital experience for licensing was not entirely an appeal for practice based upon rigorously acquired knowledge. Rather it would serve – as contemporaries well knew – to demarcate the social origins of regular medical men because such training required time and money unavailable to those from poor families.

Reformers, by their silence, apparently did not think that either lecturers or hospital men required any supervision, regulation, or central control. Disparate practitioners, whether they taught or not, shared the basic assumptions underpinning London education: the belief in free competition, individual initiative, and personal profit. None of those who demanded better qualified medical men suggested that the existing licensing bodies

80 Clark, *Royal College of Physicians*, 2: 638–9. These regulations are given in Clark's words from the Annals of the College, 30 Mar. 1807. Clark gives no record that Licentiates or Fellows at this time had to produce any certificate beyond the requirement of two years' residence at university and the MD degree. Hamilton, "Medical Professions," 154, makes an incorrect claim that "until 1812 the College of Physicians required only six months hospital practice."

81 Clark, *Royal College of Physicians*, 2: 639.

formulate requirements or guidelines to ensure that teachers would meet certain standards or cover a specific body of material.[82] The absence of such comment, especially from men who were at times exceedingly critical of the London corporations and who railed against inept, ignorant, and dangerous practitioners, reveals their general acceptance of the vitality and success of extra-apprenticeship London medical education.[83] Thus Thomas Beddoes, primarily concerned to reform physicians' training, urged that if London had a university to grant medical degrees, the capital could easily rival Paris in the excellence of its instruction; he recommended London over Edinburgh for medical training in his 1808 text.[84] Robert Kerrison, a member of both the Royal College of Surgeons and the Society of Apothecaries, wrote strongly in favor of reform in 1814. In his polemical pamphlet, he stressed the fact that London had better opportunities for medical education than theory-oriented universities, and as evidence he listed the names of lecturers, such as Cline, Abernethy, Dr. Pearson, and Dr. Denman, who made the metropolis a mecca for practical knowledge.[85]

Such implicit acceptance and explicit praise of London's advantages in medical education rested upon practitioners' social as well as technical concerns. As an anonymous reviewer in 1810 pointed out, Harrison's reforming goals openly linked suppressing "empirical practice" with preventing "the admission of mean and low persons, by a fine on all certificates of qualification."[86] Castigating the "exclusive monopolizing spirit" that inspired the medical reformers, the reviewer concluded that Parliamentary regulation of medical practice "would invade the rights of citizens and rivet the chains of monopoly." He argued that patients have the right to choose their nostrums and medical attendants; that reputation, status, and education would sufficiently guide the public in its judgments.[87] A free market for medical care, for this reviewer, meant an open market in education and talent:

82 The Association of Apothecaries and Surgeon–Apothecaries, in their January 1813 draft for a bill, did suggest that an all-professional committee should be established to regulate medical practice in England. This committee would also have authority to "appoint persons to teach, and to give lectures," but the presumed extent of its authority and jurisdiction was vague. This proposal did not last long, and other bodies, reviews, and critiques do not refer to similar plans. Newman, *Medical Education*, 66.

83 Clark, *Royal College of Physicians*, 2: 614, also notes this point.

84 Beddoes, *A Letter*, 72–81; for more on Beddoes and reform, see Porter, *Doctor of Society*, 140–53.

85 Robert Masters Kerrison, *An Inquiry into the Present State of the Medical Profession in England* (London: Longman, Hurst, Rees, Orme, and Brown, 1814), 23–4; see also Thomas Champney, *Medical and Chirurgical Reform Proposed from a Review of the Healing Art . . . with Considerations on Hospitals, Dispensaries, Poor Houses and Prisons* (London: J. Johnson, 1797).

86 Anonymous, Review of Edward Harrison's "An Address to the Lincolnshire Benevolent Medical Society" (1810) and Jeremiah Jenkin's *Observations on the Profession* (1810), in *Critical Review*, 3rd. ser., 21 (1810): 191.

87 Anonymous, Review of Edward Harrison . . . and Jeremiah Jenkin, *Critical Review*, 197.

The apothecary is therefore bound to show how he has gained any knowledge of medicine which the other [a chemist] may not possess. Is it from books? They are open to all mankind. From lectures and attendance in hospitals? These advantages too can be possessed by those who have not served apprenticeships as well as by those who have.[88]

For reformers to require apprenticeship in addition to books, lectures, and hospital experience thus exposed their fallacious claims. Aspiring practitioners would not be "mean and low persons" because such men could not afford this cumbersome route to certification.

The ambivalence over apprenticeship – whether it retarded the reach for upward status by connecting practice with craft and trade or served to support the rank and file by legitimizing their experience and excluding irregulars – continued well into the nineteenth century.[89] In the early 1800s, in contrast, courses and hospital experience became the rallying points for both reformers and the corporations. As noted, the RCP acknowledged their importance when certifying extra-Licentiates, who did not need to have MD degrees. For the Royal College of Surgeons, fresh from the controversies that had dissolved the previous Company, such extra-apprenticeship work increasingly identified the path to appropriate certification.

War and the Company/Royal College of Surgeons

During the early nineteenth century, the Royal College of Surgeons faced considerable pressure to enhance their supervisory role over the certification of surgeons. Public concern over military practice, which intensified during the long wars with France, had a more immediate effect on the College's internal regulations than reformers' voices arguing about appropriate medical education. In contrast to the controversy generated by plans for Parliamentary bills, the Royal College of Surgeons' Court of Examiners gradually and quietly introduced educational requirements for those seeking full membership and military certificates.[90]

The Royal College of Surgeons inherited the responsibility of certifying army and navy surgeons from the previous company. Lower-ranking military medical men – hospital mates, assistant surgeons, and the like – were regularly given easier examinations than men seeking the "grand diploma" for civilian practice or hoping to become full surgeons in the forces.[91] Even in times of peace before 1815, the Company of Surgeons regularly granted more military certificates than full diplomas. In 1790, for example, of the

---

88 Anonymous, Review of Edward Harrison . . . and Jeremiah Jenkin, *Critical Review*, 195.
89 Loudon, *Medical Care and the General Practitioner*, 176–80.
90 See Wall, *Surgeons' Company*, 120–4, for a discussion of the other functions of the Court of Examiners.
91 Wall, *Surgeons' Company*, 108, 118, 124–5.

371 men successfully examined at the Hall, only 109 (29 percent) applied for full diplomas; the rest sought military or East India Company certificates.[92] The high demand for medical men during the wars with France soon meant that standards fell to a bare minimum.[93] Hopes for well-educated military surgeons clashed with the reality of low pay, lack of respect, and physical dangers facing most recruits. Furthermore, while there was intense interest within England about events of the war there was also a general assumption that, since war naturally meant deaths, wounds, and disease, military leaders knew best what to demand or expect from medical care. The public rarely confronted – if it even perceived – the problem of inadequate medical facilities or attendants.[94]

The war, with its desperate need for both medical and regular enlistments and commissions and the obvious deleterious effects of sickness on the English troops, troubled the military and its medical officers from 1793. New pressures arose between 1806 and 1811, however, that account for the Royal College of Surgeons' being badgered both to raise their licensing standards and to make them explicit. First, British involvement in the war intensified in 1808. Although the kingdom had been fighting in the colonies, in the Mediterranean, and briefly on the Continent before 1808, new campaigns in Portugal and Spain required a larger, more intensive effort than the earlier conflicts. Second, in the summer of 1809 a massive expedition in support of Austria was sent to the Scheldt. The mission was disastrous, in part because of the ravages of several epidemics at Walcheren. By late summer hundreds were dying daily and thousands of sick were being transported back to England.[95] This military failure certainly touched the public: when Parliament opened in January 1810, the members immediately demanded an inquiry, and, after much debate, the House of Commons considered the affair as a Committee of the House.[96]

While the House of Commons ultimately voted to condone the govern-

---

92 Company of Surgeons, Examination Book, 1745–1800, entries for 1790.
93 Neil Cantlie, *A History of the Army Medical Department*, 2 vols. (London: Churchill Livingstone, 1974), I: 180, 197–200. The low entry standards were partially justified at the time by the claim that such young men were pupils and were only to serve under other medical men, who could teach them. For details on the numerous problems, in-fighting, and periods of near-chaos in the medical care of soldiers during the far-flung battles and campaigns from 1793–1815, see Cantlie, *Army Medical Department*, I: chs. 7–13.
94 For the period before 1793, see especially Harold J. Cook, "Practical Medicine and the British Armed Forces after the 'Glorious Revolution,' " *Medical History* 34 (1990): 1–24; Paul E. Kopperman, "Medical Services in the British Army, 1742–1783," *Journal of the History of Medicine* 34 (1979): 428–55.
95 Cantlie, *Army Medical Department*, I: 395–405; for the interconnections between war and disease in these conflicts, see also Michael Duffy, *Soldiers, Sugar and Seapower: The British Expedition to the West Indies and the War against Revolutionary France* (New York: Oxford University Press, 1987).
96 For the original bare report of the government's activity, see the *Journals of the House of Commons* 65 (1810): 13–4, 35, 38, 45–6, 68, 83, 235–7. A much fuller account of the debates exists in *The Annual Register* 52 (1810): 2–26, 41–85. See also Cantlie, *Army Medical Department*, I: 404–5.

ment's expedition and did not criticize the medical men for having to deal with epidemics beyond their control, the intense public scrutiny and dismay at the high mortality and morbidity rates produced indirect pressure on the Royal College of Surgeons to ensure that the young men replacing the dead or incapacitated military medical attendants were better prepared to face similar crises.[97] Since the 1790s, the Company/College had also encountered attacks on their monopoly to certify surgeons for the army and navy from Dublin's and Edinburgh's colleges of surgeons. From 1808 to 1810 Edinburgh particularly renewed its assault on London's privileges, claiming that its own College certified better-qualified men than did its southern counterpart. With pressure in the government to allow Edinburgh equal licensing power, the Royal College of Surgeons of London was forced to show it held high standards, in order to justify its negative response to Edinburgh's petition.[98]

The Court of Examiners left the first direct record of their policies in 1809.[99] The Royal College of Surgeons of Dublin had apparently requested that the Royal College in London enact stricter regulations on surgical education. The Court answered that they carefully examined certificates of lectures and hospital practice presented by the candidates, which they then judged on their "merits."[100] In May of 1810, the Army Medical Board officially requested a list of the RCS requirements for army surgeons, specifically asking "if any particular Schools of Surgery and Medicine [or] Hospitals are considered preferable or indispensable to entitle persons to be examined and passed." The reply of 15 June 1810 indicated that candidates did, in fact, have to have certificates of lecture and hospital attendance, but

97 The numbers of sick, with unavoidable references to the lack of medical care they received, were reported in the public press throughout the spring of 1810. See also *Observations on the Documents . . . on the subject of the late Expedition to the Scheldt* (London, 1810). This was belatedly reviewed by the *Edinburgh Review* 17 (1810–11): 330–9, early in 1811, and, once again, attention was called to the final estimate of 36,500 men whose health was affected by the expedition (p. 338).

98 RCS, Minutes of the Court of Assistants, 27 Apr. 1810; W. N. Boog Watson, "Four Monopolies," 311–22.

99 The early records are sketchy, but suggest that some criteria were in place for candidates by 1800. See Company of Surgeons, Examination Book, 20 Mar. 1800; RCS, Examination Book, 6 Nov. 1800: William Smith was "not exam^d having no Anat^y." Whether the candidates were required to bring certificates of courses is unclear, since no explicit mention is made of certificates prior to 1810. It is probable, therefore, that young men who managed to learn enough anatomy from books and by personal dissection, could still have passed any anatomy questions posed by the Court. This assumption is further supported by noting the existence of popular "cram" books, such as *Anatomical Examinations: A complete series of Anatomical Questions, with answers. The Answers arranged so as to form an elementary system of Anatomy, and intended as preparatory to Examinations at Surgeons' Hall* (London, 1807). See the short review in *Critical Review*, 3rd ser., 10 (1807): 215–6.

100 RCS, Minutes and Resolutions of the Court of Examiners, vol. 1 (1763–1825), 26 Apr. 1809. Notes from prior to 1800 were copied into this volume, but primarily deal with relations between the Company of Surgeons and the military boards, whose candidates they examined. No regulations concerning educational requirements are described.

the Court refused to specify which courses, length of practice, or hospitals they preferred. Instead, they stated that they examined in anatomy, physiology, accidents, and diseases "which are the objects of surgery and chirurgical operations."[101]

Confusion continued over what the Royal College of Surgeons actually wanted. When the Transport Office wrote to the College six months later asking about the requirements for assistant surgeons in the Royal Navy, it described Dublin's Royal College of Surgeons' expectations. The London College's answer was, again, vague regarding lectures, but the examiners claimed that they demanded six months' hospital work. They obviously wished to retain their power to be "satisfied" with certificates for the candidate to be examined.[102] Finally, in October 1811 the examiners relaxed their secrecy and ordered one hundred copies of a notice to be printed and sent to all senior surgeons of hospitals and teachers of anatomy and surgery. In it they set forth the requirements for the College's examination: attendance at lectures on anatomy, physiology, and surgery; performance of dissections; and attendance (duration unspecified) at a hospital.[103] Their final resolution before 1815 was to demand an entire year's attendance at a hospital for the College diploma or for ranking as a "principal Surgeon" in the military, a requirement which they established on 6 August 1813.[104]

The RCS Examination Books show that the Court enforced their emerging regulations. On 16 February 1810, for example, well before assuring the Army Medical Board that evidence of appropriate education was necessary, the Court refused to examine Thomas Lunsden, because he had no certificates, and David Williams, because he had not attended a hospital.[105] While the Court declined to examine candidates when they lacked proper testimonials of age, insufficient education appears to have been the most frequent reason for deferring certification, especially for those seeking the lowest military accreditation.

Whether or not the RCS requirements produced more qualified military surgeons or, for that matter, the "respectable" general practitioner that reformers dreamed of, they acknowledged the central role of courses and hospital ward-walking in distinguishing regular from irregular medical men. Such recognition tacitly legitimized the reformers' arguments for training beyond the apprentice's service to his master. These seemingly minor corporate innovations documented how London's elite surgeons

101 RCS, Minutes and Resolutions of the Court of Examiners, 15 June 1810.
102 RCS, Minutes and Resolutions of the Court of Examiners, 7 Dec. 1810.
103 RCS, Minutes and Resolutions of the Court of Examiners, 4 Oct. 1811.
104 RCS, Minutes and Resolutions of the Court of Examiners, 6 Aug. 1813. This account replaces that of Cope, *Royal College of Surgeons*, 43, and Wall, *Surgeons' Company*, 86, note.
105 RCS, Examination Book, 10 Feb. 1810. By 18 May 1810 the Court clearly required hospital work for those trying to become naval assistant surgeons. To what degree they asked for official printed certificates is unclear, however.

were prepared to institutionalize the free market in lectures and clinical experience, quite apart from the reformers' more radical proposals to license all surgeon–apothecaries, create a separate college, and register all practitioners.[106] They also underlie not only the formal provisions of the Apothecaries' Act, which was, as historians have remarked, an extremely conservative plan, but also the way that the Society of Apothecaries actually implemented its new-found powers, a point that has been insufficiently appreciated in historians' discussions of the orgins and meaning of the Act.

The Apothecaries' Act

After drawn out negotiations among the Association of Apothecaries and Surgeon–Apothecaries, the Royal College of Physicians, the Royal College of Surgeons, and the Society of Apothecaries, a bill was prepared that managed to pass Parliament on 11 July 1815. It required that all apothecaries henceforth entering practice throughout England and Wales hold the Society of Apothecaries license (LSA), and as such was a minor victory for those hoping to curtail irregular practice. That it excluded chemists and druggists, who were left unlicensed; kept medical qualifications distinct from surgical ones; maintained the colleges' traditional authority; and embarrassed provincial MDs who compounded their own medicines immediately frustrated those hoping for more powerful and comprehensive legislation.[107] Whatever disappointment reformers felt when faced with the Act's final form, however, power over de facto general practitioners had been granted to the Society of Apothecaries, whose recent concerns had laid much more stress on its role as a City trading company than as a licensing corporation.[108] When George Man Burrows, a leading reformer and member of the Society, was asked to join the twelve-member Court of Examiners in July 1815, he was dismayed to discover that several of his colleagues "did not know such an Act was in existence."[109]

The Society's near obliviousness to reform and its passive acceptance of the supervisory role over all apothecaries, essentially thrust upon it by the Royal College of Physicians, have been amply discussed elsewhere.[110] As

---

106 Loudon, *Medical Care and the General Practitioner*, 157–8.
107 Loudon, *Medical Care and the General Practitioner*, 159–88.
108 Society of Apothecaries, Court of Assistants, Minute Book, 1806–17, Guildhall Library, MS 8200/10; the entries from 1806 to July 1815 reveal the Court's utter lack of interest in reforming issues; Susan C. Lawrence, "Private Enterprise and Public Interests: Medical Education and the Apothecaries' Act, 1780–1825," in *British Medicine in an Age of Reform*, ed. Andrew Wear and Robert French (London: Routledge, 1991), 45–73.
109 George Man Burrows, *A Statement of the Circumstances connected with the Apothecaries' Act and its Administration* (London: Callow, 1817), 9; also quoted in Loudon, *Medical Care and the General Practitioner*, 169.
110 Loudon, *Medical Care and the General Practitioner*, 162–5; Holloway, "Apothecaries' Act," 121–4.

expected, the Act made both apprenticeship and a licensing examination obligatory for certification. Significantly, however, it included a clause that the newly instituted Court of Examiners could require candidates to produce "Testimonials to the Satisfaction of the said Court of Examiners, of a sufficient Medical Education, and of good moral conduct."[111] This subtle phrasing gave the Apothecaries the same power that the Royal College of Surgeons' Examiners had already appropriated. The Society's Examiners could interpret "sufficient Medical Education" as they chose and alter their criteria without further legislative action, so long as they did not infringe on the rights and prerogatives of the other corporate bodies. This open-ended mandate gave the Society, like the RCS, both the ability to recognize London's existing system of medical education and, in the succeeding decades, to influence it subtly.[112]

The twelve new Examiners of the Society of Apothecaries were clearly convinced that lectures and hospital work were important adjuncts to apprenticeship. The first Court of Examiners, appointed by a Special Court of Assistants on 19 July, quickly formulated the prerequisites needed to proceed to examination. These went into effect on 1 August. The Society required certificates of a five-year apprenticeship, attainment of the age of majority, competence in Latin, and good moral conduct. In addition, they demanded documentation of having attended two courses of anatomy and physiology, two courses in the theory and practice of medicine, one course of chemistry, and one course of materia medica. Finally, the Society of Apothecaries asked for proof that the applicant had attended six months of medical practice at a hospital, infirmary, or dispensary.[113] Far from radical innovations or even spurs to medical teaching in the metropolis, these provisions simply marked the contemporary standards and expectations among practitioners eager to mark themselves off from druggists and chemists, standards that were finally recognized by the one corporate body that Parliament and the royal colleges deemed suitable to shelter the amorphous rank and file.

In 1815, the medical occupations looked, on the surface, much as they did a century before. The tripartite division of physicians, surgeons, and apothecaries remained enshrined in the London corporations and in the London hospitals. But this division had long been an illusion for all but the

---

111 "An Act for the better regulating of the Practice of Apothecaries throughout England and Wales [12 July 1815]," *The Statutes of the United Kingdom of Great Britain and Ireland,* 55 George III (1815), Statutes at Large (London, 1815), 33: 1114.

112 S. C. Lawrence, "Private Enterprise and Public Interests," 45–73.

113 Printed notice, 31 July 1815, inserted into the Society of Apothecaries' Court of Examiners' Entry Book of "Qualifications of Candidates," Guildhall Library, MS 8241, vol. 1 (1815–19). The notice was printed for circulation to all hospitals and lecturers, in order to reach as many candidates as possible. See also Barrett, *Society of Apothecaries,* 180–2.

elite, who held tenaciously to their chartered privileges and public claims to status and knowledge. Of course irregulars still flourished, druggists still prescribed, and scores of surgeon–apothecaries still protested, albeit more frequently adorned with both LSA and MRCS after their names. The regulars, those respectable practitioners who could afford to attend courses, walk hospital wards, or observe dispensary practice, could hope that, because they had such marks of expertise, patients would choose them over the ignorant and untrained.

Whether through conscious policy or not, the Royal College of Physicians, Company/Royal College of Surgeons, and Society of Apothecaries acted not in apathy and ignorance, but in tacit acceptance of the medical marketplace as an open, competitive arena. Their failure to prosecute for irregular practice, disinclination to sponsor complete courses of introductory lectures, wariness over reform, and cautious response to military demands reveal this. Certainly they looked after their own narrow interests, but, after all, their courts were made up of successful men. Why should they worry about their less fortunate colleagues, threatened by commercial forces?

4

Walking the wards: From apprentices to pupils

"Sir," wrote John Wood of Sittingbourne, Kent, on 28 May 1788, to George Neale, surgeon,

> I take the liberty in writing to you beging [sic] the favor of a Certificate from you & the other Surgeons of the London Hospital of my being your Dresser in the Above Hospital for twelve Months, my being a Member of the Benevolent Medical Society for the County of Kent I find a Certificate from the Hospital &c may be necessary and that I could wish to have it by the 6 of June. . . . P.S. the time of my entrance in the London Hospital was October 3 1769.[1]

Nineteen years after walking the London's wards, John Wood found that evidence of that experience might "be necessary" for his practice in Kent. His brief request suggests the little ways that hospital training crept into the making of regular medical men in the eighteenth century. In 1769, Wood chose to pay to watch and assist elite surgeons in their charitable work, spending twelve months engaged in an activity hardly required for a surgeon, or surgeon–apothecary, to start treating patients in Britain. Yet it mattered. In 1788 the "Certificate from the Hospital" was valuable. It marked Wood as a practitioner with an appropriate background, whatever he actually learned under Neale and the other surgeons.

For the emergence of hospital teaching in London, Wood's decision to enter the wards evokes part of the story, the demand side, as it were, of institutional change. Equally important choices occurred when the hospital governors let him in and staff surgeons let him follow them. This chapter

---

1 Letter from John Wood to George Neale, LH/A/23/10 (loose sheet), London Hospital Archive; Neale was surgeon to the London from 1753 to his death in 1797. P. J. Wallis and R. V. Wallis, *Eighteenth Century Medics (Subscriptions, Licenses, Apprenticeships)*, 2nd ed. (Newcastle-upon-Tyne, UK: Project for Historical Biobibliography, 1988), 664, have two entries for "John Wood" of Sittingbourne, both as a "surgeon etc." near the same date, the first as a master of John Beckett, apprenticed to Wood for two years for £50 in 1787. The second entry gives John Wood, born 1766[?] and died approximately 1787, but unfortunately without a specific reference to the biographical source. "John Wood" does appear in the Pupil Register for the London (LH/X13/9) entering on Oct. 3, 1769. I am extremely grateful to Claire Daunton for providing me with a copy of this letter.

examines how and when men like John Wood gained access to the general hospitals of the metropolis. From the perspective of London practitioners and hospital governors around 1700, ward-walking was *not* an obvious sign of either educational progress or charitable care. Yet 11,059 pupils between 1725 and 1815 signed up to walk hospital wards. Eleven thousand students – do note – was hardly negligible by eighteenth-century standards. Lisa Rosner has discovered from her analysis of records at the University of Edinburgh, for example, that of the 7,784 men who matriculated there for medical courses between 1763 and 1805, 4,966 signed up to follow the practice at the Royal Infirmary; at least 5,921 pupils registered to attend the London hospitals during the same period. (Some of these, of course, were the same men, as better-off students perambulated between London and Edinburgh for knowledge, reputations and a possible MD degree.)[2]

The students whose names provide a numerical profile of London teaching officially followed either the physicians, the surgeons, or the apothecary in their respective rounds. Maintaining the formal tripartite division among the pupils supported the way that elite practitioners worked not only within the hospitals, but also outside them, as members of the London corporate bodies and as attendants and consultants to patients among the upper ranks. Whatever pupils *did* on the wards or intended for their own careers, they managed under the well-established labels of the traditional medical occupations. Within these broad categories, ward students also had a range of responsibilities for patient care that varied widely over time and among the hospitals. I define the common names and duties for those with access to the wards in Table 4.1, showing the ascending hierarchy of privileges among each sort. This is the basic vocabulary for eighteenth-century hospital training. I use "pupil" as a generic term, therefore, in the sense that dressers, house pupils, and apprentices had all of the advantages of walking pupils. Similarly, I use "pupilage" to denote the overarching *form* of instruction centered on payment for the short-term privilege of learning about practice within the medical charity, in contrast to instruction among private patients with a single practitioner. Shifting relationships

2 Lisa Rosner, "Students and Apprentices: Medical Education at Edinburgh University, 1760–1810," Ph.D. dissertation, Johns Hopkins University, 1986, 394; Wallis and Wallis, *Eighteenth Century Medics,* estimate their current register contains the names of 35,000 practitioners for the eighteenth century; their list does not include names from the London hospitals' pupil registers. Considering that 2,019 men received MDs from Edinburgh between 1726 and 1815 and a mere 439 were granted either medical degrees or licenses to practice from the University of Oxford from 1701 to 1800, London's hospitals saw a considerable number of students seeking clinical experience. *List of the Graduates in Medicine in the University of Edinburgh, from 1705 to 1866* (Edinburgh: Neill & Co., 1867), iii; Charles Webster, "The Medical Faculty and the Physic Garden," in *The History of the University of Oxford,* vol. v, *The Eighteenth Century,* ed. L. S. Sutherland and L. G. Mitchell (Oxford: Clarendon Press, 1986), 685.

Table 4.1. *Pupils on the wards in the London hospitals*

Signed up with	Privileges and duties	Fees
Physicians		
Walking pupil	Attend rounds with physicians Access to the "physicians' books"	£21-£26 per year
House pupil	Write cases into "the books"	
Surgeons		
Walking pupil	Attend rounds with surgeons Visit patients off rounds (limited) Watch operations, postmortems	£21-£32 per year shared among all staff surgeons
Dresser	Bandage wounds; perform bleeding; minor operations; assist at capital operations	£50 per year to individual surgeon
House pupil House surgeon	On hand for emergencies; responsible for patients in the absence of staff surgeons; teach pupils	£25 per year for hospital board (1781)
Apprentice	Access to full range of surgeon's hospital and private practice; assist at operations; perform operations	£200-£600 per indenture to master
Apothecary		
Walking pupil	Attend ward rounds with apothecary (and other staff); access to the "physicians' books"	£21-£32 per year (possibly shared with the surgeons)
Boarding pupil House pupil Apprentice	On hand for emergencies; responsible for patients in the absence of the apothecary; noting prescriptions; making up medicines	Unknown £100-£300 per indenture to master

among hospital governors, their "objects" of charity, staff men, and pupils over the century defined the privileges, duties, and behavior expected of hospital medical students. The vast majority of such expectations arose, moreover, when a hospital community confronted quite specific problems and came up with immediate solutions that, over time, became new traditions about how ward-walking worked. I stress this point because eighteenth-century hospital teaching arose from scores of local decisions, taking place at seven different hospitals, in six distinct neighborhoods, with three disparate administrative structures, and a bewildering array of staff interests, personalities, and skills.

The transition from one or two apprentices and university men to dozens of short-term pupils accompanying staff practitioners on their rounds grafted instruction onto the purpose of charities for the sick poor. This shift, moreover, embedded pupilage into the hospital economy, for pupils became sources of income for surgeons and physicians and of free labor on the wards. In less tangible ways, pupilage confirmed and strengthened hospital men's prestige and influence as the arbiters of medical knowledge. Well before the eighteenth century, staff physicians and surgeons had practiced publicly, in the sense that their apprentices, private students, staff colleagues, visiting governors, and, of course, hospital patients observed their work. Yet having increasing numbers of pupils on the wards extended hospital men's interpretations of disease and treatment to ever larger circles. Ward-walking opened hospital practice to those who already had some medical knowledge, allowing more medical men to witness, discuss, and (potentially) praise or criticize the bedside decisions of these elite practitioners.

The figures for ward-walking pupils, the regulations devised to manage them, the ways students and practitioners juggled the boundaries between physic and surgery, and the means by which pupils acquired clinical knowledge all reveal what it meant for the London hospitals to introduce students on the wards. Near the end of the century, John Hunter, then a disgruntled surgeon at St. George's, asked the hospital governors to "consider how far a numerous class of pupils increases the reputation of an Hospital."[3] What seems a nearly rhetorical question – deserving a promptly positive response among Hunter's peers – has a serious past.

APPRENTICES AND PUPILS, CHARACTER AND CASH

At St. Thomas's and St. Bartholomew's in the late seventeenth century, staff surgeons took their apprentices onto the wards to observe their chari-

---

3 Letter from John Hunter to the Governors of St. George's Hospital, 28 Feb. 1793, quoted in George C. Peachey, *A Memoir of William and John Hunter* (Plymouth: William Brendon & Son, 1924), 281.

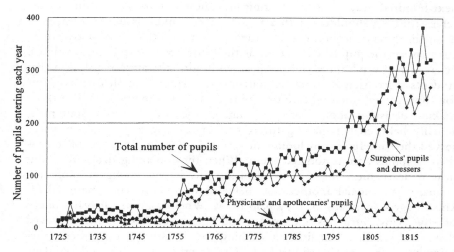

Figure 4.1. Pupils signing ward-walking registers at the London hospitals, 1725–1820 (see Table 4.2 for the names of the hospitals with registers and their dates).

table practices. On busy days, at most two or three trailed after their master, perhaps meeting one or two "young university schollers" attending rounds with the staff physicians. In 1800, 223 men signed up to see the surgeons', physicians', or apothecary's practice at St. Thomas's, Guy's, the London, the Middlesex, and St. George's, plus an unknown number at St. Bartholomew's and the Westminster, for a year (more or less) of clinical experience. Anecdotal evidence has long placed "cubs" and "schollers" in the hospitals at the start of the century, just as a few complaints about crowding in the early nineteenth century have established a textual awareness of an increase in the number of students on the wards. The figures culled from hospital and medical school records, however, reveal the magnitude of the growth that beset London's general inpatient charities. I have summarized the data from the pupil registers in Figure 4.1 (for the details on particular hospitals, see Appendix II). The appearance of a sweeping rise in the 1740s to 1760s marks the period when new hospitals opened and more pupil registers began. The story of hospital ward-walking in the metropolis over the eighteenth century rests on such basic quantitative changes in the number of those with access to charity patients and opportunity to see staff men practicing their occupations.

In the following sections I elaborate on the meaning and implications of these data. The numbers of pupils display a fundamental expansion of the models of hospital instruction available at the start of the eighteenth century, that of the "apprentice" and the "scholar." Neither disappears in the next hundred years, but men fitting into these old archetypes find themselves rubbing shoulders with a peculiar set of hybrids who increasingly define hospital education through their presence on the wards. Governors' concern for the pupils' characters, as they came to a hospital or, at times, behaved badly within it, intertwined with administrative perception that students were useful sources of staff income, labor, and rhetorical claims for "improving" medical care for the rich as well as the poor. When those making decisions about ward teaching, be they governors or staff men, actually believed that having three, ten, or seventy pupils on the wards served their interests – including an appropriate image of charitable care – then hospitals accommodated them. When those making decisions about how to learn medicine, be they aspiring physicians, young London surgeons, or provincial apothecaries, believed ward experience mattered for knowledge or reputation, they paid for it. When London's Royal College of Physicians, Surgeons' Company, and Society of Apothecaries believed that ward-walking had little or nothing to do with licensing their practitioners, a free market flourished. The emergence of hospital pupilage happened as, over and over again, governors explicitly or implicitly allowed the hospital porter to open the gates to students already waiting there.

"The apprentice shall faithfully serve his master"

By 1700, most medical practitioners learned their craft and trade by apprenticeship, formal or informal. This time-worn way for surgeons and apothecaries to gain their skills was a process for learning an occupation that was deeply embedded in early modern culture.[4] Apprenticeship, as I explained in Chapter 3, remained a staple of medical training well into the nineteenth century in Britain, however much tempered by additional coursework, charity experience, or reading. Formal apprenticeship involved a written agreement that bound the two parties in a complex moral, legal, and financial relationship. The medical apprentice, like any other articled youth, promised obedience, loyalty, secrecy, moral probity, and labor for his or her master or mistress; the practitioner–master vowed to impart knowledge, skill, moral guidance, and appropriate care for his or her charge. With the contract, a premium exchanged hands, sized according to local custom, possible family connections, and the master's prestige not only in skill but also in social influence, both of which were valuable for the apprentice's future success. Usually for five to seven years, starting at

---

4 The heading quotation comes from a 1705 apprenticeship indenture to a surgeon, quoted in Joan Lane, "The Role of Apprenticeship in Eighteenth-Century Medical Education," in *William Hunter and the Eighteenth Century Medical World,* ed. William Bynum and Roy Porter (Cambridge: Cambridge University Press, 1985), 100.

about the age of fourteen, the aspiring surgeon, apothecary, or surgeon–apothecary learned his art through experiencing whatever his master's daily practice included, from making up pills to assisting at operations. Medical masters might have several apprentices over a lifetime, sometimes with overlapping indentures, yet never took on a cluster of those at the same level. A premium was paid for individual attention, whether that meant a serious commitment to teach good practice or an opportunistic chance to get cheap help sweeping out the shop.[5]

The relationship between apprentice and master introduced teaching into hospitals well before the eighteenth century, as an apprentice to a hospital surgeon followed him as he would any master to see patients deemed suitable for the youth's level of knowledge and experience. At St. Thomas's, for instance, the surgeons took their apprentices with them onto the wards as a matter of course from at least the sixteenth century.[6] The traditions and expectations of apprenticeship define the baseline for hospital instruction in the late seventeenth century, although with an important alternate style for physicians' pupils that I discuss further later. The rules and rituals surrounding ward-walking as it emerged and changed over the eighteenth century constantly played off the elements of apprenticeship that those manipulating pupilage held on to, ignored, or modified to suit the complex claims of charity, status, demand, and "progress." In sweeping terms, the introduction of pupils into the hospitals transformed the bonds among the master, the apprentice, and the apprentice's family into a detached relationship of staff, student, and hospital administrators, while retaining the root notion that the neophyte learns practice by watching practice. While hardly a revolutionary assumption, shifting the terms of how, when, and where watching practice took place literally created the London teaching hospital.

From the first mention of hospital pupils in London, their crucial characteristic was a *short-term* cash relationship with a staff surgeon. A pupil paid for the privilege of watching a hospital surgeon, presumably to observe a

5 By far the best recent discussions of eighteenth-century medical apprenticeship are Joan Lane, "Apprenticeship," 57–104; Irvine Loudon, *Medical Care and the General Practitioner, 1750–1850* (Oxford: Clarendon Press, 1986), 39–48; and Mary Fissell, *Patients, Power, and the Poor in Eighteenth Century Bristol* (Cambridge: Cambridge University Press, 1991). In addition to the primary accounts offered by these historians, see Samuel England, Two Notebooks containing prescriptions and case notes, 1730–3, Royal College of Physicians (RCP) MS 5–6, for a glimpse of a hard-working apprentice's attempts to structure the clinical training he received under his master.

6 E. M. McInnes, *St. Thomas's Hospital* (London: George Allen & Unwin, 1963), 74–5; Frederick G. Parsons, *The History of St. Thomas's,* 3 vols. (London: Methuen & Co., 1932–6), 2: 140. As I explained in Chapter 1, the vast majority of medical apprentices and pupils were male. Certainly – except for a very few female pupils learning midwifery at the Middlesex Hospital – all of the hospital pupils were men. I thus use "he" consciously. To broaden this pronoun to "he or she" would, I believe, distort the dominant presence of men.

range of surgical conditions and operations that occurred infrequently in common practice. When and how such transitory arrangements appeared are still obscure, but by the late seventeenth century, staff men at both St. Thomas's and St. Bartholomew's had begun to take men who were not their bound apprentices onto the wards, and, it appears, to let such relative strangers assist them. Since part of the whole process of apprenticeship involved the master's giving the young practitioner responsibility for patient care when ready, apprentices had a recognized – but circumscribed – authority to practice in some situations. It was the delegation of tasks to those with unknown amounts of experience that led the governors at St. Thomas's to pronounce restrictions on the surgeons' decisions. In 1691, they ruled that any young man who helped the surgeons, by dressing wounds for instance, had to be a London apprentice – although not necessarily a staff surgeon's – bound for seven years and registered at the Barber–Surgeons' Company. They had to have served, moreover, at least two years of their apprenticeships before entering the hospital. As the governors expressed no concern for those simply watching ward practice, their status – even existence –remains ambiguous.[7]

Watching or briefly assisting a hospital surgeon on the wards challenged apprenticeship only when such experience became grounds to assert expertise *apart from* the traditional route that the Barber–Surgeons' Company controlled. Such subversive claims did not take long to surface. In 1695, the Barber–Surgeons' Company received complaints that the St. Thomas's surgeons, among others, were "breeding soe many Illiterate and unskillful pretenders to Chyrurgery."[8] The petitioners objected that

contrary to ye oath of our Company and of ye Citty of London ye Chyrurgeons pretend to qualifie any person how unfitt soever in half a year or a year for the expert practice of our art. Which injustice in them being attended with a considerable profitt is maintained by a pretence of service to the publick, Whereas in reality itt is directly contrary, and an absolute overthrow to our Company, subverting the very fundamentalls of ye Legall Education by way of apprenticeship.[9]

The St. Thomas's men immediately defended themselves by declaring that they accepted students from the country who "for bettering their Judgments in the Art came to London to see the practice of the Hospitall." They then promised, nevertheless, to take only students who could pro-

7 St. Thomas's Hospital, Minute Book of the Court of Governors, 1677–1735, 26 May 1691, Greater London Record Office (GLRO) H1/ST/A1/6; Parsons, *St. Thomas's*, 2: 124, 134. This rule was repeated in 1699. For references to pupils at St. Bartholomew's, see John L. Thornton, "The Medical College from Its Origins to the End of the Nineteenth Century," in *The Royal Hospital of Saint Bartholomew's, 1123–1973*, ed. Victor C. Medvei and John L. Thornton (London: St. Bartholomew's Hospital Medical College, 1974), 44–6.

8 Quoted from the records of the Barber–Surgeons' Company in John Flint South, *Memorials of the Craft of Surgery in England*, ed. D'Arcy Power (London: Cassell & Co., 1886), 246.

9 South, *Memorials*, 247.

duce certificates of having served an apprenticeship or "such as had served a considerable time to a Chirurgeon in the country."[10] The hospital surgeons compromised, as they clearly intended to continue to take short-term pupils, but without threatening the traditional role of apprenticeship and hence the income and importance of their nonhospital brethren.

The petitioners' accusations laid out points of suspicion that followed pupilage throughout the eighteenth century. First, apprenticeship ideally revolved around developing *character* as well as skills. The master was responsible for teaching the young person moral principles and appropriate behavior during the apprentice's time with both the master's patients and his family. But who could ensure the same for hospital pupils, perhaps barely known to the staff practitioners and only under their supervision on the wards? If "any person how unfitt soever" could learn about practice from clearly reputable men and use such experience to assert knowledge, then a bulwark of regular men's authority – a presumed probity from being "raised" in the occupation – showed some cracks.

While it is highly probable that staff surgeons shared this concern and exercised discrimination when taking pupils, the hospitals' governors took on a weak version of the master's role. Worries about "character" impelled governors to make regulations and to become active in student discipline primarily because staff men had only a part-time commitment to hospital practice. Any claim, therefore, that a limited stay on the wards could *replace* apprenticeship was in for trouble, although the Barber–Surgeons' Company could not enforce restrictions outside London. After 1745, when the new Surgeons' Company dropped apprenticeship as a prerequisite for examination, critics could no longer charge that pupilage overthrew the "very fundamentalls of ye Legall Education." For the most part, nevertheless, hospital men refrained from stating that pupilage equaled seven years with a master; they took apprentices too, after all. Ward-walking thus emerged – at least rhetorically – as a supplement to apprenticeship, as the way to better "Judgments in the Art," but not as a promise to enhance moral fiber. Pupilage then acted as mark of a better trained practitioner, one who did more than what was usually required for satisfactory expertise.

Second, the 1695 petitioners made an extremely astute observation when they wrote that pupilage "being attended with a considerable profitt is maintained by a pretence of service to the publick." Here rest two key facets of how pupilage worked in London. Just as the master got the apprenticeship premium, staff practitioners pocketed the fees they charged short-term students. With quite rare exceptions, the hospitals in London saw none of this money. Thus, unlike the arrangements in the Edinburgh

10 South, *Memorials*, 248.

Royal Infirmary, where student fees at times contributed heavily to balancing the charity's budget and led to more direct administrative involvement with hospital teaching, the London hospitals' medical staff had nearly total control over the pupils' payments throughout the century.[11] As the numbers rose, needless to say, so did the "considerable profitt" hospital men could make during their voluntary dedication to charity.[12] Precisely why the London hospitals' governors refrained from dunning pupils separately for ward access remains a puzzle, except insofar as the surgeons' privilege of having apprentices and taking their fees became the unquestioned model for ward-walking. Yet the hospitals found other rewards. Whatever rhetorical value a "pretence of service to the publick" had over the course of the century in the quest for "good" practitioners, suitably experienced pupils provided free labor for the charities. The apprentice's duty to assist his master in any task, even when elementary and tedious, shifted to certain pupils' duty to assist at the hospital, not only in carrying out practitioners' orders, but also in coping when staff were absent.

Finally, although the 1695 petitioners omitted an explicit complaint on this point, pupilage challenged one of the primary parts of "ye oath of our Company" contained in apprenticeship indentures. The hospital practitioner lost the master's customary right to his apprentice's loyalty and vow to keep his secrets. Ward-walking became, in a subtle yet significant process, public instruction, whereas apprenticeship was private. I return to this distinction and its implications at the end of the chapter but here suggest that this shift was among the most potent for reconfiguring authority within eighteenth-century medical education and, by implication, within the ways medical men made and established new knowledge. The number of pupils signing up to attend the hospitals, to recall Figure 4.1 for a moment, speaks volumes for the belief that staff men in these charities in fact offered something that apprenticeship did not. Hospital men, too, had an influence over scores of pupils' knowledge and behavior, which no

11 Guenter B. Risse, *Hospital Life in Enlightenment Scotland: Care and Teaching at the Royal Infirmary of Edinburgh* (Cambridge: Cambridge University Press, 1986), 38, 242–9.
12 For example, the Register of Surgeons' Pupils, 1775–1799, at St. Thomas's had the following grand totals figured for the period 1769 to December 1795: from St. Thomas's surgeons' and apothecary's pupils, £22,867. 15s.; from Guy's, £8,719. 4s. The £31,586. 19s. averages to about £1,140 per year or about £146 per year for each surgeon and apothecary at the two hospitals. On top of this income were fees from dressers, at £50 for one year or £31. 10s. for six months, and from apprentices. Four dressers a year could obviously bring in £200 more per surgeon. See also St. Thomas's Hospital Register's Fees [1799–1841], GLRO H1/ST/MS/G4/6, 6a, 6b. This volume was used to tally the eleven shillings each pupil (excluding physicians' pupils) paid the "register" (the apothecary, at least from 1799) on first admission and the five shillings for extending practice or readmission to both St. Thomas's and Guy's. Account of the Surgeryman's Fees on Entering Dressers and Pupils [to St. Thomas's] from April 10th 1799, GLRO H1/ST/MS/G4/7, is a similar register for the eleven shillings that each entrant paid the surgeryman.

master with a handful of apprentices could equal, no matter how qualified, respected, or kind.

Registers and regulations

Perhaps because of the concerns expressed to the Barber–Surgeons' Company in 1695, in 1703 the Court of Governors at St. Thomas's regulated the number of young men attending the hospital. They ordered that the surgeons could take only three "servants" each (not including their own apprentices) for periods of not less than one year, each of whom had to show that he had served "five years or upwards with a Surgeon or some person practicing [*sic*] in Physick and Surgery." The young man, too, had to produce a testimonial of "sober life and conversation," thus establishing his character.[13] The governors, seemingly in a suspicious mood, further required that each pupil be introduced to the Grand Committee in order to satisfy them that their requirements had been met.[14] These were decisions to be taken seriously, for, the Court continued:

And in Case any Surgeon of this hospitall shall take any other Servant or other person contrary to these Orders Except by a Special [permission] from the Committee or Treasurer he shall for every offense forfit the sum of Twenty Pounds for the use of the poor in this Hospital to be deducted from his Sallary [£40 per year] and he shall also incurr the displeasure of the Governors.[15]

Simply introducing new pupils to the Grand Committee proved to be inadequate to monitor the surgeons' and apothecary's charges. In 1723 the hospital steward (or apothecary) began the first extant pupil register, in which he wrote each student's name (excluding those of apprentices) under the surgeon or apothecary with whom he entered.[16] When the book was "laid before the Grand Committee" on 16 November 1724, the governors discovered that the three surgeons had been exceeding their quotas, as twenty-three pupils had entered between January and October instead of the nine allowed. As noted in the register itself, the governors ordered that the surgeons take no further students until the 1703 limits had been met.[17]

13 St. Thomas's, Minute Book of the Court of Governors, 1677–1735, 17 Mar. 1702/3.
14 Parsons, *St. Thomas's*, 2: 144; McInnes, *St. Thomas's*, 76.
15 St. Thomas's, Minute Book of the Court of Governors, 1677–1735, 17 Mar. 1702/3.
16 Register of Pupils and Dressers, Pupils 1723–75, Dressers 1750–96, St. Thomas's Hospital Medical School Library, H1/ST/MS/G2. In Edinburgh, the governors of the Royal Infirmary managed pupils' access to the wards, and the numbers there, by issuing a certain number of vouchers, or tickets, for three-month (1730) and annual (1756) terms. Risse, *Hospital Life*, 242.
17 Parsons, *St. Thomas's*, 2: 183–4; St. Thomas's, Register of Pupils, 1723–75, first page. It is possible that some of the pupils stayed for only six months, instead of the required year, thus allowing a surgeon to have three to four pupils at any one time. The governors'

At some point in the 1720s, although not explicitly demanded by the Grand Committee, a similar hospital register was started for St. Thomas's physicians' pupils, for whom no official limit existed.[18] Indeed, earlier references to those attending hospital physicians for instruction suggest that such pupils did so through even more private and personal relationships with the physicians than apprentices had with surgeons. In the late 1660s, for instance, complaints surfaced at St. Bartholomew's that the physicians let young "doctors" take their rounds, rather as substitutes than as students, a practice that was forbidden. Yet the governors decided to establish a library for "young university schollers" in 1669, suggesting that they welcomed physicians-in-training into the hospital in suitable circumstances.[19] Because physicians' pupils were few in number and were associated with the universities, with their aura of gentlemanly education and presumably more genteel behavior, such students apparently did not concern the governors until later in the eighteenth century.[20] At St. Thomas's in the 1720s, no hints suggest that physicians' pupils needed an introduction to the Grand Committee or testimonials of *their* characters. The clerk who wrote the names into the register until midcentury, moreover, invested all of these pupils with the title of "Dr" whether they had such a degree already or not.[21]

For physicians' pupils, then, the first hospital register appears rather as an aide-memoire than as a book for the governors to use. Certainly pupil

reprimand did not note this abuse specifically, however. In 1726, the governors raised the quotas, allowing the surgeons four pupils each and letting the apothecary, granted one pupil in 1716, and two in 1717, take three pupils of his own. Parsons, *St. Thomas's*, 2: 166–7, 184.

18 Register, Physicians' Pupils, St. Thomas's Hospital, 1729–1832, St. Thomas's Hospital Medical School Library, H1/ST/MS/G2. This register appears to have been begun earlier, as the first entries are pages cut and pasted into this volume. The dating of entries before the 1740s is thus problematic at times, although the names are in rough chronological order. The first twenty-five pupils, all apparently dated under the year 1728, likely attended in smaller groups over the previous years.

19 John L. Thornton, "Medical College," 44–5.

20 The only formal limit on the number of physicians' pupils that I have discovered occurred at St. Thomas's in 1751 when the governors established an assistant physician's post. The Grand Committee ruled that this junior physician was "at Liberty to take Pupils yearly not Exceeding Two for his own Particular Benefit." St. Thomas's, Minutes of the Grand Committee, 6 Nov. 1751, GLRO H1/ST/A1/7.

21 St. Thomas's, Physicians' Pupils, 1728–1832. Among the early students were, for example, "Dr." Kemp, "Dr." Bigsby, "Dr." William Dade, and "Dr." Weldon. Kemp was likely the Benjamin Kemp who matriculated at Cambridge in 1727, attended St. Thomas's in 1731, and took his MA in 1735. He did not take the MD, but Venn noted that Kemp "studied medicine and surgery," and practiced as a physician in Gloucester. John Venn, *Alumni Cantabrigiensis*, Part I, 4 vols. (Cambridge: At the University Press, 1922–4), 3: 5; Thomas Bigsby, similarly, entered Cambridge in 1732, received the BA in 1734, and walked at St. Thomas's in 1736. Venn identified him as a physician practicing at Halesworth, Ipswich, with no record of an MD from any university. Venn, *Alumni Cantabrigiensis*, Part I, 1: 267. Dade matriculated at Cambridge in 1744, took his BA in 1747, the MA in 1751, went to St. Thomas's in 1753, and died in 1755. According to Venn, he was

registers took on other functions over the century, as places for the staff to record fees or keep track of pupils' seniority.[22] Yet the initial impulse at St. Thomas's to monitor the surgeons' pupils is the most telling, for at all of these inpatient charities, pupils created problems. So, while the pupil registers allowed me to quantify the number of those officially entering the hospitals (as shown in Figure 4.1), they convey only part of the story. I summarize the evidence on "when" in Table 4.2 (which is also a tidy reminder of the diversity among these institutions and the pupils' categories). At the London, for instance, the clerk did not keep a register, but entered the pupils' names directly into the Weekly Board minutes. At that time each pupil had read to him a specific charge to behave properly, which the governors soon had printed up for distribution.[23] At all the other hospitals founded between 1719 and 1750, too, staff men had to reach an accommodation with the governors about taking pupils, whatever the precedents established elsewhere.

At the Westminster in 1719 and 1737, Guy's in 1727, St. George's in 1734, and the Middlesex in 1746, the governors explicitly acknowledged the staff surgeons' right to have apprentices and pupils on the wards.[24]

the son of John Dade, an MD practicing in Suffolk. Venn, *Alumni Cantabrigiensis*, Part II, 2: 45. In contrast, "Dr. Weldon," a pupil in 1734, does not appear on any of the university degree lists that I have been able to consult. He may have obtained a Continental degree, but he could also have been the Walker Weldon who was apprenticed to John Ryder, an apothecary in Brignorth, Salop, in 1730. Wallis and Wallis, *Eighteenth Century Medics*.

22 See n. 12. At St. George's surgeons' pupils became dressers according to seniority, so the registers established a chronological hierarchy available for consultation. Register of Pupils and House Officers, 1756–1837, St. George's Hospital Medical School Library.

23 London Hospital, House Committee Minutes, 1741–1815, 28 June 1743, LH/A/5, London Hospital Archives. The names of the pupils introduced to the Weekly Boards were twice extracted from the Minutes by nineteenth-century compilers. See Register of the Students at the London Hospital from its foundation, extracted from the Minute Books of the House Committee of the Hospital, London Hospital Medical College, LH/MC/S/1/3 and Register of Surgeons and Pupils of The London Hospital from the foundation in 1740 to 1846, c. 1846, LH/X/13/9. This later volume was the primary source for the analysis of the number of hospital pupils. The only contemporary list of pupils is the Surgeons' Pupils Book [1780–1830], London Hospital Medical College, LH/MC/S/1/2.

24 J. G. Humble and Peter Hansell, *The Westminster, 1716–1766* (London: Pitman Medical, 1966), 27, 66; Guy's, Minute Book of the Court of Committees, 21 July 1727, GLRO H9/GY/A3/1; H. C. Cameron, *Mr. Guy's Hospital, 1726–1948* (London, New York: Longmans, Green, 1954), 87–91, relies only on Warner's 1792 account that surgeons' pupils were in place by 1734; Laws and Regulations of St. George's Hospital extracted from the Minute Books of that Institution . . . by Joseph Gunning (1805), 129, MS, St. George's Hospital Medical School Library; Rules and Orders [of St. George's Hospital], 193, MS, St. George's Hospital Archives. See also George C. Peachey, *The History of St. George's Hospital (1733–1753)* (London: J. Bale, Sons & Danielsson, 1910), 269. Peachey claims the surgeons were limited to two apprentices each, but I did not find this regulation in the manuscript records. St. George's appears not to have allowed the apothecary to take a pupil until the 1770s: Laws and Regulations, 113; London Hospital, Court of Governors' Minutes, 22 Apr. 1741, LH/A/1; Clark-Kennedy, *The London*, 1: 47; W. J. E. Wilson, *The History of Middlesex Hospital during the First Century of its Existence, Compiled from the Hospital Records* (London: John Churchill, 1845), 246.

Table 4.2.   *Ward-walking at the London hospitals*

Hospital	Pupils known from			Registers
	Surgeons'	Physicians'	Apothecary's	
St. Thomas's	1551[a] 1691[b]	1728	1716	Surgeons'-1723 Physicians'-1729 Apothecary's-1723
St. Bartholomew's	1660s[a] 1730s?[b]	1660s?	?	No extant registers
Westminster (1719)	1719[a] 1737[b]	1770s	1738	No extant registers
Guy's (1724)	1727[c]	1770s?	1727	Pupils-1727 (not extant) Surgeons'-1768 (at St. Thomas's) Surgeons'-1778 (at Guy's) Physicians'-1784 Apothecary's-1778
St. George's (1734)	1734[c]	1730s?	1779?	Surgeons'-1756
London (1740)	1741[c]	1743	1753[a]	Surgeons'-1741 Physicians'-1743 (in Weekly Board Minutes)
Middlesex (1745)	1746[c]	1766	1765	Surgeons'-1763 Physicians'-1766

[a]Apprentices
[b]Pupils
[c]Apprentices and pupils
Sources: Guy's Hospital, Minute Book of the Court of Committees, 9 Dec. 1728, GLRO H9/GY/A3/1 and 11 Nov. 1768, GLRO H9/GY/A3/3; London Hospital, House Committee Minutes, 1741-1815, LH/A/5, London Hospital Archives; Register of Surgeons and Pupils of the London Hospital from its foundation in 1740 to 1846, compiled c. 1816, London Hospital Archives; Surgeons' Pupils Book [1780-1830], London Hospital Medical College, LH/MC/S/ 1/2; Entry of Physicians, Surgeons Pupils and Dressers, vol. 1, 1778-1813; vol. 2, 1814-27, Guy's Hospital Medical School, Registrar's Office; Register, Apothecary Pupils, 1753-9, Pupils [Surgeons' and Apothecary's], 1760-8, Pupils St. Thomas's and Guy's 1768-1801 [Surgeons' and Apothecary's pupils], St. Thomas's Hospital Medical School Library, H1/ST/MS/G4/2; Boards of Governors Minutes; Register of Pupils and House Officers, 1756-1837, St. George's Hospital Medical School Library; Parsons, *St. Thomas's*; Wilson, *The Middlesex*; Medvei and Thornton, *Saint Bartholomew's*.

Only at Guy's did the clerk record a formal application from Cross and Cooper, the surgeons, and Mr. Callaghan, the apothecary, who "prayed leave to entertain pupils in order to instruct them in their respective Arts." The Court, all but one of whom were also governors of St. Thomas's, decided

that the said surgeons be permitted leave to have and entertain three pupils each and the Apothecary two pupils they not taking more with such pupils than twenty guineas for each pupil and that no person be entertained as a pupil by the said surgeons or Apothecary but such as have first served five years to a regular surgeon or to an Apothecary practicing Surgery and produce a certificate of good behavior during that time.[25]

The Guy's men clearly adopted St. Thomas's rules outright, although the express limit on the price the staff could charge and the requirement of a surgical background for the apothecary's pupils were unusually explicit decrees compared with those of the other general hospitals. By 1737, Guy's, St. Thomas's, the Westminster, and St. George's all allowed the surgeons four pupils each, although the most junior surgeon at St. George's could take only two.[26] At the London and the Middlesex, established in the 1740s, however, the governors placed no official limit on the number of hospital pupils.[27]

That the two newer hospitals broke with the pattern previously accepted across the metropolis suggests that pupilage was beginning to move further away from the model offered by apprenticeship, where masters were expected to instruct only a few young men simultaneously. Yet throughout the 1740s and 1750s the number of ward-walking students remained relatively small, generally in accordance with the regulations imposed by the

---

25 Guy's, Court of Committees, 21 July 1727; There were twelve members of the Court of Committees present for this decision, including Charles Joy who was then treasurer of both Guy's and St. Thomas's.

26 Guy's, Court of Committees, 9 Dec. 1728; St. Thomas's, Court of Governors, 26 May 1726; Humble and Hansell, *The Westminster*, 66; St. George's, Laws and Regulations, 129, for 6 Feb. 1734; St. George's also required that pupils attend for at least a year.

27 In 1751, the London's governors decided that the newly established assistant surgeon was "not in our present situation to be allowed the benefit of Pupils or Dressers in this Hospital," although pupils could attend him on his rounds "with the same Respect & Obedience as upon the ordinary Surgeons." The London, Court of Governors Minutes, 6 Feb. 1750/1. In 1753, the London's governors decided that the senior surgeon "be allowed two dressing and two walking Pupils before the other Surgeons be allowed to take any. [But after that condition] there was to be no limitation or prescription of numbers whatever." Quoted in Clark-Kennedy, *The London*, 1: 99. The number of pupils entering in the early years at both the London and the Middlesex was generally less than three or even four per surgeon; this number suggests a relative lack of demand for hospital experience at these institutions. During the first ten years of the London (1741–50), for example, only twenty-nine students were listed in the House Committee minutes, scarcely three a year; at the Middlesex in its first decade (1745–55), only fourteen pupils and apprentices are named in the Weekly Board minutes. Wilson, *The Middlesex*, 246–7.

governors.[28] From at least 1727, nevertheless, the St. Thomas's surgeons began to ignore the rule that pupils enter for at least a year, taking some students for less than twelve months while only having four each at any one time.[29] During the 1750s at St. George's and after 1768 at St. Thomas's and Guy's, the surgeons clearly began exceeding their quotas as well as taking pupils for less than a year, although no formal permission to dispense with the limits appears in their governors' minutes.[30] The decades between 1750 and 1770 thus saw the major shift away from the control that the governors exercised in the first half of the century. After 1770, the number of ward-walking students primarily corresponds to open demand, not to institutional fiats, except for apothecaries' pupils and surgeons' dressers, both of whom had more direct responsibility for patient care than walking pupils did.

The early regulations on the number of hospital pupils channeled entrants through the governors' weekly boards, the committees which oversaw the routine work of the charities. There the aspiring students had their testimonials examined, were instructed in the hospitals' rules, and were usually warned that misbehavior would lead to dismissal.[31] At the London, the first pupils were simply charged "to be constant in . . . attendance, Tender and careful to the patients."[32] In 1758, St. Thomas's Grand Committee ordered that pupils must leave the wards by 1:00 p.m.[33] In 1761, the Middlesex governors proclaimed pointedly:

28 At Guy's, where the early pupil registers have vanished, it appears that the surgeons likely kept well within their limits of four pupils each, or twelve per year. The Court of Committees reviewed the Steward's salary and benefits in 1763, noted that he received about £3. 10s. a year from the combined 10s. fee for entering pupils and writing their certificates, "about 7 or 8 in a year." Guy's, Court of Committees, 16 Nov. 1763.

29 St. Thomas's, Register of Pupils, 1723–75. In 1741–2, the registrar began to note the name of the pupil that a new student replaced, likely to keep closer tabs on the surgeons' and apothecary's students. This information shows that, for example, the surgeon Paul had eight students enter under him between 15 Apr. 1741 and 17 June 1743. Of these, one served for two months, one for four months, one for nine months, three for a year, one for fourteen months, and one for twenty months.

30 Parsons, *St. Thomas's*, 2: 184; Warner to Gunning, 1792, in Cameron, *Guy's*, 91; St. George's, Register of Pupils.

31 At Guy's in 1768, the governors also required that a pupil entering either Guy's or St. Thomas's obtain a ticket on admission "which will be his Introduction to both Hospitals & shall be given up on signing his certificate and no person shall be admitted without such a Ticket." Guy's, Court of Committees, 11 Nov. 1768.

32 Clark-Kennedy, *The London*, 1: 47; London, House Committee Minutes, 28 June 1743. Pupils attending the London had to be introduced by the surgeon or, in some cases, by another governor, who attested to their qualifications. See, for example, 6 Nov. 1744, where the chapalin, Rev. Audley, recommended Jeffrey Lang as a dressing pupil; 18 Dec. 1744, where a governor, Mr. Henry Woodfall, introduced John Sherwood, "late apprentice to Mr. Robert Turner of Wakefield in Yorkshire, to be registered as a dressing pupil for one year."

33 Parsons, *St. Thomas's*, 2: 215.

Whereas several inconveniences attended the not having any rules for the conduct and behavior of the last house pupil, and also the apprentices and pupils attending the hospital, the following [were decided upon]: [1] That no apprentice or pupil is to enter the women's wards but at the time of dressing the patients, nor to enter the apothecary's shop or the laboratory on any account whatsoever. [2] That no apprentice or pupil is to stay in the hospital after the business of the day is finished. [3] That during the time they are in the hospital, there be no swearing or noise made, or any kind of indecency committed, nor the medicines, &c., of the hospital wasted or embezzeled, and that every offender in these particulars be reported to the weekly board by the house pupil, and be liable to be suspended, or even expelled from the hospital, at their discretion.[34]

After these rules were read to him, each pupil was given a copy and instructed to "enter his own name at the same time in the Book of Orders & Regulations for Apprentices & Pupils as a Witness of his Knowing the said Rules & his obligation to observe them."[35]

The hospitals' governors contined to pass measures to manage ward pupils throughout the century.[36] Their rules conjure up images of unruly, swearing, noisy students disrupting equally ill-mannered patients and nurses on the wards.[37] Popular caricatures of medical students in the early nineteenth century have only reinforced the judgment that the hospital pupil "was not [a] gentleman."[38] And certainly the charities' governors discovered disorder, rudeness, carelessness, and rebellion among those walking the wards over these decades.[39] Mr. Braithwaite, the apothecary's

---

34 Middlesex Hospital, Minutes of the Weekly Board, Court of Governors, 20 Jan. 1761; also quoted in Wilson, *Middlesex*, 249–50.

35 Middlesex Hospital, Minutes of the Weekly Board, Court of Governors, 20 Jan. 1761. This instruction implies that a volume of pupils' signatures existed before the surviving register of 1763 began. In the early years at the London, as well, the Weekly Board regularly called upon the surgeons to attest to a pupil's regular appearance on the wards whenever students asked for certificates to document their attendance at the hospital. London, House Committee Minutes, 27 Feb. 1744/5, 5 June 1745; notices of certificates granted appear throughout the minutes. Middlesex, Minutes of the Weekly Board, Court of Governors, 28 Apr. 1778; Guy's, Court of Committees, 9 Dec. 1728; McInnes, *St. Thomas's*, 79.

36 See, for later disciplinary rules, Warner to Gunning (1793) in Cameron, *Guy's*, 91; St. George's Hospital, Board of Governors' Minutes, 14 June 1793. See also Peachey, *Memoir*, 299, where identical wording exists in the surgeons' report to the committee investigating education at St. George's. In 1815, the governors at St. Bartholomew's similarly repeated or articulated the common injunction that house surgeons and dressers had to be formally introduced to the house committee. Moore, *St. Bartholomew's*, 2: 381.

37 In 1691, for example, the St. Thomas's governors reiterated a rule forbidding swearing by patients and all hospital servants. St. Thomas's, Minute Book of the Court of Governors, 26 May 1691.

38 Morris, *The London*, 170; Clark-Kennedy, *The London*, 1: 104; Charles Newman, *The Evolution of Medical Education in the Nineteenth Century* (London: Oxford University Press, 1957), 41–6.

39 Clark-Kennedy, *The London*, 1: 103–5; Morris, *The London*, 171–2.

apprentice, was expelled from St. Thomas's in 1718 when bodies from St. Saviour's Churchyard were found in his room. At Guy's, the Court of Committees refused to allow John Potter, an apprentice to the surgeon Andrew Cooper, back into the hospital after they decided that "he has been guilty of great insolence and indecency and behaved himself very disorderly with respect to the Patients and also to the Steward one of the sisters and the Keepers of the Lunatic House."[40] Mr. Hill, one of the governors on an inspection visit to the Middlesex in July 1755, discovered the dresser John Hart "behaving himself in a very improper manner on the Bed with one of the Patients in the Women's Sick Ward." A full investigation ensued and Hart explained that he had been removing a splinter from the woman's finger. He was reprimanded, nevertheless, for not accounting for his actions to Mr. Hill.[41] In 1795, the Westminster's governors elliptically observed "that on account of some disagreeable Circumstances which have lately happened, the Surgeons' Pupils can not be permitted to be in the Hospital, except when the Principal Surgeons are in the House."[42]

As well as enforcing discipline, the governors occasionally intervened with the organization of ward-walking. In 1734, the Weekly Board at St. George's ruled that all apprentices and pupils in the hospital entered under the command and care of *all* of the staff surgeons. A similar regulation appeared at the London in 1763, while an agreement between Guy's and St. Thomas's in 1768 also required that the surgeons and apothecaries of both hospitals share in the instruction of all surgeons' and apothecaries' pupils and split the pooled fees equally. At all of the hospitals where the shift from personal to public, or shared, pupilage was made explicit, the arrangement had the approval of most of the voluntary staff.[43] In effect, by the 1760s (and earlier in some hospitals), the surgeons' students could follow any surgeon on his rounds, whether they had signed up with him or not. At the London, at least, this development emerged explicitly because pupils thought "themselves subject only to the orders of the particular Surgeon with whom they are entered" and so were more difficult to discipline.[44] In breaking down this remnant of apprenticeship, the governors' decisions effectively created "hospital" students, shifting personal loyalty away from a single staff man

40 McInnes, *St. Thomas's,* 78; Guy's, Court of Committees, 2 Mar. 1732. Potter was readmitted to the hospital after petitioning and, presumably, apologizing, on 19 May 1732.
41 Middlesex, Minutes of the Weekly Board, Court of Governors, 29 July, 5 Aug. 1755; see also 26 Mar., 2 Apr. 1811.
42 Proceedings of the Trustees of the Westminster Hospital, 9 Sept. 1795; see also 28 May 1788.
43 St. George's, Rules and Orders, 192. This regulation was reiterated in the review of rules passed by a Special General Court: Minutes of the Board of Governors, 14 June 1793; Morris, *The London,* 171; Guy's, Court of Committees, 16 Nov. 1763; Cameron, *Guy's,* 89; Parsons, *St. Thomas's,* 2: 223–4.
44 Quoted in Clark-Kennedy, *The London,* 1: 102; Morris, *The London,* 171; London, Minutes of the House Committee, 14 Mar. 1758.

and to the institution.[45] Pedagogically, moving the students' relationship from a "master" to the institution distributed the teaching loads of individual surgeons and allowed pupils to see various surgical techniques; both actions undermined the traditions of craft instruction.

John Hunter, surgeon to St. George's, experienced the results of the institutions' taking over the entitlements of the master in a bitter dispute that he had with his colleagues in 1792–3.[46] The flurry of accusations and counteraccusations about the quality of teaching at St. George's began over ward pupils and their fees. As Hunter told his fellow staff surgeons in July of 1792, he had decided "not to account in future with the surgeons of the hospital for the money I receive [from pupils], but consider it wholly my own." He had done most of the ward rounds, with the most pupils, for years, Hunter claimed, and would no longer let the other surgeons benefit from his fame, especially as he needed to pay much less attention to his hospital work. Hunter's attempt to embarrass his peers about what he viewed as a remarkable sign of their lack of character did not work. The Board of Governors, which at St. George's included all of the hospital practitioners, considered their charity's teaching at various meetings over the next year. In April of 1793, the governors created a committee of nonstaff medical and lay men to examine the "Laws relative to the Surgeons's Pupils, to consider the best methods of improving their Education."[47] Ironically, the "Laws" finally passed (14 June 1793) not only kept

45 See Warner to Gunning, 29 Dec. 1792: "The pupils [at Guy's and St. Thomas's] are considered as belonging to the hospitals, not to one particular Surgeon." Quoted in Cameron, *Guy's*, 92. "[St. George's] Surgeons' Reply to Hunter's Address," 1793, printed in Peachey, *Memoir*, 284.

46 George C. Peachey wrote the now-classic account of Hunter's dispute with the other St. George's surgeons in his *A Memoir of William and John Hunter* (1924), 204–22; he printed copies of the manuscript correspondence and reports in his appendix IV, 272–303. All biographies of John Hunter included a discussion of this argument, as it has been repeatedly stated that it led to Hunter's fatal heart attack on 16 Oct. 1793. Peachey suggested (216–8) that the hospital surgeons, particularly John Gunning, designed regulations that would force Hunter to resign, as one demanded that all the full surgeons attend the wards regularly. Hunter had cut back on this task, letting his assistant surgeon, Everard Home, do it. The already angry Hunter (from this perspective) tried to get the new entry rules waived for a few pupils at the October Weekly Board meeting, became enraged, and died (218–9). That Hunter was angry was undoubtedly true, but the events surrounding the whole dispute have been heavily skewed toward showing Hunter as a near-martyr for hospital education, when he seems to have fulminated about regulations that he had implicitly supported and that were customary practices across the metropolis.

47 St. George's Hospital, Board of Governors' Minutes, 17 Apr. 1793; present at the Weekly Board meeting of 17 Apr. 1793, when the committee was formed, were Rev. James Clarke, Chaplain and Chairman; Mr. Aisley, Esq., Treasurer; Drs. Baillie, Ford, and Robertson, hospital physicians; John Gunning, Mr. Keate, and John Hunter, hospital surgeons, with Everard Home, assistant surgeon to John Hunter; D. Gibb, nonstaff surgeon; Mr. Yateman, nonstaff apothecary; and C. Warren, Richard Little, and S. Payne, unidentified governors. Peachey, in his otherwise thorough account, did not mention that John Hunter was in fact present at the meeting creating the committee. The committee itself consisted of three former hospital physicians and six nonstaff governors.

the division of pupils' fees among all the surgeons, but also laid out, for the first time in much detail for St. George's, the regulations covering access to the wards. Several of these closely resembled the rules in place at other London hospitals, including the necessity for pupils to present certificates "of having been bred up to the Profession, and of their good Behavior," to the surgeons and to the Weekly Board of Governors.[48] Hunter's threatening strategy of claiming autonomy by keeping *his* pupils' fees thus resulted in the governors' strengthening the institutional organization of pupilage at the hospital.

Despite undoubted incidences of staff disputes, body-snatching, unauthorized dissection, "indecencies," and insolence, however, confrontations with pupils rarely appear in the governors' minutes. More important than some students' misbehavior was the perception that pupils might disturb the delicate balances of propriety and authority which the governors tried to impose upon the patients and hospital servants. The administrators thus developed rules that would remind the pupils that the governors had the ultimate control over hospital discipline, even though the pupils' fees passed directly to the medical and surgical staff men. As the hospitals' physicians, surgeons, and apothecaries were not officially held accountable for their students' behavior in any of the regulations passed during the century, the governors took on and retained the moral and physical authority that the master had over the apprentice.[49] However free the medical officers were to profit from teaching and to shape the clinical instruction in the hospitals, by the 1760s (if not obvious before) they clearly did *not* have the power to construct distinct institutions in which pupils would answer only to them within the charities' walls.

Servants to charity: the pupils' hierarchy

For the vast majority of pupils during the eighteenth century, their primary duty was to behave well. Obedient, respectful, and, perhaps, "tender," they could walk unobtrusively between the humble orders in the beds and the more exalted – or at least more prosperous, if not necessarily more refined – in the boardrooms. Yet from the inception of pupilage, letting young men into the wards to observe the sick carried with it the potential to use their labor for patient care. Just as apprentices served their masters as

48 Board of Governors Minutes, 14 June 1793. The Board's minutes give the resolutions as passed, usually worded identically to the surgeons' report to the "education" committee submitted on 27 May 1793, which Peachey printed in his *Memoir*, 297–303.
49 Only one reference has as yet been discovered to a staff man's being responsible for his pupils' actions. In 1716, when St. Thomas's governors allowed the apothecary one pupil, they noted that he "is to be Answerable for his Miscarriages [?] or Imbezillments [*sic*]." St. Thomas's, Court of Governors, 1 Mar. 1715/16. It is likely that the medical staff informally disciplined students if they found them disrupting the wards, as suggested by the 1795 Westminster rule limiting pupils' hours to times when the surgeons were in the hospital.

shop assistants and aides during treatment and operations, so could hospital pupils and dressers perform some of the mundane chores beneath the staff men's interests and above the nurses' capabilities. Over the decades, the hospitals' governors thus found their pupils a necessary evil: a possible threat to order, yet a supply of increasingly indispensable free work. For the most part, ward-walking pupils, even with testimonials of previous education and good character, were too transient to be trusted with regular duties. On rare occasions, however, hints indicate that they were expected to contribute to the smooth running of the hospitals. At the Middlesex, the Weekly Board ruled in 1749 that surgeons' apprentices "or other Assistant[s]" were not to leave the hospital until the physicians had finished taking in patients.[50] The governors at the London demanded in 1744 "that the Physicians Pupils do as usual enter the Names of the several Petitioners [to become outpatients] in the Book kept for that purpose, That the House Steward may soley attend the Business of the Committee."[51]

Dressing pupils, in contrast, paid for the privilege to change bandages, attend to wounds, perform minor operations, and generally assist a surgeon in his work, next to the surgeon's apprentices.[52] From at least 1750, to be a dresser at St. Thomas's, for example, cost £50 for a year's instruction. Such fees, unlike those of the walking pupils, were not divided among all the surgeons.[53] At Guy's and St. Thomas's in 1768, the governors ruled that the surgeons could take only four dressers (including apprentices) at any one time, for a minimum of six months, probably in order to limit the number of students who could handle the patients.[54] Dresserships were so popular at Guy's and St. Thomas's that in 1783 both hospitals required that "one or more of the four [dressers] be an apprentice or apprentices," apparently trying to shore up the traditional source of surgical assistants in the face of more profitable short-term students.[55] The

50 Middlesex, Minutes of the Weekly Board, Court of Governors, 31 Oct. 1749, 28 Jan. 1766. On 24 Oct. 1749, a stronger motion had passed (modified on 31 Oct.) that demanded all "the Pupils and Apprentices to the Surgeons" not leave the hospital "without leave from the Physicians and Surgeons"; see St. George's, Laws and Regulations, 130, for a 1739 rule requiring pupils to leave the wards after rounds unless the House Pupil gave them tasks to do.

51 London Hospital, House Committee Minutes, 26 June 1744.

52 See the description of a dresser's privileges given by an anonymous student in a late-eighteenth-century letter, quoted in Parsons, *St. Thomas's*, 2: 249–50.

53 Parsons, *St. Thomas's*, 2: 188, 204. Pupils, in contrast, paid only twenty-four guineas (£25. 2s.) for twelve months on the wards in 1768. Cameron, *Guy's*, 92.

54 Parsons, *St. Thomas's*, 2: 243–4; Cameron, *Guy's*, 92; Guy's, Court of Committees, 11 Nov. 1768. Although most of the dresser's fees went directly to the surgeon, the 1768 agreement specified that the surgeon was to pay the apothecary six guineas for each dresser he entered. In 1730, the governors at Guy's had denied the surgeons' request that "they might have liberty to Lett one Pupil each dress the patients in this house in Common Cases." It is likely, however, that they soon acquired this privilege, as it existed at St. Thomas's. Guy's, Court of Committees, 4 Aug. 1730.

55 Guy's, Court of Committees, 21 Oct. 1783. In June, 1783, St. Thomas's Court of Governors passed a similar rule, requiring that each surgeon could have only two dressers

surgeons at St. George's established a quite different system, deciding in 1734 that pupils (and apprentices in the hospital) would be allowed to dress patients after serving for at least three months.[56] At the London, the House Committee in 1758 had to reiterate that only those who had "received [the Chairman's] Charge" to do so could dress patients. They were "ordered to wear the dress of their office" on the wards between 11:00 a.m. and 2:00 p.m. to distinguish them from other pupils, marking both their relative status and their duties.[57]

Students who chose such hands-on experience provided the hospitals with valuable services, since many of their tasks were routine accompaniments to surgical conditions. Not surprisingly, some hospitals' governors added to the dressers' regular duties under their surgeons, using them to attend in the wards outside the surgeons' rounds. Complaints from patients at the Middlesex in 1767 suggest that dressers were to take turns waiting for any emergency cases, which they did not always treat satisfactorily. In one incident, the Weekly Board called in Mr. Falkner, a dresser, for failing to show up for his Sunday duty. He claimed that he had delegated this chore to another pupil, Jesse Foote.[58] At Guy's and St. Thomas's, "one of the dressers is in waiting for a week by rotation, to take the care of accidents."[59] The London also used a "pupil of the week" (likely a dresser) to take care of emergencies.[60] In 1767, the House Committee decided that this pupil should be instructed on how to write up descriptions of incoming accidents, so that notices could be sent to the *Public Advertiser* on the London's philanthropic efforts.[61]

without taking an apprentice. Parsons, *St. Thomas's*, 2: 243. If a surgeon had four dressers a year he could pocket £200; over seven years, this would amount to £1,400, with no costs for food, lodging or clothes. Even the highest apprenticeship fees for London hospital surgeons in the late eighteenth century rarely exceeded £800. Lane, "Apprenticeship," 69–72; in 1800, for example, Benjamin Travers was apprenticed to Astley Cooper for £630. Royal College of Surgeons (RCS), Examination Book, 1800–20, 7 Aug. 1800.

56 St. George's, Laws and Regulations, 129. In 1781, this rule was modified to specify that only pupils who signed up for at least a year would be allowed to dress patients after three months' experience in the hospital (p. 85). The Middlesex Hospital likely imitated St. George's, as dressers are only distinguished from surgeons' pupils in the register in 1811. St. Bartholomew's had dressers from at least the 1760s, but the surgeons also used patients as salaried "box-carriers" throughout the century. Moore, *St. Bartholomew's*, 2: 368, 381.

57 London, House Committee, 14 Feb. 1758; the "dress" was not specified.

58 Middlesex, Minutes of the Weekly Board, Court of Governors, 9 June 1767.

59 Warner to Gunning, 29 Dec. 1792, quoted in Cameron, *Guy's*, 91. No reference to this practice has been discovered in the governors' minutes, however, so it perhaps was an arrangement agreed upon between the dressers and the hospitals' surgeons. For an account of the dressers' numerous duties at St. Thomas's in 1813–14, see Charles Lett Feltoe, comp., *Memorials of John Flint South* (London: John Murray, 1884), 24–6.

60 London, Minutes of the House Committee, 14 Feb. 1758; Clark-Kennedy, *The London*, 1: 104.

61 London, Minutes of the House Committee, 13 June 1769; the Board of Governors discussed sending reports of accidents to the *Public Advertiser* in 1756, resolving that the admitting surgeon should write these notices. Mr. Woodfall, a governor and, quite usefully, editor of the paper, promised that they would be published. London, Minutes of the Board of Governors, 24 Mar. 1756, 17 June 1757.

While St. Thomas's and Guy's relied entirely upon dressers to give immediate care to accident victims and messengers to summon the charities' practitioners in emergencies, the staff and governors at the London and the three West End hospitals, the Westminster, St. George's, and the Middlesex, created yet another category of student assistants.[62] These men clearly existed to free the voluntary surgeons from overlong duties on the wards and too-frequent calls for skilled medical advice. In February 1736, soon after the hospital opened, the governors of St. George's hospital decided to admit Thomas Clare as a "House Pupil." He was to live in the hospital, to follow the surgeons' directions in their absence, and to take care of emergencies.[63] In 1737, William Cheselden, then surgeon and governor to the hospital, suggested that "any Pupil offering to reside in this House shall be Examined by all the Principall Surgeons for the future," and the Board agreed.[64] The Quarterly General Court of St. George's resolved in 1741 that the house pupil could stay for a maximum of eighteen months, thus clearly establishing the position as a training post and not as an extended junior office.[65] The Westminster, in 1738, and the Middlesex, in 1757, followed St. George's example, creating house pupils' posts with nearly identical requirements.[66] From the 1740s, the London also appointed an annual house pupil from those who had served as dressers, although his qualifications and duties were not discussed.[67]

62 The existence of house surgeons at St. Bartholomew's is more problematic. In 1813, nevertheless, the governors ruled that "house surgeons" from then on needed the recommendation of the surgeons and the approval of the house committee. When this post began is unknown. Moore, *St. Bartholomew's*, 2: 381.

63 St. George's, Laws and Regulations, 129.

64 St. George's, Rules and Orders, 197. It should be noted that "Principal Surgeon" was an honorary office; the other surgeons actually attended the sick and only they were allowed to have pupils. The designation of "Principal Surgeon" lapsed by 1750. See Peachey, *St. George's*, 271, 278.

65 St. George's, Laws and Regulations, 131.

66 Humble and Hansell, *The Westminster*, 66. The Westminster likely followed St. George's example in this innovation, since William Cheselden also served the Westminster as a governor and consulting surgeon from 1733 to 1739. By 1811, the post of assistant house surgeon existed at the Westminster. This pupil, who was to succeed the full house surgeon, both received extra training and shared the duties of residing in the hospital. See Westminster Hospital, Proceedings of the Trustees of the Westminster Hospital, 4 Mar. 1812, GLRO H2/WH/A1/24. Wilson, *The Middlesex*, 247–49; Middlesex, Minutes of the Weekly Board, Court of Governors, 21 June, 4 Aug. 1757. Henry Watson, surgeon and governor to the Middlesex in 1757, attended these meetings and may have been the instigator of this post. In the report to the Weekly Board, St. George's model was mentioned explicitly. The Middlesex governors required the House Pupil to have served a five-year apprenticeship and to be "examined and approved as qualified for the Trust, by the Surgeons of this House."

67 Students called "House Pupils" simply appeared in the minutes and their role within the charity is unclear (see, for example, London, Minutes of the House Committee, 5 June 1745, 5 May 1778). A few years later, the surgeons requested that "one of their Pupils . . . be always resident at the Infirmary" (26 Jan. 1747/8). References and regulations about these pupils, especially their duties compared with those of the "weekly pupils," seem not to exist until 1827, when the Board of Governors agreed to have a senior pupil reside in

By the 1770s, the "House Pupil" had been recast as the "House Surgeon," suggesting both the scope of his duties, in contrast with those of the resident apothecary and his pupils, and a titular increase in status from the days when, at least at St. George's, the house pupil was classed as an "upper servant."[68] Throughout the century, most of the house surgeons were selected from the surgeons' pupils and dressers, with an occasional apprentice. Some of these young men served as pupils for as little as three months before immediately becoming house surgeons; others waited several years between walking the wards and taking on the responsibility for dozens of hospital patients.[69] Unlike dressers and pupils, the house surgeon did not give any of the staff a fee for training him. Instead, the governors expected that he pay only for his board, which ranged from ten to fifteen guineas per year at midcentury, while they provided lodging and coals within the hospital.[70] Thus the house surgeon was neither a pupil nor a full-fledged member of staff, but a newly skilled practitioner willing to immerse himself in hospital duties without pay in order to gain additional experience and, at least in a few cases, perhaps an inside edge during the competitions for election to hospital posts.[71]

As a hospital resident, the house surgeon soon had numerous duties heaped upon him. The house surgeons, like the apothecary, could not leave the hospital without permission and faced the governors' disciplinary action if he were negligent.[72] He was to attend to all emergencies and

the hospital for three-month periods. He was, when the surgeons were absent, to "take the superintendance [*sic*] of the House Pupils and be their guide & instructor in their employment and opportunities for improvement." London, Minutes of the Board of Governors, 30 May 1827.

68 St. George's, Laws and Regulations, 130.

69 At the Middlesex, for example, of the forty-six House Surgeons listed from 1763 to 1815, forty appear in the pupil registers, one of whom, G. Neville Wyatt, was given as apprenticed to John Wyatt, Middlesex surgeon from 1765 to 1797. Jesse Foote entered the Middlesex in March 1766 as a surgeons' pupil; in June he became the house pupil. In contrast, Holland Fowke started as a pupil in May of 1768 and is listed as house surgeon in 1772. The procedure for choosing house surgeons is still obscure, but it likely involved a combination of recognized ability, seniority among the candidates, and the patronage of a staff surgeon.

70 In 1736, Thomas Clare paid £12 for his board at St. George's; in 1781, the cost had risen to £25 per year, and in 1821 it was £50. At the Westminster in 1776, the house surgeon paid £15. 14s. a year, while the Middlesex governors demanded fifteen guineas in 1757. Receiving about seven to ten pence per day from the house surgeon hardly gave the charities much cash profit from these "pupils." St. George's, Laws and Regulations, 86, 92, 130; Westminster, Proceedings of the Trustees, 3 July 1776; Middlesex, Minutes of the Weekly Board, Court of Governors, 4 Aug. 1757.

71 In the seven elections for surgeons at the Middlesex between 1763 and 1815, four positions were won by former pupils, John Chafy (1763), John Wyatt (1765), Henry Witham (1778), and John Joberns (1801), two of whom (Chafy and Joberns) had also been house surgeons; of the other three, one success went to Daniel Minors, son of the staff surgeon Isaac Minors. The others were Richard Cartwright (1806) and Charles Bell (1814).

72 In 1788, for example, Mr. Bellett, the house surgeon at the Westminster, was dismissed for being "frequently irregular," but most especially for "an instance of secreting the Body

provide needed care for the surgical patients whenever the surgeons were absent. While banned from performing major operations, he was responsible for deciding when to summon the staff surgeons. When the physicians and surgeons appeared in the wards, he was to follow their directions precisely. At the Middlesex and St. George's, the house surgeon shouldered the burden of overseeing the pupils for the governors and directing the dressers' tasks after ward rounds. Finally, he also served as a general note-taker and medical messenger. In rules laid down at the Middlesex in 1761, for instance, the governors instructed the house pupil to "carry pen, ink, and paper, to minute down all messages to the physicians, or instructions relating to the patients."[73] From hospital servant, the house surgeon became a linchpin in hospital management and teaching by the end of the eighteenth century at the West End hospitals. That he acted (at least in the regulations) as a barely acknowledged assistant in clinical instruction, moreover, highlights the use that both staff and administrators could make of men willing to pay for such experience and indicates the evolution of an ad hoc hierarchy among pupils on the wards.

Hospital surgeons, with the threat of accident victims appearing at their charities at any hour, had good reasons to support the "weekly pupils" or house surgeons delegated to deal with crises. But other resident pupils roamed the wards off and on during the 1700s, answering to the hospitals' apothecaries and physicians. The governors' policies on boarding apothecaries' pupils varied widely, both between institutions and over the century, often giving rise to controversy. As the apothecary was required to live at the hospital, if he took an apprentice or resident pupil, clearly the student needed to stay there too. Apothecaries allowed to take short-term students, moreover, appear to have pressed to be able to offer them board, again placing them within the institutions day and night. Some governors dealt with the issue simply: at the London, except for a special dispensation in 1753–4, the apothecary had no pupils or apprentices, although in 1775 he acquired a paid assistant elected by the governors.[74] At St. Thomas's and Guy's, the governors granted their apothecaries both apprentices and yearly pupils early in the century, and these medical men managed to have

of a Poor Man who died in the house last week." Westminster, Proceedings of the Trustees, 28 May 1788. At the Middlesex in 1812, the Weekly Board repeatedly discussed the plan to have the house surgeon and the apothecary's pupil sign in and out of the hospital for any absences, specifying who allowed them to do so. Middlesex, Minutes of the Weekly Board, Court of Governors, 10 Mar. 1812.

73 Middlesex, Minutes of the Weekly Board, Court of Governors, 20 Jan. 1761, also quoted in Wilson, *The Middlesex*, 248. For other duties, see 22 Jan. 1765, 29 Oct. 1771; Middlesex, Minutes of the Medical Committee, 1773–78 [1783], 31 Jan. 1778; St. George's, Laws and Regulations, 86, 130.

74 London, Minutes of the House Committee, 31 Dec. 1753; Minutes of the Board of Governors, 20 June 1753, 25 Sept. 1754, 1 June 1775; Morris, *The London*, 53; Clark-Kennedy, *The London*, 1: 101.

at least some of their pupils board privately with them.[75] When the Guy's Court of Committees agreed in 1806 with the cryptic advice of Benjamin Harrison, the treasurer, that "it would be for the advantage of the Hospital" for the apothecary, Mr. Stead, no longer to have boarding pupils or apprentices, they increased his wages to compensate.[76] He continued to take ward-walking students, however, and to share in the combined surgeons' fees. In general, St. Bartholomew's, the Middlesex, the Westminster, and St. George's all let the apothecary take pupils and apprentices, although they limited him to one or two each year and demanded a charge to cover hospital board, as for house surgeons.[77]

By the 1780s at St. George's and the Westminster, the apothecary's boarding pupil officially had duties similar to his surgical counterpart's. Required to remain in the hospital, to serve on the wards when the apothecary was absent, and to note down orders on the physicians' rounds, he became another fixture in the charities' routines.[78] To prevent possible conflicts with the surgeons, the Board at St. George's decided that the student could attend surgical operations, but forbade him to "act in the chirurgical department at all."[79] The apothecary's pupil became a pawn in some minor skirmishes for medical authority within the hospitals, for, like the salaried apothecary, he needed to bow to the physicians' control over

---

75 The St. Thomas's apothecary had both "regular" ward-walking pupils, as the surgeons did, and more private ones, apparently equivalent in status to the surgeons' dressers, several of whom may have boarded with him. This separate group of apothecary's pupils was explicitly noted in a new register, begun in 1796. It is labeled "Dressers" (St. Thomas's Hospital Medical School Library), and each dresser was entered with a specific surgeon, with an equivalent section for certain apothecary's pupils.

76 Guy's, Court of Committees, 30 Apr. 1806, 4 Mar. 1807; in 1807, the governors raised Stead's wages from £50 to £100 per year, plus £100 per year for the loss in pupils' fees.

77 Middlesex, Minutes of the Weekly Board, Court of Governors, 12 Feb. 1765, 25 July 1769, 5 Aug. 1773, 5 May 1814. In 1773, the Weekly Board decided that the house surgeon should pay fifteen guineas a year for board, the apothecary's apprentice twenty, and the apothecary's pupil twenty-five. These charges may well reflect either the charity's cost for each, or a measure of profit for the apothecary's charges; Wilson, *The Middlesex*, 251–3 lists the names of all the apothecary's annual pupils and apprentices in 1767–1819; St. George's, Laws and Regulations, 113–16, suggests that the apothecary was granted a pupil in 1779; in 1799 the governors decided to try a three-year apprentice to the hospital, with the student paying 200 guineas to the charity, 100 guineas to the apothecary, and 100 guineas for board. This experiment ended in 1802; Humble and Hansel, *The Westminster*, 66; Westminster, Proceedings of the Trustees, 22 Jan. 1783, 15 Feb. 1792, 23 Nov. 1803, 5 Nov., 12 Oct. 1806.

78 St. George's, Laws and Regulations, 113; Westminster, Proceedings of the Trustees, 22 Jan. 1783. For a description of the tasks a boarding apothecary's pupil had to take on at St. Thomas's, see John M. T. Ford, ed., *A Medical Student at St. Thomas's Hospital, 1801–1802: The Weekes Family Letters* (*Medical History*, Supplement No. 7, 1987).

79 St. George's, Laws and Regulations, 113–14, from minutes of 31 May 1779, 25 Jan. 1782. The 1779 reference contains the first mention of the apothecary's pupil, in which the apothecary was instructed to take the recommendation of the surgeons, if they gave him three months' notice. This rule, whether enforced or not, shows the surgeons' dominance in teaching in the hospital.

treatment for the strictly medical patients. At St. George's, for example, the physicians in 1797, Matthew Baillie, George Pearson, and William Heberden, Jr., demanded the right to approve the apothecary's pupil before he was admitted to the house. A series of disputes ensued between the physicians and the apothecary, Mr. Kelly, ending with Kelly's dismissal in 1802 and the decision in 1803 that the "office of Pupil to the Apothecary was unnecessary."[80]

The physicians at the Westminster in 1792, George Hicks, George Paulet Morris, and the newly elected William Blackburne, took a different course.[81] They suggested, and their fellow governors agreed, that the apothecary not be allowed to have a boarding pupil, and that his assistant be forbidden to attend lectures. Essentially eliminating the apothecary's teaching presence on the wards, they decided instead that a physicians' pupil could live in the hospital, paying £35 for his keep. While he would be under the apothecary's direction when the physicians were absent, they specifically ruled that "his duty [is] to take cases and keep a Register in which they may be faithfully recorded."[82] The Westminster's physicians may have looked to the Middlesex for their initial inspiration, since a physicians' pupil, Dr. Ciceri, had been allowed to board in the hospital in 1789.[83] However revolutionary the Westminster physicians hoped to be, their innovation closely follows the precedents set for surgeons' and apothecaries' house pupils. More important, at least in the short term, it suggests the tensions between hospital practitioners over the appropriate status for the medical house pupil. Certainly the Westminster's apothecary did not

---

80 St. George's, Board of Governors Minutes, 25 Oct. 1797, 13 Feb., 6 Nov., 9 Dec., 23 Dec. 1801, 15 Jan. 1802, 15 Apr. 1803. After cancelling the post of apothecary's pupil or apprentice, St. George's began to elect assistant apothecaries, like those at the London.

81 William Blackburne joined the staff in June 1791 with a 1781 MD from Edinburgh. In 1802, he was on the committee of the Associated Faculty, which demonstrates his more radical leanings. He left the staff of the Westminster in 1794. Dr. George Paulet Morris joined the staff in 1788, with a bachelor's degree in Physic from Cambridge, and did not get his MD until 1793. He was thirty-three in 1792 and may have had a youthful interest in supporting clinical training for other young physicians. The last, George Hicks, had been on staff from 1775, with an Edinburgh MD from 1768. He died, likely in his forties or early fifties, in 1792. As a group, then, the physicians were fairly young – not hampered by an elderly Fellow of the Royal College of Physicians who might object to or stand aloof from changes in hospital teaching. William Munk, *The Roll of the Royal College of Physicians of London*, 2nd ed., 4 vols. (London: Royal College of Physicians, 1878), 2: 287, 363–4, 437; Clark, *Royal College of Physicians*, 2: 631.

82 Westminster, Proceedings of the Trustees, 15 Feb. 1792. Unfortunately, as the boarding medical pupil did not have to introduce himself to the Weekly Board, as the surgeons' pupils did, it is impossible to know how many – and who – took advantage of the Westminster's position.

83 Middlesex, Minutes of the Weekly Board, Court of Governors, 19 Sept. 1789. Dr. Ciceri paid the Weekly Board £10 for his board and lodging for three months. Although he was introduced as a physicians' pupil, his name does not appear in the register. No further references to boarding physicians' pupils were discovered; hence this incident may well have been an isolated courtesy to a foreign visitor.

rest content with the physicians' monopoly. By 1803, he had gained the full support of the governors again to take on resident apprentices, who would be able to attend both the physicians' and surgeons' practices.[84] In 1806 they reinstated the apothecary's privilege to take a boarding pupil, noting that this step had been recommended by the physicians and surgeons.[85] Two out of the three physicians (Blackburne and Hicks) who originally suggested the abolition of this pupilage were gone; that, and the support of the surgeons, and probable pressure from the apothecary himself, led to a renewal of past practice. The position of boarding physicians' pupil was never formally abolished but vanishes in the minutes' silence. Tainted, perhaps, with the aura of being a hospital "servant" and creating an awkward division of authority between the physicians and apothecary outside ward rounds, the post embodied a shift too radical for applicants ambitious to declare themselves "physicians."

The vagaries of resident physicians' and apothecaries' pupils compared with the easy entrenchment of house surgeons or rotating dressers at all the London hospitals by the close of the eighteenth century captures the governors' ambivalence toward blending the need to care for patients as cheaply as possible with the use of the hospital as a twenty-four-hour training ground for medical practitioners. Surgeons had a strong case for requiring a resident pupil with enough experience to handle accidents; the governors generally agreed – most notably at the hospitals where staff surgeons sat on the boards. Apothecaries and physicians, however, had a less evident claim, since the apothecary already lived in the hospital specifically to be on hand for emergencies among the physicians' patients. Whatever labor their pupils could offer often seemed suited to the supervised hours of the physicians' and apothecary's rounds. Casting pupils as servants to charity thus in part accounts for the differing opportunities for resident clinical practice available to surgeons', apothecaries', and physicians' students throughout the century. House pupils were not there to learn (although they did), but to labor.

ON THE WARDS: INCREASING NUMBERS,
BLURRY BOUNDARIES

As I emphasized at the outset of this chapter, when a student went to the one of the London hospitals he signed up to follow a practitioner according to the traditional divisions among medical occupations. The vast majority (75–80 percent from the 1760s) chose to follow the surgeons on their

84 Westminster, Proceedings of the Trustees, 23 Nov. 1803.
85 Westminster, Proceedings of the Trustees, 5 Nov. 1806. The fee set was forty guineas "to the charity" presumably for a year's boarding; on 12 Oct. 1808 this was reduced to twenty guineas. The house surgeon in 1803 had paid only £21 for his annual board (21 Oct. 1803).

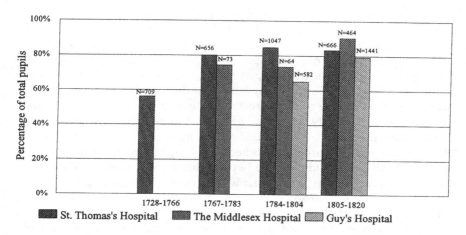

Figure 4.2. Surgeons' pupils at St. Thomas's, the Middlesex, and Guy's hospitals, 1728–1820, as percentages of the total number of pupils in the hospital's registers each period (N = number of surgeons' pupils).

rounds (Figure 4.2). After the 1750s and 1760s, when the hospitals abandoned limits on the number of surgeons' pupils, their numbers reflect a free market demand. Similarly, the number of physicians' pupils also seems to have been as extensive as the demand for such experience, while the number of apothecaries' pupils remained constrained by the different charities' various regulations. Probing the conditions of this "free" market suggests some of the social and occupational influences on London pupilage. A few factors are so global that gauging their effects requires great caution. The growth in the number of hospital pupils, for instance, correlates roughly with the estimated population increase in England and Wales during the 1770s and 1780s. Pupilage took off at a greater rate than population expansion only from the mid-1790s (see Appendix II). Clearly mere population growth does not account for the increase in ward-walking for the entire period – even with the grossly simplistic assumption that all other circumstances remained static. In contrast, some of the "free" market elements are so obviously local and contingent that they demand attention to the particular nuances that influenced personal decisions, such as location, cost, family traditions, or religious concerns, not to mention staff reputations and access to lectures.

Taken together, such details go a long way to make sense of ward-walking in London. But they do not quite suffice to explain Figure 4.1. The broader impulse underlying the growth in the number of surgeons' pupils, and the relative stasis among physicians' and apothecaries' pupils, rests on the dynamic interchanges between the accessibility of hospital teaching and the fundamental belief that it *mattered* for eighteenth-century practice. Spending some time on hospital wards, following men engaged in "pure" surgery or "pure" physic, and observing treatment open to public scrutiny clearly offered pupils something that they could not, did not, or would not get through apprenticeship, university study, or clinical experience elsewhere. For most, at least according to the numbers, hospitals promised an intense exposure to surgical conditions and operations not only seen less frequently in private practice, but also diagnosed and performed with the most current methods. As more and more practitioners labeled themselves as surgeon–apothecaries, hospital work enhanced their claims to have surgical knowledge beyond that learned during the routine rounds of apprenticeship. As historians have repeatedly noted, presumably the relative economic prosperity of the middling sorts during the eighteenth century (and their willingness to accept hospitals as a source of "good" knowledge) increased the consumer demand for care by regular men with this training.[86] Paying for "educated" treatment figures as a mechanism for change in this argument, by the way, whether or not eighteenth-century patients (or historians) could establish that London-learned therapy worked, much less that the sick made rational choices.[87]

Consumer demand does help to explain Figure 4.1 at a level somewhere between the overwhelmingly global and the numbingly local. Yet "demand," that amorphous catch-all of modern market life, still requires much more detailed investigation before its causal aura is shown working in particular circumstances. I have found two questions about the demand for practitioners to be particularly suggestive in exploring the broad patterns of hospital ward-walking in eighteenth-century London. As these center on what went on in the hospitals and among hospital pupils, however, they illuminate responses to outside conditions, not yet full stories of consumer hopes and expectations. First, along with the pocketbook-based choices of middle-ranking patients, state interests also influenced the patterns of medical training. As I explained in Chapter 3, it was partly the military demand for practitioners that kept the Surgeons' Company busy

86 This point has been convincingly argued by several historians: see, among others, Ivan Waddington, "General Practitioners and Consultants in Early Nineteenth Century England: The Sociology of an Intra-Professional Conflict," in *Health Care and Popular Medicine in Nineteenth Century England,* ed. John Woodward and David Richards (New York: Holmes and Meier, 1977), 169. Roy Porter, *English Society in the Eighteenth Century* (Harmondsworth: Penguin, 1982), 91–100; Loudon, *Medical Care and the General Practitioner, 1750–1850* (Oxford: Clarendon, 1987).
87 The appeal to "educated" knowledge, whether "better" or not, has particularly been used and discussed in the history of midwifery. How and why men started practicing midwifery – and the associated issue of why women chose them over female midwives – center on such claims for knowledge and expertise. See Jean Donnison, *Midwives and Medical Men: A History of Inter-Professional Rivalry and Women's Rights* (New York: Schocken Books, 1977); Judith Leavitt, *Brought to Bed: Childbearing in America, 1750–1950* (New York: Oxford University Press, 1986).

examining applicants for certification in surgical expertise, and military pressure that led the Royal College of Surgeons to make its expectations on appropriate education more explicit and public. Did Britain's state of peace or war drive men away from or toward the hospitals? Second, where do physicians' and apothecary's pupils fit into the hospital marketplace, when so much contemporary attention praised London as a place for surgical training? Here the adherence to the tripartite divisions for ward-walking has obscured changes that began in the late eighteenth century to accommodate pupils seeking, as Richard Kay put it in 1743, to practice as "both Surgeon and Physician."[88]

Surgeons' pupils: the call of war?

The connections among military needs, the requirements of commercial empire, and the number of surgeons' pupils at the London hospitals illustrate some implicit points about the relationships of ward-walking, status, and skills. Not surprisingly, at the most prestigious level of military service for medical men, such as Surgeon General or Physician General, hospital practitioners enjoyed the authority and perquisites of government patronage.[89] But the military definitely needed medical practitioners for far more prosaic duties, and wanted neither to pay them very much nor to require more entry criteria than absolutely necessary. For most entry positions, as mate or assistant of various types, the hopeful practitioner only had to pass a cursory examination at the Surgeons' Company. The armed services may have hoped that regimental and military hospital surgeons had a company diploma, but neither the army nor the navy required one.[90] While the forces took on a modest number of practitioners in peacetime, it was war, of course, that spurred demand. Army medical commissions, for instance, clearly track the major mid- to late-eighteenth-century British conflicts: the

---

88 Richard Kay, *The Diary of Richard Kay, 1751–61, of Baldingstone, near Bury: A Lancaster Doctor*, ed. W. Brockbank and F. Kenworthy (Manchester: The Chetham Society, Manchester University Press, 1968), 80; see also p. 61.

89 John Hunter (St. George's) and Thomas Keate (St. George's) were two of the better known hospital surgeons who served as Surgeon General; for Keate's career, see *Commissioned Officers in the Medical Services of the British Army, 1660–1960*, comp. Alfred Peterkin and William Johnson, 2 vols. (London: Wellcome Historical Medical Library, 1968), 1: 51. Among the physicians, Sir Lucas Pepys, physician to the Middlesex from 1769 to 1775, later became Physician General to the army, although rather quickly replaced as he knew very little about the medical problems that concerned the military; Munk, *Roll*, 2: 305–6.

90 For detailed accounts of military medicine and its practitioners, see Sir Neil Cantlie, *A History of the Army Medical Department*, 2 vols. (Edinburgh: Churchill Livingstone, 1974), vol. 1; Christopher Lloyd and Jack L. S. Coulter, *Medicine and the Navy, 1200–1900*, Vol. III, *1714–1815*, 4 vols. (Edinburgh and London: E. & S. Livingstone, 1961); Lloyd G. Stevenson, "A Note on the Relation of Military Service to Licensing in the History of British Surgery," *Bulletin of the History of Medicine* 27 (1953): 420–7; W. N. Boog-Watson, "Four Monopolies and the Surgeons of London and Edinburgh," *Journal of the History of Medicine* 25 (1970): 313–14.

Seven Years' War (1756–63), the War of American Independence (1775–83) and, most important, the wars with France (1793–1815).[91] Yet hospital enrollments do not correlate very neatly with these obvious sources of demand. While the numbers of pupils increased during each war (albeit modestly for the War of American Independence), they also rose before these conflicts and, more significantly, did not drop afterward, when the number of available military posts plummeted. Indeed, among all those commissioned as army practitioners between 1750 and 1820, at most 10 percent appeared to have previously signed one of the hospitals' pupil registers. Doubling or even tripling this empirical result (to cover naval surgeons and the unknown pupils at St. Bartholomew's and the Westminster), to estimate that 20 or 30 percent of hospital pupils joined the armed services, still means that most hospital students had prospects for a more advantageous start in life, except when adventure, patriotism, or ineptitude made military service appealing.

The previously apprenticed (or experienced) surgeons' pupil able to pay to observe hospital practice (and to attend lectures, I must add) sought ward-walking as a voluntary capstone to his training. In individual cases, hospital pupils, house surgeons, and hospital surgeons' apprentices did seek the challenge of rough war surgery, particularly during the disease-ridden and bloody conflict with France that plagued Britain off and on for twenty-two years.[92] Thomas Watkins's life offers a relatively typical vignette of those passing quickly through the wards. He signed up to follow the surgeons for three months at the Middlesex Hospital on 1 January 1795, probably breaking off his 1792 apprenticeship to William Hanson, a drug-

91 See Appendix II for data drawn from Peterkin and Johnson, *Commissioned Officers*. For the navy services, see Lloyd and Coulter, *Medicine and the Navy*, 3: 19–21, 104, 114. No navy lists remain for medical appointments before 1809. Lloyd and Coulter note totals for 1793, 1806 and 1814, but provide little information on the rate of entry. For the beginning of the Seven Years' War, however, they record that in 1755, seven surgeons entered naval service, while in 1756 sixty-eight did so. This rise corresponds to the increase in army medical entrants during the same years from eight to forty-four. See also Alan Valentine, *Lord North*, 2 vols. (Norman: University of Oklahoma Press, 1967), 1: 123, 173–4, 212–14.

92 At most five (23 percent) of the twenty-two house surgeons at the Middlesex went on to try military practice, while ten (40 percent) of the twenty-five house surgeons at St. George's between 1793 and 1814 did so. Examples of hospital surgeons' apprentices include Titus Berry, apprenticed to Forster at Guy's in 1795, who became an army staff surgeon in 1806; Thomas Howden, William Cooper's apprentice at Guy's in 1786, who also entered the army as a staff surgeon in 1793; while Charles Edward Clarke, apprenticed to Howard at the Middlesex at the age of fifteen in 1785, entered as an assistant surgeon in 1801. Joseph Cooke, for example, was apprenticed to Howard in 1799, served as house surgeon to the Middlesex in 1802, and enlisted as a hospital mate in 1803. Similarly, William White, apprenticed to Lucas at Guy's in 1808, became a hospital assistant in 1813. Register of Surgeons' Pupils, Middlesex Hospital; Entry Book of Physicians' and Surgeons' Pupils and Dressers, Guy's Hospital, vol. 1 (1778–1813) and vol. 2 (1814–1827), Guy's Hospital Medical School, Secretary's Office; Peterkin and Johnson, *Commissioned Officers*, 1: 75, 152, 171, 246. A later physician who was known to have done military service specifically for surgical experience, was Dr. John R. Farre. He was a surgical

gist in Hereford.[93] He enlisted immediately after his brief spell at ward-walking, becoming a regimental mate on 24 April 1795, a hospital mate on 2 August 1796, and an assistant surgeon in 1799. Watkins retired with full pay in 1816, and perhaps began to practice, but died in 1822.[94] Watkins's climb through the ranks exemplifies the manner in which military experience provided the training ground for presumably adequate medical service. While complaints and criticisms about the poor quality of care available in the army and navy were regular refrains throughout the century, the government did little to change the initial requirements, pay, or status of military practitioners. The system managed to work well enough for eighteenth-century military organizations, for whom medical concerns were perpetual, yet often peripheral, problems in their own complex tangles of patronage, power, and politics.

While those who sought hospital training hardly flocked to military service, however, hints remain that the army preferred such recruits. In 1805 the government decided to subsidize some hospital ward-walking – the opportunity, that is, to learn "operative surgery at the Westminster Hospital" for men who promised to take on army practice.[95] The Westminster surgeon, William Lynn, obtained a commission as an army staff surgeon on 21 November 1805, and probably organized the work there.[96] A similar arrangement began at St. George's in April 1806.[97] Thomas Keate and John Gunning, Jr., and the assistant surgeon (to the elder Keate) Robert Keate held high-ranking positions as army surgeons.[98] Such plans

student at St. Thomas's and Guy's in 1792, became a member of the Company of Surgeons in 1793, and then joined up. He does not appear in Peterkin and Johnson, *Commissioned Officers*, however, so he either served below commissioned rank or was in the navy. He left before the wars ended, studying in Edinburgh for two years and taking an Aberdeen MD in 1806. Munk, *Roll*, 3: 33–4.

93 Wallis and Wallis, *Eighteenth Century Medics*, list only one Thomas Watkins for the late eighteenth century. He is given as apprenticed to Hanson for five years at £50.
94 Register of Surgeons' Pupils, Middlesex Hospital, 1 Jan. 1795; Peterkin and Johnson, *Commissioned Officers*, 1: 127. Among other examples, see Henry Randolph Scott, who spent twelve months at the Middlesex in 1806–7. He appears as an assistant surgeon in the army in June 1809. Register of Surgeons' Pupils, Middlesex Hospital, 21 Oct. 1809; Peterkin and Johnson, *Commissioned Officers*, 1: 198. Another example might be the case of John Armstrong, a twelve-month surgeons' pupil in 1802 at the Middlesex. A John Armstrong appears much later in the army list (1: 220) as a hospital mate (general services) in 1811 and became an assistant surgeon in 1813.
95 Cantlie, *Army Medical Department*, 1: 201.
96 Peterkin and Johnson, *Commissioned Officers*, 1: 167. William Lynn was also placed in charge of teaching pupils at the York hospital and a military infirmary in Chelsea until he retired on half pay in September 1814.
97 One of the "cadets," Charles Cook, appears in the list of army medical officers explicitly as a "Medical Cadet prior to being commissioned," an identification that confirms the existence of a government plan at the hospital. St. George's Hospital, Register.
98 Thomas Keate was Surgeon General and a member of the Army Medical Board, which theoretically supervised all of the army's medical affairs. John Gunning, Jr., became an army surgeon in 1793 and held various ranks until 1815, although he was not in service between 1805 and 1808. Robert Keate had also entered the army before joining St.

thus apparently began and worked through the appropriate connections between hospital surgeons and army interests. Since no mention of these arrangements appeared in either hospitals' governors' minutes or newspaper announcements during the usual rush of advertisements for ward-walking and lectures, "cadets" (as they were called at St. George's) could also have been the beneficiaries of patronage, not "public" admission. Whatever the means of access, from the perspective of hospital teaching and military demand, the brief appearance of "cadets" on the wards is significant for the army's implicit endorsement of hospital pupilage in London's voluntary charities. Somehow ward-walking worked to prepare a practitioner effectively, and perhaps efficiently, for the responsibilities of patient care.

In sum, army "demand" – the one quantifiable indicator of a market for practitioners – influenced hospital registration quite modestly. Students may well have tried ward-walking intending to enter military service and then changed their minds, but I strongly suspect that the gap between the large number of medical recruits and the small number of them who signed up for ward-walking in London reveals civilian ambitions and subtle disparities in financial, if not social, status. Pupils sought ward experience not to train for battlefield surgery, but to prepare for the exigencies of rural and urban practice, where injuries called for decisions about where, when, and how to use the surgeon's skills. Yet not *all* pupils followed the surgeons on rounds. Neither the tidy categories of a tripartite profession, nor the reasonable explanation just offered for the high proportion of surgeons' pupils, quite accounts for the range of hospital experience seen in the metropolis or the complexities of students' choices.

Physicians' pupils, apothecaries' pupils – and dual practice

Between 1728 and 1820, at least 20 percent of the ward-walking pupils in London followed the physicians and apothecaries on their rounds. They came to learn the practice of physic, the way that medical men diagnosed "internal" conditions and dealt with them through diet, bathing, and the materia medica. While knowledge of the theoretical principles of physic ostensibly distinguished scholarly physicians from trading apothecaries, much of their basic routines of practice overlapped at the bedside. It was this sense of the empirical connections between the two branches that underlay Richard Kay's remark that he would practice as "both Surgeon and Physician," after training under his father and being an *apothecary's* pupil at Guy's.

George's as assistant in 1800 and was on full military pay from 1803 to 1810. Cantlie, *Army Medical Department*, 1: 177, 182, 184, 188; Peterkin and Johnson, *Commissioned Officers*, 1: 51, 74, 92.

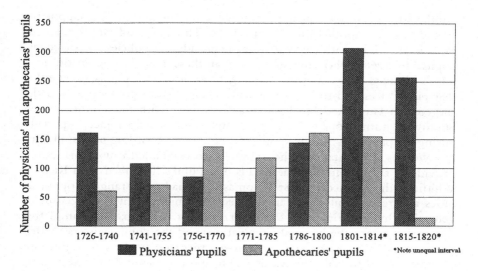

Figure 4.3. Physicians' and apothecaries' pupils, 1728–1820, who signed the registers at St. Thomas's, the Middlesex, and Guy's.

Because the London hospitals have been frequently cast as places for surgeons' pupils, I emphasize that ward instruction in physic coexisted with training in surgery for the entire century, and that – despite the criticisms of medical training rampant during discussions of medical reform and the Apothecaries' Act – students *did* have access to clinical experience in physic.[99] Whether they chose to take it is a rather different question, the answer to which is complicated by the fewer extant registers for physicians' and apothecaries' pupils than for surgeons' students. The proportion of physicians' to apothecaries' pupils actually registered, moreover, varied considerably between the 1720s and the 1810s (Figure 4.3), for a complex range of reasons, including changes in pupils' preferences and basic accessibility. Limits on the apothecary's privilege to have pupils at the London, the Westminster, St. George's, and the Middlesex quite obviously circumscribed these staff men's ability to offer bedside training for specifically "apothecary's pupils," while they may well have taught some surgeons' pupils a bit of physic anyway.

Only at St. Thomas's and Guy's, in fact, did the hospital apothecaries have groups of paying students following them on rounds in large enough

99 See Cameron, *Guy's*, 168–9, for a typical account of the classic view that opportunities for seeing physicians' practice barely existed in London until after the Apothecaries' Act forced physicians to do this. Susan C. Lawrence, "Private Enterprise and Public Interests: Medical Education and the Apothecaries' Act, 1780–1825," in *British Medicine in an Age of Reform*, ed. Roger French and Andrew Wear (London: Routledge, 1991), 51, 58–62.

numbers to break with the appearances of apprenticeship. The supportive attitude toward apothecaries' pupils at St. Thomas's and Guy's emerged early in the eighteenth century, right alongside the policies for surgeons' pupils. In 1768, when the governors at these neighboring institutions jointly decided to open ward-walking to each other's pupils, they ruled that pupils' fees had to be split equally between the apothecaries and the surgeons at Guy's and St. Thomas's.[100] Serving with the apothecaries in Southwark turned out to be a moderately popular experience, especially during the periods when the apothecary could take boarding pupils. Hampton Weekes, for instance, whose 1801–3 correspondence with his family provides a rare glimpse of the details of a pupil's life, lived with Richard Whitfield, the apothecary at St. Thomas's. He had a rich range of opportunities and responsibilities as an apothecary's pupil, yet it is dangerous to generalize his experience to the other London charities. My cumulative impression, from the hospitals' regulations and the pupil registers, is that few aspiring apothecaries or surgeon–apothecaries in the late eighteenth century wished to walk the wards where apothecaries still figured as regimented "servants," just when the rank and file's concern for status and respect grumbled at the traditional hierarchy embodied in London's tripartite system.

Throughout the second half of the eighteenth century (and probably before), moreover, aspiring surgeons and surgeon–apothecaries had no need to follow an apothecary if they wished to see physic practiced at the bedside. They could well have trailed after the physicians, in the company of university students and men with MD degrees.[101] As the number of physicians' pupils seems quite small compared to that of surgeons' pupils, of course, the ways that demand for clinical observations in physic meshed with what physicians were willing to supply remains quite ambiguous. For aspiring physicians, too, the universities had their own neighboring institutions for clinical education in the later part of the century. Edinburgh, with the Royal Infirmary and, from midcentury, its well-known clinical lectures given by physicians, had obvious advantages.[102] Addenbrooke's Hospital finally opened in Cambridge in 1766 and the Radcliffe Infirmary followed in Oxford in 1770. Both soon provided medical students at the English universities with some practical experience, although

100 Guy's, Court of Committees, 11 Nov. 1768; St. Thomas's, Grand Committee Minutes, 14 Dec. 1768. See also Parsons, *St. Thomas's*, 2: 224; Cameron, *Guy's*, 89; McInnes, *St. Thomas's*, 80–1.
101 James Johnston Abraham, *Lettsom, His Life, Times, Friends and Descendants* (London: W. Heinemann, 1933), 44–5.
102 Christopher Lawrence, "Early Edinburgh Medicine: Theory and Practice," in *The Early Years of the Edinburgh Medical School*, ed. R. G. W. Anderson and A. D. C. Simpson (Edinburgh: Royal Scottish Museum, 1976), 86–90. The two professors were John Rutherford (1726–66) and Robert Whyte (1747–66). Later, William Cullen (1773–90) joined the university and attracted dozens of pupils. See also David Hamilton, *The*

Oxbridge men certainly continued to visit other schools and hospitals.[103] Dispensaries and other hospitals, as well, took physicians' pupils, yet unfortunately have left few references to who, much less to how many, tried their clinical rounds.[104]

A brief analysis of the physicians' pupils at St. Thomas's illustrates that the *label* of "physicians' pupil" covered a multitude of practitioners (Table 4.3).[105] When counted according to possible university affiliation, particu-

Healers: A History of Medicine in Scotland (Edinburgh: Canongate, 1981), 111, 118–9, 123–4, 134–5; L. R. C. Agnew, "Scottish Medical Education" in *The History of Medical Education*, ed. C. D. O'Malley (Berkeley: University of California Press, 1970), 258–9; Risse, *Hospital Life*, 240–78. Rosner, *Medical Education*, 53–74, 97–116, 146–66, 195–206.

103 A. H. T. Robb-Smith, "Medical Education at Oxford and Cambridge Prior to 1850," in *The Evolution of Medical Education in Britain*, ed. F. N. L. Poynter (London: Pitman Medical, 1966), 44–5; F. N. L. Poynter, "Medical Education in England since 1600," in *History of Medical Education*, ed. C. D. O'Malley, 239.

104 Soon after St. Luke's, a lunatic asylum, opened in 1751, for example, its physician, Dr. William Battie, pressed for the admission of "young Physicians" to observe his care of the insane. Quoted in Charles Newman, "The Hospital as a Teaching Center," in *The Evolution of the Hospital in Britain*, ed. F. N. L. Poynter (London: Pitman, 1964), 196. For dispensaries, see Anthony Highmore, *Pietas Londinensis: The History, Design and Present State of the Various Public Dispensaries in and Near London* (London: Cradock & Joy, 1814); William Hartson, "Medical Dispensaries in Eighteenth-Century London," *Proceedings of the Royal Society of Medicine* 56 (1963): 756. There is little evidence for or against medical teaching at the dispensaries in the period before 1780. The decision to have one or two pupils to observe or assist with the outpatient work would likely have been left to the discretion and personal inclination of the attending physicians. The Westminster Dispensary did specifically allow the surgeon, Edward Ford, to have a pupil in 1776, and it has been assumed that other pupils attended as well. Sir Zachary Cope, "The Influence of Free Dispensaries upon Medical Education in Britain," *Medical History* 13 (1969): 29–30; Irvine Loudon, "The Origins and Growth of the Dispensary Movement in England," *Bulletin of the History of Medicine* 55 (1981): 341, n. 45; S. Lawrence, "Private Enterprise and Public Interests," 58–63.

105 These figures are tentative and conservative estimates, based on the identification of St. Thomas's pupils in published lists. Several, such as "Dr. Watson" and "Dr. Williams" and "Dr. John Smith," ended up under "unknown" because there were too many possibilities for any judgment to be made. Others, who had a location of origin listed in the register, were categorized by supporting evidence of their origins or practice. "Dr. Disne" from Pontefract, a pupil in 1733, for example, appears with a 1734 Cambridge MB as Gervaise Disney, who practiced in Pontefract. "Dr. Brewster" of Bath, at St. Thomas's in 1735, is likely the Thomas Brewster who matriculated at Oxford in 1724, received the DM in 1738, and was noted practicing in Bath. Finally, other identifications followed on fairly unusual names that appeared to be chronologically consistent. Theodoric Bland, for example, attended St. Thomas's in 1761 and appears on the list of Edinburgh graduates in 1763. "Bela. Lincoln," who registered as a pupil on 28 Jan. 1765, was listed as receiving an Aberdeen degree in the same year with the testimonials of Drs. Aikenside and Russel [*sic*], both physicians to St. Thomas's. John Venn, *Alumni Cantabrigiensis*, Part I, 4 vols. (Cambridge: Cambridge University Press, 1922–4) and Part II, 6 vols. (Cambridge: Cambridge University Press, 1926–54); Joseph Foster, *Alumni Oxoniensis*, 4 vols. (London and Oxford: Parker & Co., 1888); Robert W. Innes-Smith, *English Speaking Students of Medicine in the University of Leyden* (Edinburgh: Oliver and Boyd, 1932); Peter John Anderson, *Fasti Academiae Marischallanae Aberdonensis*, vol. 2 (Aberdeen: New Spalding Club, 1898); *List of the Graduates in Medicine in the University of Edinburgh, from 1705 to 1866* (Edinburgh: Neill & Co., 1867); Wallis and Wallis, *Eighteenth Century Medics*.

Table 4.3.   *University affiliations of St. Thomas's physicians' pupils, 1728-1815*

	1728-1755	1756-1815	Total
Oxford			
MD, MB, licence to practice	41	11	52
BA, MA, matriculated	14	4	18
Cambridge			
MD, MB, licence to practice	48	5	53
BA, MA, matriculated	17	4	
Leiden			
MD	26	15	41
matriculated	12	0	12
Edinburgh			
MD	13	41	54
Aberdeen, Glasgow, St. Andrews			
MD	11	5	16
Continental/Dublin			
MD	9	--	--
Unknown			
MD	2	--	--
University men (total)	193 (72%)	85 (61%)	278 (68%)
No degree/unknown	76 (28%)	54 (39%)	130 (32%)
Total (all physicians' pupils)	269	139	408

larly the number who obtained an MD (including the MB and license to practice from Oxford or Cambridge), clearly a good proportion became – or already were – physicians when they attended the hospital. That nearly two-thirds of the university men came from, or soon went to, Oxford and Cambridge in the first part of the century, moreover, highlights an interest in clinical experience not often associated with such learned practitioners in either contemporary or historical commentary.[106] After midcentury, however, only a few Oxbridge men chose to obtain clinical training at the metropolitan hospitals. George Gilbert Currey, for example, was a physicians' pupil at St. Thomas's in 1800; he was elected assistant physician at the hospital in 1802 and obtained his Oxford MD in 1804.[107] After 1760, the profile of the physicians' pupils shifts toward a more diverse, yet much smaller, group. In these later years, most of the aspiring MDs walking the wards either had, or would soon get, their degrees from Edinburgh, and went to London to enhance their contact with hospital clinicians. For instance, when Benjamin Rush was studying in Edinburgh in 1768, he revealingly commented that he intended to go south to the hospitals "as my reputation may be influenced by it."[108]

In contrast, "Dr." J. B. DeMainaudue, a physicians' pupil in 1778, is almost certainly the John Bonniot Demainaudue listed (with an MD) as a surgeon in the 1783 *Medical Register*. "Dr." John Lynch, following the physicians at St. Thomas's in 1785, had likely been apprenticed as a surgeon–apothecary in Reading in 1781.[109] Similarly, John Joberns signed up with the physicians at the Middlesex in 1783, signed with the surgeons in 1787, and joined the staff as a surgeon in 1801. These individuals, among others, suggest not only how the formal boundaries between physic and surgery blurred for students from the 1780s – already obvious in how surgeon–apothecaries practiced – but also that clinical experience with hospital physicians began to have a more obvious place in general medical training.[110] In 1788, the physicians at St. Thomas's instituted a special practice that actually institutionalized the option for dual clinical work for a few decades. In that year, Drs. George Fordyce, Gilbert Blane and Adair Crawford

106 Charles Webster, "The Medical Faculty and the Physic Garden," 683–723.
107 Munk, *Roll*, 3: 26; Register of St. Thomas's Physicians Pupils.
108 Letter of Benjamin Rush to John Morgan 27 July 1768 in *Letters of Benjamin Rush*, ed. L. H. Butterfield, American Philosophical Society, *Memoir*, 30 pt. 1, 1955, 61. See also Sylas Neville, *The Diary of Silas Neville, 1767–1788*, ed. Basil Cozens-Hardy (London: Oxford University Press, 1950), 247–8, 254, 257. Neville went to London in 1776–7, at William Cullen's recommendation after his Edinburgh MD. Physicians' Pupil Register, St. Thomas's, 1777. His good friend, Thomas Blackburne, who studied with Neville in Edinburgh, appears in the register in 1776, perhaps another influence on Neville's choice.
109 Wallis and Wallis, *Eighteenth Century Medics*.
110 William Hamilton, The first of a series of clinical lectures delivered at the London Medical College [*sic*], c. 1787–90, RCP MS 44. Hamilton, a staff physician, assumed that his audience included surgeons' pupils, as he pointed out the clinical lectures' convenience "for those who attend the practice of the Surgeons" (p. 20).

of Saint Thomas's Hospital [took] into consideration the necessity of the Surgeons' Pupils being instructed in Medicine as well as in Surgery, the Practice of most of them when they come into Business being principally in Medicine, they have therefore been induced to come to a Resolution of admitting them into the Prescribing Rooms, so that they may be able to see and understand the Physicians Practice.[111]

Although this initial statement specified practice in the "Prescribing Rooms," which likely referred to the area in which outpatients were seen, these pupils were also allowed to observe at the bedsides and to "look over their [the Physicians'] Books."[112] They got a good rate, too, for the physicians charged only £5 5s. 6d. per student, about half the cost for six months of the physicians' regular practice.

Fordyce, with an Edinburgh MD, had been physician to St. Thomas's since 1770 and had lectured since the late 1750s; he was deeply suspicious of claims to clinical expertise based on mere book knowledge. His colleagues, Adair Crawford and Gilbert Blane, both joined the hospital in 1783 with Glasgow MDs. Blane had served as a physician in the navy, while Crawford had been physician to the General Dispensary, so they had familiarity with the daily routines of general practice, even if they had served as elite physicians.[113] As I have noted, the St. Thomas's governors had previously been rather concerned to make regulations about pupilage, yet mention of this innovation never appears in the hospital minutes. Perhaps but another instance of physicians' status and presumed standards, the apparent informality with which this practice began and ended further indicates how malleable ward-

---

111 St. Thomas's, Register of the Surgeons' Dressers and Pupils entering to the Medical Practice, St. Thomas's Hospital Medical School Library, 1 Oct. 1788.

112 St. Thomas's had served outpatients since at least 1760. In 1790, the assistant physician, then William Lister, was given the duty of attending to them. See Parsons, *St. Thomas's,* 2: 217, 246. That the special physicians' pupils were given permission to watch the physicians practice at the bedsides on the wards is clear from a copy of the resolution quoted previously, which exists in the Entry Book of Physicians' and Surgeons' Pupils and Dressers, Guy's Hospital, vol. 1 (loose sheet). The words "and Bedside" have been inserted after the words "Prescribing Rooms." Furthermore, in the register at St. Thomas's, the page where pupils' names were entered begins, "The following Gentlemen have entered with the Physicians to Attend their Practice in this Hospital and look over their Books." Ironically, Charles Newman, whose views on London medical education have shaped decades of opinion, claimed that Dr. Fordyce "did not teach in the wards." Newman, "The Hospital as Teaching Center," 197.

113 Blane was thirty-nine and Crawford forty-three in 1788. Both had published well-received books. Blane's *Observations on the Diseases Incident to Seamen* appeared in 1785, while Crawford's *Experiments and Observations on Animal Heat* (1779) came out in a second, revised edition in 1788. None of these physicians was just setting out to establish a reputation, with lots of time on his hands for teaching in the hospital. Their plan seems to have arisen from a real commitment to widening medical education, rather than youthful enthusiasm. See Munk, *Roll,* 2: 326–8, 339–40.

walking was to staff interests and opportunities. The physic-for-surgeons practice stopped in 1812 when, with no further explanation, Richard Whitfield, clerk of the Register and Apothecary of St. Thomas's, noted "Drs. Lister, Wells and Turner Discontinued admitting Surgeons Dressers and Pupils to attend the Medical Practice."[114] All in all, 154, or 9 percent, of the St. Thomas's surgeons' and apothecary's pupils in these years took advantage of being "able to see and understand the Physicians Practice," most of them between 1798 and 1804.[115]

From the 1790s, the shift to nonuniversity physicians' pupils among those signing up at Guy's and the Middlesex also became quite marked. At Guy's, for instance, of the forty-six physicians' pupils who entered in 1802 and 1803, twenty came from apprenticeships, eight from universities (with and without MDs), and sixteen were, or had been, registered at Guy's as surgeons' and/or apothecary's pupils. These various aspiring practitioners, whatever their motives and career plans, not only sought clinical experience with hospital physicians, but obviously were accepted by them as appropriate pupils. The willingness to pay for broad experience, moreover, appeared among the handful of men who signed up for surgical ward rounds and displayed "MD" after their names. At St. Thomas's in 1796, Henry Hibbs, MD, entered as a surgeons' pupil; Robert Berkeley, MD, became a surgeons' pupil under Forster at Guy's in 1801; Thomas Massie, MD, served as Chandler's dresser at St. Thomas's in 1804. Some of these energetic and modestly well-off souls likely had their eyes on military

---

114 Register of the Surgeons' Dressers and Pupils entering to the Medical Practice, St. Thomas's, last page. Drs. Henry Ainslie and William Lister replaced Crawford and Blane in 1795. Ainslie had a 1793 MD from Cambridge and had served at Addenbrooke's Hospital as physician from 1787 before moving to London. Lister, with a 1781 MD from Edinburgh, was physician to the Smallpox Hospital from 1789 to 1791 and was the first assistant physician to St. Thomas's when that post was revived in 1790. William Charles Wells then replaced Ainslie, and Thomas Turner replaced Fordyce. Wells received an Edinburgh MD in 1780, after military service as a surgeon. Munk reports that he had very little private practice, as a result of his irritable character. Turner, in contrast, obtained his Cambridge MD in 1804 and became an active member of the Royal College of Physicians. He also studied as a physicians' pupil at St. Thomas's himself, in 1797. The as yet meager biographical backgrounds of the successor physicians clearly show no obvious reasons why Turner, Wells, and Lister chose to discontinue the "special" practice. Munk, *Roll*, 2: 329–30, 437–8, 382; 3: 26–8.

115 See Appendix II. In addition to the 154 from St. Thomas's, 5 Guy's pupils were admitted. The practice not only attracted potential surgeon–apothecaries, but also those among the "upper" ranks of surgeons' pupils. Chandler's apprentice, Isaac Sherwood, for instance, signed up in April 1807 for a term by the physicians' beds. A former house surgeon at St. George's, Philip Caddell, moreover, extended his education at St. Thomas's. He entered for a year with Whitfield in October 1800 and in December added the special physicians' practice to his rounds. St. Thomas's, Register of the Surgeons' Dressers and Pupils entering to the Medical Practice, Dec. 1800; St. George's, Register of Pupils and House Officers, 1799. Caddell registered as a perpetual surgeons' pupil in 1798 at St. George's.

service, although I have been able to trace only a few into the army.[116] On rare occasions an MD entered as an apothecary's pupil, as John Beamish did with George Whitfield at St. Thomas's in 1796.[117]

Beamish's choice stood the traditional hierarchy of the tripartite profession on its head: a physician followed an *apothecary* as a pupil in a hospital where real, elite physicians practiced. With less radical, but equally innovative choices, surgeons' apprentices followed physicians and MDs followed surgeons. Although they comprised a modest proportion of hospital pupils, those who crossed the formal boundaries between the branches of the medical profession demonstrate how pupils used London ward-walking to serve their own notions of appropriate training.[118] The introduction of special physicians' pupils at St. Thomas's aptly shows that staff men recognized the multiple concerns of general practitioners, not to mention that such variations on ward-walking went on within the hospitals without ever touching the governors' deliberations. By the beginning of the nineteenth century, the official labels on types of practice and rules for pupilage promulgated by the hospitals' governors and staff men shaped the outlines of ward access and behavior, but neither predicted who walked the wards with particular practitioners nor, more importantly, determined the content of that experience.

LEARNING ON THE WARDS

In 1729, William Graeme, a nonhospital physician eager to give lectures in London, remarked that, after a suitably learned education, the physician should attend a hospital to "apply what he had read to the particular circumstances of the Patient."[119] Such matter-of-fact advice dotted the pages of guides on how to become a medical man throughout the century, although by 1800 authors offered this familiar counsel to surgeon–apothecaries more than to aspiring physicians.[120] The basic way that students

116 One of these, Dr. James Barry, spent some time as a surgeons' pupil at St. Thomas's in 1812, having also received his Edinburgh degree that year, and then entered the service as a hospital mate in July 1813; Dr. Barry was promoted to assistant surgeon in December 1815. Peterkin and Johnson, *Commissioned Officers*, 1: 242. Similarly, at least two of the first MDs signing up for twelve months of surgical work at St. George's, Thomas Callander and David Maclagen (MD, Edinburgh 1805), did so in preparation for their military medical work. Peterkin and Johnson, *Commissioned Officers*, 1: 181, 184. I have been unable to trace the source of Hibbs's, Berkeley's, or Massie's MD degree.

117 Of the four MDs entering with the apothecary, I have found a probable MD degree only for John Beamish, who is likely the MD listed as graduating from Edinburgh in 1796.

118 James Lucas, *Candid Inquiry into the Education, Qualifications and Offices of a Surgeon Apothecary* (London: S. Hazard, 1800), 55.

119 William Graeme, *An Essay on the Method of Acquiring Knowledge in Physick* (London: Lawton Gulliver, 1729), 27.

120 William Heberden, "An Introduction to the Study of Physick," ed. LeRoy Crummer, *Annals of Medical History* 10 (1928): 359; D. D. Gibbs, "Recommendations of Sir John

learned on the wards seems clear. Pupils watched a skilled practitioner practice. Perhaps the physician, surgeon, or apothecary offered verbal accounts of what he observed, and why and how he decided to act; perhaps not. Perhaps the student asked questions or volunteered comments; perhaps not. Benjamin Rush captured contemporary (and a common retrospective) contempt for this amorphous London system when he wrote, while in Edinburgh, that "I am sure little knowledge can be acquired from the random prescriptions of the London hospital physicians." He was pleasantly surprised when he got to the metropolis and became a pupil with Dr. Huck: "I visit him at all hours and derive considerable improvement from him, not only from his prescriptions in the Middlesex Hospital (which I attend), but likewise from his private conversation."[121]

Hospital pupilage carried the extremes of "random prescriptions" and "considerable improvement" throughout the century, providing ample fodder for both detractors and supporters of ward-walking, and making generalizations from any single account about this form of training problematic. Students' perceptions and claims nonetheless delimit the available possibilities – and suggest intriguing nuances in how London pupilage constructed "good" clinical knowledge. First, whatever pupils learned when following staff on rounds, it appears that what mattered more for various individuals was access to the hospital at other times, whether as participants in care, quiet observers, or beneficiaries of "private conversation." In addition to the staff men, moreover, apprentices, dressers, and pupils taught each other, a point so obvious it is worth making explicit. Second, as I stated earlier, with more and more medical men on the wards, from neophytes to MDs and experienced surgeons, hospital practice became increasingly public in a way that apprenticeship, centered on the master and private patients, was not. This sense of "public," which included formal clinical lectures on hospital cases in the last third of the eighteenth century, figured in notions of how practitioners made good medical knowledge both off and on the wards. The fragmentary evidence for the ways that hospital pupils learned points to what they and their hospital mentors valued in clinical experience, and hence perpetuated as proper means to teach, to practice, and to "advance" medicine.

Floyer on the Education of a Physician," *Proceedings of the XXIII International Congress on the History of Medicine* (London, 1974), 368–9; Richard Davies, *The General State of Education in the Universities* (Bath: M. Cooper, 1759), 353–4; James Lucas, *Candid Inquiry*, 55; James Parkinson, *The Hospital Pupil, or an Essay Intended to Facilitate the Study of Medicine and Surgery in Four Letters* (London: H. D. Symonds, 1800), 53–5.

121 Letters from Benjamin Rush to John Morgan, 27 July and 21 Oct. 1768, in Butterfield, *Letters of Benjamin Rush*, 61, 66. For an example of particularly dismissive retrospective remarks, see Abraham, *Lettsom*, 157–62.

Access and initiative

In his autobiographical notes, John Flint South wrote a biting description of ward-walking at St. Thomas's in 1813–4:

[T]he visit commenced. The surgeon, accompanied by his dressers, each carrying their plaister boxes, which they considered a mark of distinction . . . visited both the male and female wards. The pupils accompanied them in shoals, if the surgeon was a favorite, and pushed and jostled, and ran and crowded round the beds, quite regardless of the patients' feelings or condition. . . . Certainly not much was to be learned at these "goings round;" they were mostly occupied with chattering and playing, and making extra-hospital arrangements.

"But," South continued, "the working pupils might be seen at other times on the wards, caretaking or watching, and assisting the dressers in carrying out the orders given by the surgeons."[122] John Coakely Lettsom, who took a Leiden MD in 1769, proudly remembered his diligence in observing the physicians' patients when he was a surgeon's dresser at St. Thomas's.

I devoted myself incessantly to the Hospital. . . . In the morning, early, before any attendance was given, I usually visited many select patients, wrote out the symptoms, and afterwards examined the prescriptions of the physicians on some particular cases. . . . At the same time, I continued to take notes of, and made reflections upon, what I saw and thus acquired a method of investigation and decision, which ever afterwards proved of the highest use in determining my medical conduct and practice.[123]

So Lettsom and South, both partly to recall their own earnest devotion even as students, testify to what "working" pupils did to gain practical experience quite aside from ward-walking. And, without requirements, examinations, or other official means to certify knowledge or skills, they had a point – actually learning something demanded "character."

Ironically, however, such accounts illustrate how the London system was *supposed* to work, just as much as they imply that only a few students chose to give it the requisite time and energy. The St. George's surgeons responding to Hunter's attack explained this, in quotable detail, to their fellow governors in 1793. Pupils

attend your hospital, they are present at our operations, at our consultations previous to these operations; they attend our dressings, the causes for our practice are assigned, we answer any questions that are asked, *we conceal nothing.* They dress in rotation and at no advanced price [unlike the procedure at other hospitals], as soon as they are acquainted with the forms of the hospital. They are present at the examination of morbid bodies, they come to see the benefit of our experience, to see our mode of practice, and by dressing the patients themselves become more

122 South, *Memorials*, 26–7.
123 Quoted from John Coakely Lettsom's manuscript autobiography in Abraham, *Lettsom*, 44–5.

intimately acquainted with the cases under their care, with the effect of external applications, and acquire an hability [*sic*] in the art of applying them. They are sent to in case of accidents and informed of operations. . . . [If they try only] to acquire a superficial knowledge in everything and no substantial knowledge in anything, it is not the fault of the surgeons to St. George's Hospital that they are not better instructed in Surgery.[124]

The details here underscore what access to a hospital could mean. Watching operations, inspecting morbid bodies, having presumably skilled prac-titioners "conceal nothing," all supplemented merely seeing the current "mode of practice." But it was *not the surgeons' fault*, do note, if pupils did none of this – a point as apt in 1793 as it had been in 1695, and would be until well after 1820.[125]

It is hardly surprising that information on what students did at the London hospitals has survived from those who were "working" pupils, not South's romping sort. And they did indeed watch operations and autopsies, and spend time on their own observing patients, as all-too-brief comments by various pupils attest.[126] Some of these dedicated folk, as Lettsom said of himself, took notes on ward cases, leaving collections of intriguing observations, prescriptions, and cryptic remarks.[127] Whether in rough form, or recopied into fair versions, with entries for a single patient neatly grouped together, these case books suggest the fundamentally prag-matic aims of their authors. Short on theory or explanations, they docu-

---

124 "Surgeons' Reply to John Hunter's Address (1793)," quoted in Peachey, *Memoir*, 292–3; my emphasis.
125 The Society of Apothecaries began to be concerned about certificates of clinical experi-ence in the 1820s. S. Lawrence, "Private Enterprise and Public Interests," 64–5.
126 Kay, *Diary*, 61–80; Betsy Copping Corner, ed. *William Shippen Jr.: Pioneer in American Medical Education*, American Philosophical Society, *Memoir* 28, 1951, 24–77; Whitfield Bell, "James Hutchison (1753–1793): Letters from an American Student in London," *Transactions and Studies of the College of Physicians of Philadelphia*, 4th ser., 34 (1966): 22–4; Cooper (?), Diary written by a student assistant physician or surgeon at the Westminster Hospital, 18 June–27 Aug. 1786 [this is an archivist's attribution; considering the internal descriptions, I believe Cooper was at most a dresser at the hospital], WIHM MS 1856; Ford, ed., *A Medical Student*; V. Mary Crosse, *A Surgeon in the Early Nineteenth Century* (London: E. & S. Livingstone, 1968); John Green Crosse, Diary 1811–14, Norfolk Record Office (NRO) MS 468. See also Samuel Clossey's references to cases and post-mortems he observed at St. George's in 1753–4 in his *Observations on Some of the Diseases of the Parts of the Human Body* (1763), reprinted in Clossey, *The Existing Works*, ed. Morris H. Saffron (New York: Hafner, 1967), 15–16, 40–1, 62–3, 91, 93–4, 118–19, 133–4, 149–67; Clossey later obtained an MD from Trinity College, Dublin.
127 For range of examples, see: E. Muirhead Little, "A Clinical Notebook of 1710," *British Medical Journal* (8 Dec. 1928): 1052; Charles Oxley, Casebook 1725–26, St. Thomas's Hospital Medical School; [anonymous], Notes, chiefly medical, taken at St. Bartholo-mew's Hospital [1778–1781], WIHM MS 4337; Widdows Golding, Commonplace Book 1786–8, RCP MS 250; Benjamin Brodie, Casebook [1805], MS 30, St. George's Hospital Medical School Library; John Gordon, Notes of Cases in the London Hospital under Mr. [Thomas] Blizard, NIMMO collection, University of Edinburgh Library; Joshua Waddington, Guy's Hospital – Clinical cases and lectures [1816–17], Wills Library, Guy's Hospital Medical School.

ment significant symptoms and the treatment at hand. Charles Oxley, an apothecary's pupil at St. Thomas's in 1725–6, followed a series of case histories in his notebook with two pages of "Doctors prescriptions taken out of their [prescription] Books," noting that "these are sufficient to Shew the practice."[128] "Mr. B[lizard] dissuades strongly from applying leeches [to bruises]," wrote Dr. John Gordon, visiting from Edinburgh in 1805, "indeed I saw their bad effect, and here the side was bruised; leeches were applied by one of the pupils and in a short time one of the wounds degenerated into a foul ulcer."[129]

Taking (and keeping) case notes was, of course, one of the ways that any practitioner – elite physician or apothecary's apprentice – could learn on or off the wards.[130] Yet various references to the physicians' "Books" and other hospital-based documents hint that pupils had access to material about patients that may have influenced what information they saw as relevant to record and how they learned to narrate it. Oxley's notes about the St. Thomas's prescriptions, for instance, read like the brief receipts for medications so common in health literature for centuries, and may well reflect the way the hospital apothecary kept records of the physicians' common decisions. As I have mentioned, the boarding physicians' pupil at the Westminster was to "take cases and keep a Register in which they may be faithfully recorded."[131] In 1793, the St. George's surgeons recommended

that a Book should be kept by the House Surgeon for the Instruction of the Pupils, wherein should be entered the material cases – the admission of the Patients, their Chirurgical Treatment, & the Event; together with the Appearances on the Examination of morbid Bodies. That each Pupil should be allowed to take a copy of such Entries at his Leisure & that Saturday in every week should be set apart for that purpose.[132]

128 Charles Oxley, Casebook 1725–26, St. Thomas's Hospital Medical School, n.p.; Oxley appears as an apothecary's pupil in the St. Thomas's Register.
129 Gordon, Notes of Cases in the London Hospital; Gordon, who obtained his Edinburgh MD earlier in 1805, does *not* appear in the register of pupils at the London Hospital; perhaps he saw the practice there as a favored visitor. For Gordon's education, see Daniel Ellis, *Memoir of the Life and Writings of John Gordon, MD FRSE* (Edinburgh: Archibald Constable; London: Hurst, Robinson & Co., 1823), 3–14.
130 James Lucas, *Candid Inquiry*, 55, 79–81; England, Two Notebooks, 1730–3; England was an apprentice near Taunton; he is not listed, however, in Wallis and Wallis, *Eighteenth Century Medics*; John Baly, Medical Case Book [1762–4], RCP MS 105. Baly, a practitioner in Chichester, took his Edinburgh MD in 1754. These are fair notes of private cases, and it is not clear why Baly took the notes or recopied them.
131 Westminster, Proceedings of the Trustees, 15 Feb. 1792.
132 Board of Governors' Minutes, St. George's Hospital, 14 June 1793; also in Surgeons' Report, Peachey, *Memoir*, 298–9; Benjamin Brodie's first extant case book, begun while he was House Surgeon at St. George's in 1805, *may* have served as this "register," although it seems to have been an arrangement of loose sheets that Brodie later had bound, and the case entries are (more or less) chronologically coherent for an individual patient.

John Green Crosse, studying in London in 1812–3, signed up as a pupil at the Lock Hospital and noted that he spent time "copying cases at the lock" in the evenings.[133] In contrast, James Macartney found, when a demonstrator of anatomy at St. Bartholomew's from 1798 to 1803, that keeping a hospital book might be fine in theory but was difficult to implement. He tried "registering the dissections made in the dead house & the corresponding cases," but he "could not get the medical men & pupils to continue to furnish [him] with the latter & the scheme was given up."[134] The process of "registering" and "copying" cases, whatever that entailed, certainly points to an intermediate set of observations and interpretations the pupil could use to replace, supplement, or test his own experience with the patient. Since none of the general London hospitals have extant clinical ward books from the period before the 1820s, however, the relationship between official registers (if there were indeed any kept) and pupilage remains temptingly speculative.

Public knowledge and clinical lectures

Samuel England, an apprentice to a provincial surgeon–apothecary in the 1730s, kept two clinical notebooks: one for surgical cases, the other for cases in physic. He copied into them, in more or less detail, interesting accounts from his master's practice, his own experience, and occasional tidbits from medical consultations. To "not be Deficient" in his knowledge, however, England stated,

I have Collected the Following Hystorys; and Ransacked ye most Approved Authors I have been able Yett to come att, the Better able to Illustrate them, Comparing their Definitions, Causes, Signs & Method with what I have Learn't and Seen in My M[aste]rs.[135]

To expand his experience, in short, England turned to books. In London, hospital pupils turned to watching several different staff men practice to extend their clinical knowledge. Especially eager surgical students traipsed from one institution to another to observe operations.[136] "Carious bones are dressed with the calx viv: & dry lint in St. Thomas's Hospital," noted Widdows Golding, "with Tinct. Myrrhi in Guy's."[137] The hospitals offered an empirical immediacy for a variety of both conditions *and* methods

---

133 Crosse, Diary 1811–14, 7 May, 27 May 1812.
134 Quoted from James Macartney's manuscript diary in John L. Thornton, "A Diary of James Macartney (1770–1843) with Notes on His Writings," *Medical History* 12 (1968): 167.
135 England, Two notebooks, 1730–3, 1: 5.
136 Kay, *Diary*, 83–7; Corner, *Shippen*, 11–14, 21, 28; Bell, "Hutchison," 24; James Ware, Notes of Lectures, 1763, MS St. Thomas's Hospital Medical School.
137 Golding, Commonplace Book, first section, 13.

and augmented the stock of "public" knowledge in print with the "public" cases at the charities. Hospital pupils could question the practitioners they watched in the process of making decisions. Samuel England had no such opportunities with his "Approved Authors."

Historians of clinical and hospital medicine have frequently observed that inpatient and outpatient services allowed medical men and women to see a greater variety of conditions than that available among the common ailments of private patients. Large hospitals, in this view, thus allowed – even compelled – increasing discernment in clinical diagnosis and morbid anatomy, and the potential for a numerical analysis of cases, both well-recognized signs of the medical revolution in Paris during the late eighteenth and early nineteenth centuries.[138] The notion that hospital wards in London offered access to diverse diseases efficiently gathered in one place clearly became part of the rhetoric of hospital experience by the late eighteenth century. "Here is the Practice of two large Hospitals before you, in which you may observe cases of every description," Astley Cooper told his St. Thomas's and Guy's pupils in 1808.[139] From the evidence of students' notebooks of both ward and lecture material, however, the availability of numerous patients mattered far less for a quantitative experience than as a source for appropriate demonstrations of disorders and treatments, at least those worth bothering to talk and to write about for one reason or another. This point is crucial to remember, for, as I have stressed, taking case notes was neither part of hospitals' official administrative functions nor a routine element of pupilage.[140] What made a case useful to a pupil depended intimately on the way it fit into a complex system of perceptions and knowledge. Hospital experience, in short, did not teach simply because it was there, however large the institution or busy its postmortem rooms. Hospital staff, apprentices, house surgeons, dressers, and walking pupils, not to mention the patients themselves, all constructed the perception and meaning of an illness or injury, from entry to discharge or burial. And *most* of this occurred within the oral culture of the wards, prescribing rooms,

---

138 See Chapter 1; Erwin H. Ackerknecht, *Medicine at the Paris Hospital, 1794–1848* (Baltimore: The Johns Hopkins University Press, 1967), 15–28; N. D. Jewson, "The Disappearance of the Sick-Man from Medical Cosmology, 1770–1870," *Sociology* 10 (1976): 225–44; A. J. Youngson, *The Scientific Revolution in Victorian Medicine* (London, New York: Holmes & Meier Publishers, 1979).

139 Astley Cooper, Lectures on Surgery, 1808, St. Thomas's Hospital Medical School Library, 5.

140 In contrast, the Royal Infirmary at Edinburgh had a more organized system for keeping case records that pupils could consult. Risse, *Hospital Life,* 5; Hamilton, Clinical lectures, 19, mentions a "register" at the London for the cases to be discussed in the clinical lectures, which "will be kept in a convenient part of the Hospital constantly open to the inspection of the pupils who attend the lectures." It clearly seems to have been a book specifically for selected cases, rather than a more general hospital document.

lecture theaters, medical societies, and student haunts, a point I develop in later chapters.

During the second half of the eighteenth century, nevertheless, hospital men began to articulate in medical lectures the connections between the abstract or general knowledge of physic and surgery and hospital patients. In many instances, lecturers simply directed their auditors to the wards. James Moffat (surgeon, Middlesex, 1759–65), for example, promised in an advertisement for his anatomy course in 1765 that

Lectures will also be given upon the Practice of Physick and Surgery, to his House Pupils and Hospital Pupils; the Principles of which they will see confirmed by the Treatment of the Patients in the Hospital, and of a great Number of Poor that daily apply at Mr. Moffat's House.[141]

Pupils would "see" principles "confirmed" by treatment of the poor in various circumstances, presumably pointed out with verbal explanations. Similarly, several surgeons used cases from their own experience, including those from previous and current ward patients, to illustrate points in their general lectures, a practice which probably served to make ward-walking intelligible to attentive hospital pupils in the audience.[142]

Physicians, in contrast, rarely discussed specific cases in their courses on the principles and practice of medicine, preferring a more "learned" style, one with diseases and disorders detached from the possibly idiosyncratic individual.[143] Hence, when physicians began to take explicit note of hospital patients, they did so in clinical *lectures,* clearly introducing an Edinburgh ritual to London. The Edinburgh Royal Infirmary had offered formal clinical lectures since 1748, when Dr. John Rutherford, professor of the practice of medicine at the university, began a series modeled after Her-

141 *Daily Advertiser,* 19 Sept. 1765; since the hospital governors forced Moffat to resign in October, during a dispute with the other practitioners, he hardly had a chance to implement his promises. Middlesex Hospital, Minutes of the Weekly Board, Court of Governors, 24 Sept., 22 Oct., 31 Oct. 1765; I have found no further advertisements for Moffat's course.

142 See, for example, Percival Pott, Lectures on Surgery, Given at the Theatre at Bartholomew's Hospital [*sic*], ca. 1770, taken down by an anonymous pupil, WIHM MS 3957, p. 28; Joseph Else, Lectures on Anatomy, ca. 1770, taken down by an anonymous pupil, NLM MS B5, 269–70. According to his nephew, when planning his surgical lectures in 1792–3, Astley Cooper "selected the cases of disease, and the casualties admitted into the two hospitals, and bringing such of them before the notice of his pupils, as would illustrate the subject on which he was treating, he first pointed out to them the nature of the disease or accident, described the appropriate treatment, and afterwards inculcated the theoretical views which indicated it." B. B. Cooper, *Cooper,* 1: 229.

143 See, for example, Theophilus Lobb, *A Compendium of the Practice of Physick: or the Heads of a System of Practical Physick contained in twenty-four lectures* (London: James Buckland, 1747); William Saunders, Lectures on the Theory and Practice of Physic, 1788, taken down by William Savory, MS St. Thomas's Hospital Medical School; George Fordyce, Lectures on the Theory and Practice of Physic, 1787, taken down by William Lambe, WIHM MS 2401.

mann Boerhaave's earlier clinical teaching at Leiden.[144] William Saunders, the first to advertise clinical lectures in London, had studied at Edinburgh, taking his MD there in 1765. Saunders joined Guy's as a physician in 1770 and immediately took the lectures he had been giving in London on medicine, chemistry, and materia medica to the hospital, but adding "Clinical lectures."[145] In 1780, Saunders's advertisement spelled out the details. The physician

proposes to illustrate his Subject [the Theory and Practice of Medicine] by explaining to his Pupils the cases of Patients in the Hospital, etc. and giving them the Opportunity of inspecting his Books. This is the most approved method of instruction by clinical lectures.[146]

In subsequent announcements, he continued to refer to "regular Reports . . . taken every Day in a Book," and, by the late 1780s, offered his clinical lectures on specific hospital cases twice a week in the winter.[147] Unlike the practice at Edinburgh, however, where the governors started a separate teaching ward with ten or so patients transferred into it for clinical scrutiny, Saunders presented cases spread out all over Guy's, probably as they appeared on his regular ward rounds.[148]

Most of the other London physicians who started clinical lectures also had Edinburgh degrees and, presumably, experience with the clinical courses at the Royal Infirmary (Table 4.4). By the end of the century, some hospital surgeons had followed suit. Anthony Carlisle and William Lynn, for example, advertised "Clinical Lectures on every Operation, or important Case which falls under their care" in 1794, during a valiant attempt to start a school at the Westminster.[149] From the way they were advertised, and from the few surviving sets of pupils' notes, clinical lectures were *not*

144 John Rutherford, Clinical Lectures, MS 1, St. George's Hosptial Medical School Library; Risse, *Hospital Life*, 240–6, 301–2; C. Lawrence, "Early Edinburgh Medicine." The clinical lectures were recognized as part of the official university curriculum for medical studies in 1777 and required for the MD in 1783; Rosner, *Medical Education*, 53–5.
145 *Gazetteer and New Daily Advertiser*, 19 Sept. 1770; Wilks and Bettany, *Biographical History of Guy's Hospital*, 190.
146 *Daily Advertiser*, 25 Sept. 1780.
147 *Daily Advertiser*, 26 Sept. 1785; 18 Jan., 30 Sept. 1788.
148 Chavasse, Dr. Saunders's Clinical Lectures, MS D.k.5.2, University of Edinburgh Library.
149 *Times*, 20 Sept. 1794. See also Mr. Turnball's advertisement for clinical lectures on the surgical cases at the Eastern Dispensary, to begin in November, *Times*, 1 Oct. 1794. In Paris, in contrast, the physician adopted a form of clinical lecturing first introduced by a surgeon. Pierre-Joseph Desault's innovation, the "clinical surgical lesson," in the 1780s inspired Corvisart to try a new method of clinical instruction in medicine (in 1788) at the Charité. Toby Gelfand, *Professionalizing Modern Medicine: Paris Surgeons and Medical Science and Institutions in the Eighteenth Century* (Westport, CT: Greenwood Press, 1980), 119–25, 144–5. Astley Cooper visited Paris and saw Desault teach in 1792. He noted that Desault "was a good anatomist and an excellent manipulating surgeon; but, as far as I could judge, not possessing the higher scientific principles which are necessary to consti-

Table 4.4. *Introduction of clinical lectures at the London hospitals, 1770-1815*

Hospital	Lecturer(s)	Practice and advertised date
Guy's	William Saunders, MD Edinburgh Astley Cooper	Physic, 1770 Surgery, 1800
St. Thomas's	George Fordyce, MD Edinburgh	Physic, 1780
London	James Maddocks, MD Edinburgh William Blizzard	Physic, 1783 Surgery, 1805
St. George's	George Pearson, MD Edinburgh	Physic, 1792
Westminster	Thomas Bradley, MD Edinburgh ⎫ Alexander Crichton, MD Leiden ⎬ Michael Morris, MD Cambridge William Lynn ⎫ Anthony Carlisle ⎬	Physic, 1794 Surgery, 1794
St. Bartholomew's	John Latham, MD Oxford	Physic, 1798
Middlesex	Richard Satterly, MD Cambridge	Physic, 1809

Note: These dates do not mark the start of continuous course offerings.
Sources: *Gazetteer and New Daily Advertiser*, 19 Sept. 1770; *Daily Advertiser*, 16 Sept. 1780; *Daily Advertiser*, 6 Oct. 1783; *Medical Register* (1783); *Daily Advertiser*, 10 Sept. 1790; *New London Medical and Surgical Journal*, 1 (1792): 422; *Times*, 20 Sept. 1794; *Times*, 17, 20 Sept. 1795; *Morning Chronicle*, 19 Sept. 1798; *Times*, 12 Sept. 1800; *Times*, 22 Sept. 1803; *Times*, 16 Sept. 1805; *Times*, 22 Sept. 1809.

the same as ward-walking. Indeed, they gave the "academic" case report to London pupils, as the student focused on all the details of how to prepare a case history, from the initial account by the patient of his or her condition, through the ongoing entries for symptoms and treatment, to the final commentary elucidating the case's particular peculiarities and general import. Thus in 1785–7 George Fordyce presented narratives of cases that

tute a surgeon of the first order." He did not comment, however, on Desault's teaching methods, so I hesitate to suggest that Cooper imitated a Parisian model when he advertised clinical lectures in 1800; see B. B. Cooper, *Cooper*, 1: 219–20.

he had seen in 1781–3, yet *called* them clinical lectures. His auditors learned a clinical *style* from appropriate models, without necessarily needing to see the patient for themselves. Yet at the same time Fordyce insisted on the importance of ward experience to actually learning how to diagnose and treat the sick and worked to make the physicians' hospital practice more accessible to pupils.[150]

The clinical lecture offered an intense, explicated account of specific cases. It was, as James Parkinson put it in 1800, "to the practice of medicine, what dissection is to anatomy – it is demonstration."[151] Yet, in contrast to the growth in ward-walking, hospital men's clinical lectures did not seem particularly popular. When William Hamilton, for example, introduced a course of clinical lectures at the London in the late 1780s, he told those who appeared at the first session that only "if a sufficient number of pupils" came the following week would "clinical patients . . . be selected & taken in." Hamilton hastened to say that "private pecuniary emolument could not possibly have had any influence with us," for demanding a reasonable enrollment. The hospital physicians just could not see spending "a considerable share of hours (for which we have abundant occupation otherwise) if a very inconsiderable number only, is to have the share of improvement from it."[152] A pencil scrawl on the manuscript by his son-in-law noted, "The Clinical Lectures were soon abandoned as the pupils who were at that time all [surgeons? . . .] would not attend."[153] Hampton Weekes, soon after his arrival at St. Thomas's as a boarding apothecary's pupil, told his father that, among other courses, he did *not* plan to sign up for "Saunder's Clinical Lectures." Perhaps smarting from a snub, he continued

I myself do not know if they will be of real benifit, if you think I should hear any of the preceding Lectures write me word, they are all for the money, I am shure; if you are introduced to any of them, they mearly bow & bow again, but they think nothing of you after, unless you put money in their pocketts.[154]

150 Clinical Lectures by George Fordyce, Physician to St. Thomas's Hospital, 2 vols., 1785–6, taken down by Henry Rumsey, RCP MS 138–9, and see pp. 137–8 in George Fordyce, The Substance of Two Courses of Clinical Lectures Delivered by Dr. Fordyce partly in 1785, 1786 & 1787, by Henry Rumsey, RCP MS 140; William Saunders, Clinical and Physical Lectures, 2 vols., 1785, WIHM MS 4371–2, taken down by an anonymous student: vol. 1 contains the clinical lectures; Chavasse, Dr. Saunders's Clinical lectures. There are several examples of students' notes from Edinburgh, discussed in Risse, *Hospital Life,* and Rosner, *Medical Education.*
151 James Parkinson, *Hospital Pupil,* 53, 55.
152 William Hamilton, Clinical lectures, 21–2.
153 According to Dr. Little, who apparently donated the manuscript to the Royal College of Physicians, Dr. Archibald Billing, who married "one of the daughters of Dr. Hamilton," penciled in the remarks found in the text. Billings ascribed the report that the clinical lectures were soon given up to "Mrs. Hamilton" (presumably his mother-in-law). Hamilton, Clinical lectures, 16.
154 Hampton Weekes to his father, 28 Sept. 1801, in Ford, ed., *A Medical Student,* 47–8.

Instead of listening to Dr. Saunders, Hampton attended the elderly Dr. Fordyce's (unadvertised) "Clinical Lecture" that he gave on his taking-in days. Indeed, Hampton noted that Fordyce was "a Man of few words," and offered his father an example of the physician's case style – at most two dozen Latin terms for clinical description and prescriptions. It was these concise remarks that Hampton decided to write in his "book," which "if it serves no other purpose it will serve to make me conversant in reading Physicians praescriptions."[155] At least for Weekes, Fordyce's pragmatic information outweighed Saunders's potential insights into case narratives.

Other pupils may well have thought that lectures on the theory of physic, ward-walking, texts, and previous experience provided all that clinical lectures did, without the added expense. Whatever the degree of their popularity, however, such lectures made hospital teaching "public" in the sense that learning to arrange and to talk about case reports transferred observations and experience into a form designed for communication, be it oral or written, that imitated a well-known university-centered format to convey the practice of medicine. They also made the use of hospital patients for teaching *literally* public, moreover, for, with curious reticence, hospital men did not advertise ward-walking in the daily newspapers until after 1815. The notices for clinical lectures, such as Saunders's statement quoted previously, were the first to remark, quite matter-of-factly, that "Patients in the Hospital" came under medical scrutiny for more than just their care. Perhaps everybody in the 1720s to 1770s already knew that the poor entering London's hospitals might find gawking pupils at their bedsides or watching their operations. From the 1770s on, however, hospital teaching appeared at the newspaper level of common knowledge. Even casual readers of the *Daily Advertiser,* the *Morning Chronicle,* or the *Times* could discover that physicians and surgeons had expanded charitable service into a business. In the process, some lucky – or unfortunate – patients in hospital beds joined the ranks of "the most instructive Cases," with the details of their conditions "read once a week" until discharge or death.[156]

Owen Evans, a pupil at St. Bartholomew's in 1797, expressed an appropriate concluding complaint for this chapter. "We have a great deal too much to attend to," he wrote to his friend Hampton Weekes.

I am of opinion [sic] for a Man to make himself a good Anatomist shd. attend only to that subject; I would the next Course if I could, attend only to this, but in the situation in which I am I cannot; as I must attend to the Patients in the Hospital &

155 Hampton Weekes to his father, 1 Nov. 1801, in Ford, ed., *A Medical Student,* 59–60.
156 *Daily Advertiser,* 18 Jan. 1788, advertisement for William Saunders's clinical lectures at Guy's.

go round with the Physicians as well as the Surgeons which takes up a great deal of time. ——[157]

Evans's brief letters have the familiar tone of a student swamped with work. He rather matter-of-factly notes that he went "round" with both physicians and surgeons, doing dual practice. Yet as central as this experience was for his education in London, he evokes the way that pupilage had become one routine among the many demands on his time, not least of which was going to other lectures and wanting to become "a good Anatomist." At the turn of the century, ward-walking, "which takes up a great deal of time," had become so thoroughly ensconced in London training that, ironically, students started griping about it.

Eighteenth-century hospitals opened their doors to students to serve the demands of medical training as well as the needs of charity. The pupil registers, along with the governors' minute books, show that practical instruction and free labor were understood as parts of hospital life by the latter half of the century, even if a mixed blessing for those concerned with order and decorum on the wards. Apprentices, dressers, short-term pupils, boarding students, or resident physicians' pupils would not have found a place among the sick poor unless they appealed to the governors' interests as much as to those of the medical practitioners on their rounds. In conjunction with administrative tolerance and, at times, overt support, staff men transformed medical training on the wards by reconfiguring the traditional relationship that bound apprentices to their masters with long-term legal and moral responsibilities. Pupilage started with modest numbers, blending into both apprenticeship and university study as means for supplemental experience, but expanded rapidly during the last decades of the century. By the 1790s, ward-walking catered to hundreds of men distinguishing themselves from their irregular and untrained competitors. So when the Royal College of Surgeons explicitly required six months' surgical attendance at a hospital in 1810 and the Apothecaries' Examiners ruled that candidates had to hold certificates of six months' work on medical cases at a hospital or dispensary, neither body had outrageous expectations. They confirmed and codified what they saw around them – especially the Royal College of Surgeons' Court of Examiners, many of whom were hospital men themselves.

The tripartite division of pupils under the physicians, surgeons, and apothecaries provided traditional labels for a vast range of students, from Oxbridge MDs to men about to go off to war as lowly medical mates. Such diversity captures the complexity of eighteenth-century medical experience, for as much as the official categories still worked for the hospital elite, students' choices and ward-walking opportunities illustrate the com-

157 Owen Evans to Hampton Weekes, 2 Jan. 1797, in Ford, ed., *A Medical Student*, 35.

mon concern to prepare for general practice and highlight how physic and surgery appeared as distinct subjects, but not distinct occupations. The students who went to London – whatever their previous education or later career choices – became the respectable rank and file evoked by medical reformers. They read the new professional periodicals, swelled the meetings of medical societies, and found themselves still competing with irregular practitioners. In the fees they paid, as well as the audience they provided for the techniques, knowledge, and values disseminated on the wards, pupils constantly reinforced the centrality of hospital practice and hospital practitioners in medical education during the later eighteenth century.

The notion of learning by watching and doing, so basic to apprenticeship, remained the core assumption of how pupils assimilated information on the wards. Whatever they obtained for their fees was primarily their responsibility; hospital staff men basically showed up and displayed themselves in action. How hospital physicians and surgeons structured and interpreted their observations and decisions for the pupils attending them thus depended upon both the particular staff man's interest and the pupils' initiatives. Ward-walking, in short, maintained an empirical diversity that, in its very spontaneity, was a training "system" that resisted medical "systems." *Doing* it promoted, quite pragmatically, an emphasis on discrete observations, on the primacy of direct experience, that supported the eighteenth–century focus on case accounts as the wellspring of medical knowledge so apparent in London men's work. Physicians offered clinical lectures in attempts to give hospital experience a narrative rigor suitable to learned perception and communication. That these were only moderately popular strongly suggests that pupils found other ways to embed the particularity of ward cases into explanatory frameworks meaningful to their previous training and expectations of future practice. Hospital pupils and practitioners did so, as I explain in the next chapter, through lecture courses on the theory of physic, the principles of surgery, or other topics offered in an academic style that gave medicine, as William Hamilton put it, "all the graces of science."[158]

158 Hamilton, Clinical lectures, 4.

5

London lecturing: Public knowledge and private courses

In September of 1769, Mr. Horsley paid for a notice in the *Daily Advertiser*, one of the newspapers devoted to announcing the wares of the commercial metropolis:

Young Gentlemen desirous of acquiring a competent Knowledge in Anatomy and Surgery, may be privately instructed in each Branch, both scientifically & practically, by Mr. Horsley, Surgeon & Man-Midwife, at Houghton-St., near Clare-Market. As one single course of lectures cannot answer the Student's purpose, Mr. Horsley therefore intends to continue his instruction till his pupils have made sufficient proficiency, by which means, and a regular attendance on the Hospitals, they may soon be initiated into these sciences, without being subject to seven years servitude; a consideration well worthy of the attention of parents or Guardians. For terms enquire as above.[1]

Mr. Horsley's appeal to "Young Gentlemen" encapsulates the themes of this chapter. He offered *private* instruction that, together with hospital ward-walking, would free "the Student" from the "seven years servitude" of apprenticeship. He promised to teach "both scientifically & practically," casting anatomy and surgery as "sciences" into which students were "initiated." Mr. Horsley couched his advertisement for a competitive market. He sold more than "one single course of lectures" at a time when medical lectures had become familiar items in newspaper notices. While it is impossible to estimate Mr. Horsley's success in his teaching career, in 1769 he appeared as a quintessential entrepreneur in the knowledge market of mideighteenth-century London.[2]

---

1 *Daily Advertiser*, 30 Sept. 1769; newspaper advertisements were fairly expensive, although clearly not beyond the means of the middling sort. The *Daily Advertiser* charged three shillings for a notice, as printed in the paper, without specifying how many times the advertisement would appear.

2 I have no idea how successful Mr. Horsley was as a private teacher, although he advertised again fourteen years later – this time to teach "Female Pupils" in midwifery. *Daily Advertiser*, 2 Oct. 1783. Horsley referred to himself as "Dr." in this advertisement, claiming that he had taught "Anatomy, Surgery and Practical Midwifery for 22 years." A Theodore Horsley appears in the *Medical Register* of 1783 as a member of the Corporation of Surgeons.

The emergence of medical lecturing in London was part of a much larger transformation of metropolitan society, urban education, and consumer opportunities.[3] Like the purveyors of publications, tutors and lecturers spoke to those seeking alternatives and supplements to schools, apprenticeship, or universities for self-improvement and entertainment. Medical lectures, whether or not combined with hospital ward-walking, further disengaged medicine from the university or apprenticeship routes to regular medical practice which had characterized previous centuries. With neither the expense nor the elitism of university matriculation, London's individualistic style of lecturing presented medical knowledge to the lower ranks of practitioners: to the apothecaries, surgeons, and man-midwives providing much of the medical care in England. To attend, moreover, a student needed only cash – no evidence of prior training, no testimonials of good character. Where short-term pupilage in the hospitals reconfigured the relationship between apprentice and master to one among pupil, staff men, and hospital, medical lecturing ignored it altogether. Nothing, except perhaps a certificate of attendance, verified that the student had this experience, much less that he learned anything. The students who entered, nevertheless, presumably left hoping that they had acquired attributes distinguishing themselves as "Gentlemen" from those "subject to . . . servitude."

From a broad perspective, eighteenth-century London lecturers' claims to provide appropriate and useful knowledge were far more market-oriented in England's metropolis than in cities with universities which had formal medical curricula, even when students did not pursue an MD degree or took private classes outside such institutions. London lecturers presented what they believed pupils should know. Students paid because they believed that the lecturers knew what they were talking about. Neither party needed a university's stamp of approval or licensing requirements to define what constituted material for good practice. London's lecturing system embodies the emerging values of eighteenth-century medical culture, both occupational and lay. New expectations and opportunities gave lecture pupils faith in the professional and social advantages to be had by exposure to the public knowledge and practice available in private courses.

London medical lecturing appeared and flourished entirely as an adventure in private enterprise, an exemplary illustration of Adam Smith's invisi-

---

In P. J. Wallis and R. V. Wallis, *Eighteenth Century Medics (Subscriptions, Licenses, Apprenticeships)*, 2nd. ed. (Newcastle upon Tyne, UK: Project for Historical Biobibliography, 1988), "Theodore Horsley" is listed as an apothecary in London. None of the other "Horsley"s seems a likely candidate for this lecturer/tutor.

3 Roy Porter, *Health for Sale: Quackery in England 1660–1850* (Manchester: Manchester University Press, 1989); Neil McKendrick, John Brewer, and J. H. Plumb, *The Birth of a Consumer Society: The Commercialization of Eighteenth-Century England* (Bloomington: Indiana University Press, 1982).

ble hand at work in Enlightenment England.[4] As explained in Chapter 3, the Society of Apothecaries, the Company of Surgeons, and the Royal College of Physicians each had a responsibility to certify qualifications, not to educate aspiring practitioners – except for the public anatomy lectures and dissections at Surgeons' Hall. "Private" and "public" are such useful and ubiquitous adjectives for understanding medical teaching that I start this chapter by briefly clarifying the different work they do when applied to economic relationships, knowledge, and institutions in the medical marketplace. I then provide an overview of the supply side of London lecturing, looking at the number of medical courses advertised in London newspapers throughout the century, and the ways that these were organized across the metropolis. Historians have already shown that London had a reputation as a center for the study of anatomy and surgery, not to mention natural philosophy and chemistry. But it offered far more than that.[5] Well before the 1790s, when the number of ward-walking pupils started to increase dramatically, aspiring practitioners could choose from courses on materia medica, the principles of physic, the practice of physic, midwifery, anatomy (with or without a separate dissection course), the principles of surgery, the practice of surgery, chemistry, natural philosophy, and clinical lectures on medical cases. In the breadth of its ad hoc curriculum, London offered opportunities in medical education that clearly rivaled those of its Scots competitor, the University of Edinburgh, by the mid-1770s.[6]

The outline I provide on London lecturers and their courses constructs the London system that the rest of this chapter explores. Examining the first decades of medical lecturing in the metropolis shows how medical men started private teaching and the strategies they used to promote their

4 Susan C. Lawrence, "Entrepreneurs and Private Enterprise: The Development of Medical Lecturing in London, 1775–1820," *Bulletin of the History of Medicine* 62 (1988): 171–92. For an account of those who have previously characterized London teaching as "private," see pp. 174–5, esp. n. 11.
5 An underestimation of medical teaching in London appears in most of the classics on the subject. See S. W. F. Holloway, "The Apothecaries' Act, 1815: A Reinterpretation," *Medical History* 10 (1966): 107–29, 221–36; idem, "Medical Education in England, 1830–1858: A Sociological Analysis," *History* 49 (1964): 299–324; Frederick N. L. Poynter, "Medical Education in England Since 1600," in *The History of Medical Education*, ed. C. D. O'Malley (Berkeley: University of California Press, 1970), 240; Zachary Cope, "The Private Medical Schools of London (1746–1914)," in Frederick N. L. Poynter, *Evolution of Medical Education in Britain* (London: Pitman Medical, 1966), 97. Hospital historians have equally ignored or downplayed the extent of medical teaching, other than courses in anatomy and surgery. For example, see A. E. Clark-Kennedy, *The London: A Study in the Voluntary Hospital System*, 2 vols. (London: Pitman Medical, 1962), 1: 166–8, where he describes Blizard's work but passes over courses given by Drs. Healde, Cooke, Hamilton, and Buxton, all of whom he mentioned in other contexts (1: 163–4, 174–6, 201); Hector Charles Cameron, *Mr. Guy's Hospital, 1726–1948* (London, New York: Longmans, Green, 1954), 95.
6 Lisa Rosner, *Medical Education in the Age of Improvement* (Edinburgh: University of Edinburgh Press, 1991).

courses. Medical lecturers drew inspiration and audiences from those involved in the "rise of public science" in England before 1750. Broad curiosity about the natural world and fascination with instruments and experiments marked early-eighteenth-century urban culture – enough, at least, to create markets for the books, lecturers, and objects promising secular revelation.[7] Yet the men offering medical courses in these years could not simply ride on the coattails of natural philosophers and cunning chemists. They had to convince aspiring practitioners to pay for *their* wisdom and expertise in addition to, or in place of, apprenticeship, university matriculation, and the Barber–Surgeons' public and private anatomies.

By the 1770s, private lectures had joined ward-walking as one of London's familiar advantages for those seeking medical training. I turn my account, then, to how private lecturers managed to give their courses *on* hospital grounds, those public institutions established to care for the sick poor. From the perspective of some governors and staff men, this was not necessarily an obvious idea, much less a good one, especially for anatomy courses. The construction of purpose-built lecture theaters at St. Thomas's, Guy's, the London, and St. Bartholomew's between 1770 and 1800 shows that lay governors eventually accepted the academic side of medical teaching as an appropriate, even useful, part of their charities' interests and reputations. In this process, hospital lecturers gradually acquired collective identities and status derived from their institutional homes. By the 1820s, they had laid the foundations for claims to authority over good knowledge that, consolidated in hospital schools, gave them a competitive advantage over other private lecturers – at the cost, however, of autonomy.

PRIVATE AND PUBLIC: BUSINESS, KNOWLEDGE, ACCESS, AND AUTHORITY

The notions of "private" and "public" play off each other throughout this chapter, since each evokes the other for its meaning in particular situations. I rely upon the eighteenth-century connotations for these paired adjectives, albeit reflected through a twentieth-century perspective. When applied to lecturing in London, these terms cluster around four interconnected ways to think about the dissemination of medical knowledge.[8] First, there is the familiar meaning associated with commerce and property. Lecturers sold their private courses to the student, who paid for them up front. Thus, when Dr. Denman advertised "a publick lecture on the Study of Medicine,

---

7 Larry Stewart, *The Rise of Public Science: Rhetoric, Technology and Natural Philosophy in Newtonian Britain, 1660–1750* (Cambridge: Cambridge University Press, 1992).
8 I do *not* touch on all the rhetorical force of "private" and "public" in eighteenth-century England. These terms were used extensively in discussions of politics, moral reform, domestic life, manners, and the law.

adopted to the Opportunities of acquiring medical knowledge in London,"
in 1775, he doubtless meant that hearing *this* one was free.[9] I presume that
most lecturers felt, as William Hunter certainly did at midcentury, that the
lectures themselves were personal property, even if occasionally given
without charge. In various priority disputes that Hunter had with his
rivals, he considered reading his lectures as the equivalent of publishing
them in establishing a claim to original discoveries.[10]

Other connotations for private and public must be distinguished from
the narrowly economic one, although they intertwine considerably at
times. First, consider how these modifiers apply to knowledge itself. "Private" implies restricted information, the knowledge that masters might
share with apprentices sworn to keep their secrets; "public" implies material more openly known or available for knowing. In this sense, *all* the
medical knowledge printed in books circulating among eighteenth-century
readers, discussed in lectures, and announced on wardrounds was public
knowledge. Second, "private" and "public" also refer to locations, and
therefore to access to knowledge. Sites for medical lectures fell within the
spectrum that lay between the obvious extremes of private places like a
gentleman's closet, where domestic manners (and servants) protected
him from outsiders, and public spaces, such as Tyburn field, where condemned felons were executed in the open for anyone to watch.[11] Medical
men lectured in private rooms that they rented in coffeehouses; they lectured, too, in the public theater at Surgeons' Hall. The difference is not
simply about ease of entry for the stranger off the street, but about the
criteria required to get in and who chose them. The lecturer at the coffeeshop, at home, or in his own theater could discriminate as he pleased. In
contrast, the designated anatomy lecturer at Surgeons' Hall spoke to the
Company's members, their apprentices, their guests, and whomever else
the Company's officers deemed appropriate. It is from this perspective that
private locations seem potentially more open to diverse audiences than
public ones at the corporations or colleges. Yet it also means that a private
lecturer's personal standards for students – their manners, for instance, or

9 *Daily Advertiser*, 23 Sept. 1775.
10 Roy Porter, "William Hunter: A Surgeon and a Gentleman," in *William Hunter and the Eighteenth-Century Medical World*, ed. W. F. Bynum and Roy Porter (Cambridge: Cambridge University Press, 1985), 24–8. In 1825, in contrast, John Abernethy lost his suit against Thomas Wakley, who had published Abernethy's lectures at St. Bartholomew's verbatim in the *Lancet*, without Abernethy's permission. Abernethy tried to claim the protection of copyright. Wakley's counsel basically won with the argument that (as Wakley later put it), "Of course Abernethy's lectures are public property. [T]hey are delivered in his public capacity as surgeon to a public charity." Quoted in S. Squire Sprigge, *The Life and Times of Thomas Wakley* [1899] (New York: Robert E. Krieger, 1974), 101.
11 Steven Shapin, "The House of Experiment in Seventeenth Century England," *Isis* 79 (1988): 373–404.

their religion, politics, or career plans – figured in ways that I cannot assess.

Lastly, as my examples already suggest, "private" pairs with "public" to contrast personal concerns and experience with collective interests and approbation. In this sense the universities, the licensing corporations, and the hospitals were public bodies in the eighteenth century. When these terms modify "lecturer," they point to the basis of his authority to teach. Every lecturer spoke, of course, from his own previous education, reading of texts, consultations with other practitioners, and experience with patients. But the private lecturer was a self-proclaimed expert on this material. Even when he relied upon the authority of famous authors to compile his lectures, in the marketplace his success depended upon getting and keeping students. Pupils granted a lecturer authority when he convinced them that he gave them good knowledge. The label of "public" lecturer, in contrast, carried an institutional weight, for it meant that some public group – such as the Court of Assistants at the Surgeons' Company – appointed him. His peers granted him the umbrella of their collective standing to fulfill a public duty and convey information for the public good. He had authority by virtue of his position, however well or poorly he managed to deliver his knowledge.

THE LONDON SYSTEM: AN OVERVIEW

For the most part, biographical vignettes, lecturers' comments in texts and articles, and students' lecture notes provided historians with evidence about the formation of private and hospital schools in the eighteenth century. As George Peachey demonstrated in 1924, however, newspapers are a far better source for discovering lecturers too obscure or too transient for contemporary commentary, much less for the relative fame of historical remembrance. Peachey concentrated on finding the men who foreshadowed William Hunter's famous anatomy course in 1746 (a moment to which I return later) and ended his broad survey of medical lecturers with Hunter's innovation. Yet lecturers throughout the century used the new medium offered by daily papers to advertise their courses, placing their notices among those for the other commodities readily for sale in the metropolitan marketplace.[12]

---

12 For a general overview of newspapers and advertising, see Arthur Aspinall, *Politics and the Press, ca. 1750–1850* (London: Home & Van Thal, 1949), ch. 1; *The History of the Times*, 3 vols. (London: Macmillan, 1935), I: 33–46. Newspapers researched: *Postman, Daily Courant, London Evening Post, Daily Post, London Daily Post, Daily Advertiser, Morning Chronicle, The World, Lloyd's Evening Post and British Chronicle, Gazetteer and New Daily Advertiser*, the *Times*. Years checked: 1700–6, 1708, 1710–15, 1717, 1719–22, 1724–7, 1729, 1730, 1732, 1733–6, 1738–44, 1746, 1747, 1749, 1750, 1752–5, 1757, 1759–66, 1768–72, 1774–85, 1788, 1790–1, 1793–5, 1797–1800, 1802–5, 1807, 1810, 1812–25.

In Figure 5.1, I have summarized the number of course advertisements for sampled years between 1755 and 1820 (see Appendix III). It displays only the number of "core" medical courses, grouped into three main categories, excluding the interesting, but irregular, announcements for lectures on natural philosophy, botany, veterinary medicine, and teeth. "Surgical" refers to all the courses on the principles and practice of surgery, anatomical lectures, and practical anatomy, one of the euphemisms for courses of dissection. "Medical" denotes, in this case, the topics associated with learning physic: the theory and practice of medicine, chemistry, and the materia medica, or theoretical pharmacy. Lastly, "midwifery" obviously covers lecture courses in midwifery, which usually included the diseases of women and children as an associated subject.[13] The overlapping graphical representation of the numbers of these courses makes a basic point. After the mid-1750s, lecturers advertised courses in all three general categories every year. These fields emerged together in eighteenth-century London, and they stayed together as staple parts of a London-wide curriculum, from the slow growth of the 1760s and 1770s through the rapid increase in advertisements in the 1790s.[14] London pupils nearly always had courses available that could help to prepare them for de facto general practice.

As I have already remarked, London lecturers worked in an open market for medical education. The material underlying Figure 5.1 supports five major points that clarify just what these market conditions meant over the century. First, as "open market" implies, medical lecturing centered on cash and competition. Except for the public anatomy lectures at Surgeons' Hall, and the occasional courses and demonstrations that the Society of

---

The number and kinds of courses advertised do not necessarily correspond to those actually given, for some men lectured without announcing their projects in the daily press and others may well have found empty rooms when they arrived to teach. Medical lecturers also distributed printed syllabi to booksellers, druggists, and hospital apothecaries, where pupils might see them. Some of these are the only surviving clues about lectures given. See, for example, William Cheselden, *Syllabus sive Index Humani Corporis partum Anatomicus, in xxxv Praelectiones distinctus in usum Theatri Anatomici* (London: For the Author, 1711); Nicholas Robinson, *A General Scheme for a Course of Medical Lectures Intended for the Improvement of Young Physicians and Gentlemen* (London, 1725?). For references to printed syllabi advertised along with courses, see, for example, *Daily Advertiser*, 27 Dec. 1765; *Times*, 15 Sept. 1815, 21 Sept. 1818; George C. Peachey, *A Memoir of William and John Hunter* (Plymouth: William Brendon & Son, 1924), 32.

13 For an introduction into midwifery for *male* practitioners, see Jean Donnison, *Midwives and Medical Men: A History of Inter-Professional Rivalry and Women's Rights* (New York: Schocken Books, 1977), 21–2, 35, 37, 42. Donnison primarily discusses licensing controversies, the education of female midwives, and the relative status of male and female practitioners. She does not note the concurrent rise in formal educational opportunities for men, which certainly helped men take on their new role at the expense of female practitioners. The outburst of midwifery lectures and the sometimes explicit advertising of simultaneous practical experience strengthen her argument.

14 S. Lawrence, "Entrepreneurs and Private Enterprise."

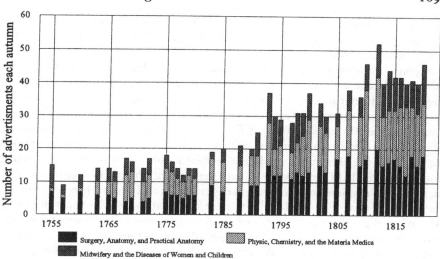

Figure 5.1. London lectures, 1755–1820.

Apothecaries sponsored, medical lecturing rested on a simple cash relationship between the lecturer and the student. London's lecturers directly received the fees they charged their auditors. Early in the century, courses stabilized at a cost of between £3 and £4 each and remained there for the next hundred years.[15] For aspiring practitioners, such fees were high enough to discourage marginal men from attending, especially with the cost of hospital pupilage and dresserships in addition to the expense of visiting London.[16] Would-be lecturers, in turn, took the risks of investing in material and they gathered the profits – or debts. And, at least according to historical gossip, profits there were. Dr. William Saunders, for example, is said to have earned £1,000 a year from his medical courses at Guy's.[17]

15 London lecturers usually charged about three guineas for each new course. In 1738, for example, William Bromfield's anatomy course cost three guineas for the first attendance, with reduced fees thereafter; *London Daily Post*, 2 Mar. 1738/9. In 1810, Anthony Carlisle's course on surgery was still three guineas for the first attendance. *Times*, 24 Sept. 1810.

16 Provincial students probably found that going to London cost about as much as studying (but not graduating) in Edinburgh. The 1775 estimate that it took £150 per year to study medicine in Edinburgh would have comfortably served a London student. Belt-tightening could make the cost much less, and London pupils at least did not have to pay matriculation fees or graduation expenses, as those proceeding to the MD faced in Edinburgh. Lisa Rosner, "Students and Apprentices: Medical Education at Edinburgh University, 1760–1810," Ph.D. dissertation, The Johns Hopkins University, 1985, 58–9, 65, 72.

17 Samuel Wilks and G. T. Bettany, *A Biographical History of Guy's Hospital* (London: New, Ward, Lock, Bowden & Co., 1892), 109; Munk states that Henry Clutterbuck, physician to the General Dispensary in 1807, also made over £1,000 per year from lecturing in the early nineteenth century. William Munk, *Roll of the Royal College of Physicians of London*,

Lecturing probably appealed to many men with a wide variety of motives, including sincere desire to influence their fields and their occupations. But it was, at root, a business.

Second, those who chose to lecture had considerable freedom over how, when, and where they gave courses. Lecturers had no restrictions (other than, of course, those of common decency and common law) on what they said, no corporate interests concerned with their courses' appropriate content or certification, no hopes for state grants of teaching monopolies or Parliamentary favoritism. At a bare minimum, the practitioner who lectured on the theory of medicine required only a room and his own knowledge, culled from texts and experience. The chemistry lecturer who pledged to illustrate his lectures with experiments and "actual preparations" needed rather more space for equipment and materials. The practitioners who offered practical anatomy needed access to corpses for demonstrations and student dissections. They, too, required enough room to prepare specimens, to supervise student work, and, with improved methods for preserving body parts, to store useful preparations.[18] In part to deal with the necessary investments in space, time, and material, lecturers collaborated with colleagues teaching the same subject (an especially common practice among midwifery lecturers) and, more noticeably from the 1790s, with those lecturing on different topics. These co-lecturers jointly advertised their courses and usually shared the same location.[19] Under the vagaries of

2nd ed., 4 vols. (London: Royal College of Physicians, 1878), 3: 15. Joshua Brookes supposedly had 5,000 pupils in his forty years of teaching. If his fees were similar to Charles Bell's, who advertised a basic charge of £3. 3s. for dissection and £5. 5s. for his anatomy and surgery lectures in 1809 [*Edinburgh Medical and Surgical Journal* 5 (1809): 489–90] then, assuming an average of £7 per student, Brookes could have grossed £35,000 or £875 a year. A lecturer in chemistry, medicine, or midwifery with a class of twenty and a fee of £3 could gross £60 a season or £180 a year (including summers).

18 William Lewis, for example, promised "the actual preparation of the Chymical and Galenical Medicines now in use" during his course "at the Elaboratory, in New Street," *The Literary Courier of Grub-Street*, 26 Jan. 1739; Nathaniel St. Andre promised several skeletons, among other preparations, in his anatomy course, *Daily Courant*, 5 Oct. 1721. Peachey, *Memoir*, 33, 49–51. Later anatomists' collections, particularly John Hunter's, William Hunter's, and Joshua Brookes', became treasures for display as well as teaching devices. With such collections turning into "museums" for appreciation and study, they became overtly institutionalized. For examples of physicians' lecturing at home, at a "hotel," or in other rented rooms, see *Public Advertiser*, 25 Sept. 1755; "Sketch of the Life of Hugh Smith," in his *Formulae Medicamentorum Concinnatae* (London: J. S. Barr, 1791), iv; *Daily Advertiser*, 13 Oct. 1760; *Daily Advertiser*, 1 Oct. 1772.

19 The single early exception to this generalization is the brief 1746 collaboration between William Bromfield and Dr. Robert James, who announced a course of anatomy, surgery, and medical lectures; Peachey, *Memoir*, 37. Other collaborations began with lecturers on closely related topics. John Hunter, for example, announced his course on surgery at his brother William's Theatre of Anatomy on Great Windmill Street in 1776 and 1777, in between lecturing at other places; *Daily Advertiser*, 23 Sept. 1776, 6 Sept. 1777, see also Peachey, *Memoir*, 163. William Saunders, a Guy's physician who gave courses on physic, materia medica, and chemistry at the hospital in the early 1770s, let Dr. William Keir

the open market, moreover, partnerships and nascent schools dissolved as readily as they formed.[20]

Third, pupils, as consumers, had considerable freedom to tailor their lecture choices to their own backgrounds, interests, incomes, and ambitions. From midcentury on, open competition among lecturers for pupils narrowed to competition primarily between lecturers in the *same* subjects, with conventional times for lectures on physic, anatomy, chemistry, surgery, and midwifery. I sketch out a typical day (circa 1800) in Table 5.1, using information pieced together from various advertisements. Whatever specific conditions encouraged lecturers to adhere to a time schedule in which they competed within, and not across, disciplines, the result was a remarkable underlying coherence for London's system.[21] Students in London, as at university, could take a full range of subjects, with the added advantage of periods for both hospital ward-walking and dissection. Biographical information about particular students, such as Richard Kay, who visited London from 1743 to 1744, and William Fairchild, who attended courses in 1811 and 1812, confirms that would-be regular medical men indeed went to lectures in several branches of medicine.[22] Fairchild, an apothecary's apprentice who became a surgeon, chose Dr. Squire for midwifery; Joshua Brookes for anatomy; Anthony Carlisle for surgery;

share the chemistry lectures there from 1778 to 1783, when Keir suddenly died; *Public Advertiser*, 26 Sept. 1778; *Daily Advertiser*, 14 Sept. 1779. From 1779 to 1780, Keir also gave a chemistry course on his own at No. 7, Adam St., Adelphi; see *Daily Advertiser*, 14 Sept. 1779. Keir was elected physician to St. Thomas's in 1780; by 1783 he alone gave the chemistry lectures, although still at Guy's; *Daily Advertiser*, 22 Jan. 1783.

20 In 1772–3, for example, William Hewson stopped working with William Hunter at the Great Windmill Street Theatre apparently over a dispute about the ownership of the anatomical preparations made there; Peachey, *Memoir*, 122; Stewart Craig Thomson, "The Great Windmill Street School," *Bulletin of the History of Medicine* 12 (1942): 385–6. Bransby Cooper, in his biography of his uncle, Sir Astley Cooper, mentioned the abortive "negotiations" between John Hunter and John Haighton to form a lecturing partnership. His account stressed the importance of personalities and ambitions as key elements in this case. The potential relationship fell through because Haighton felt "mortification" at the idea of being "second-best to John Hunter." Bransby B. Cooper, *Life of Sir Astley P. Cooper*, 2 vols. (London: J. W. Parker, 1843), 1: 121–4.

21 Dr. Maddocks noted that he had planned to start his course on the theory and practice of medicine at 11:00 a.m., but changed it to 9:30 when told that "an earlier hour would be more agreeable and convenient." *Daily Advertiser*, 1 Oct. 1772.

22 Richard Kay walked the wards as an apothecary's pupil at Guy's. He heard lectures on anatomy and surgery from Samuel Sharp, Guy's surgeon, and John Girle, St. Thomas's surgeon, and on midwifery (with practical experience) from William Smellie, a nonhospital man. Proximity to Sharp and Girle might have influenced his choice, as others offered anatomy in London in that year. Kay, moreover, could have paid for chemistry lectures and (perhaps) for a series in physick, but did not. Richard Kay, *The Diary of Richard Kay of Baldingstone, near Bury, 1716–51*, ed. W. Brockbank and F. Kenworthy (Manchester: Chetham Society, 1968), 68–89; see also, Joan Lane, "The Role of Apprenticeship in Eighteenth-Century Medical Education in England," in Bynum and Porter, *William Hunter*, 77, 83–5, 101.

Table 5.1. *The London timetable for the core subjects, ca. 1800*

Hours	Subjects
7:30/8:00-9:00 a.m.	Materia medica/medicine (on alternate days)
9:00-10:00 a.m.	Chemistry
10:00/10:30-11:00/11:30 a.m.	Midwifery & the diseases of women and children
11:00 a.m.-1:00 p.m.	Hospital/dispensary rounds
1:00-2:00 or 2:00-3:00 p.m.	Anatomy
3:00-5:00 p.m.	Practical anatomy (dissection)
5:00-6:00 p.m.	Midwifery & the diseases of women and children
7:00-8:00 or 8:00-9:00 p.m.	Surgery

Dr. George Tuthill for pathology, the practice of physic, and the materia medica; and the Westminster hospital for six months of surgical ward-walking. Considering the rich array of courses given at various locations and the contemporary prestige of other lecturers – such as Astley Cooper at Guy's – Fairchild made modest decisions.[23] That is, of course, the point. Students kept on paying the now-obscure men, as well as those still famous, to suit their needs.

Beyond accounts of certain individuals' experiences, very little information exists on how many – or which – pupils attended eighteenth-century courses. What does remain often has a rhetorical intent. John Hunter claimed, for instance, that about fifty to sixty pupils attended his brother William's lectures in the early 1750s, compared with competing anatomy classes that attracted only about thirty students, an obvious testimony to William's skill.[24] The rise in the number of courses in the mid-1790s clearly parallels the surge in the number of hospital pupils (compare Figure 5.1 with Figure 4.1) and points to mutually reinforcing market connections between courses and ward-walking pupils. A rare list of early-nineteenth-century lecture students, moreover, shows that at least half of the twenty-four stu-

23 Cecil Wall, *The History of the Surgeons' Company, 1745–1800* (London: Hutchison's Scientific and Technical Publications, 1937), 85–6, gives this information on William Fairchild from the details of a case of slander brought in 1819. Fairchild used them to convince the court that he was a well-qualified medical man.

24 Samuel Foart Simmons and John Hunter, *William Hunter, 1718–1783, a Memoir,* ed. C. H. Brock (Glasgow: University of Glasgow Press, 1983), 5; Jesse Foot, *The Life of John Hunter* (London: T. Becket, 1794), 72.

25 This is the only list of lecture attenders I have found for the period before 1820. In 1814,

dents who paid for Francis Ramsbotham's midwifery lectures at the London hospital in 1815–16 walked its wards.[25] Hospital students were undoubtedly a major audience for lecturers, yet the medical lecturers' technical topics and obvious customers did not then make all of those who attended into future practitioners of regular medicine. The open, cash-based London system had plenty of literal and conceptual room for curious laity to pay to hear medical men expound on the body, disease, and therapies.[26]

Fourth, evaluating the place of hospital practitioners and of hospitals' facilities in the London lecturing market demands restraint. I later emphasize the ways that hospital men grafted lecturing onto their charitable institutions, in part because hospital involvement left hints about the process of legitimizing such medical instruction. Physicians and surgeons with hospital posts, moreover, lectured outside their charities, for hospital grounds were but one of many sites that eighteenth-century entrepreneurs used for giving courses. Yet hospital lecturers always comprised a minority of those presenting courses before 1820, a pervasive reminder that lecturing thrived without any institutional sanction (Table 5.2). Indeed, on average nearly half of London's instructors had no connections with hospitals, dispensaries, or lying-in charities, although the overall proportion of nonaffiliated lecturers declined in the late eighteenth and early nineteenth centuries.

Lastly, practitioners who gave courses participated in "advancing" medical knowledge by disseminating up-to-date ideas and treatments at the same time that they promoted themselves as medical authorities. Dale Ingram, for example, noted in 1756 that he "added many curious Cases, practical Observations, and the late improvements in Surgery" to his anatomy "lectures read some Years since."[27] To offer lectures marked a claim to expertise. To have them succeed, advertised season after season, demonstrated that others (if only students) accepted and confirmed such claims through their market choices. When John Hall, a fairly obscure nonhospital lecturer, identified himself as a "Teacher of Anatomy" in an article published in 1786, the label placed him on the occupational map as a person with a certain credibility.[28] The rough profile of London's lecturers shown

Dr. Francis Henry Ramsbotham began an account book for his "Lectures with Cases on Midwifery . . . at the London Hospital." He had lectured outside the hospital, at No. 9, Old Jewry, from 1810 (see, for example, *Times*, 3 Oct. 1814), but any registers from that time have not survived. Of the twenty-four students he listed from October 1814 through January 1816, *at least* thirteen (54%) were, or had been, pupils at the London Hospital. Ramsbotham, A List of the names of Gentlemen entered as pupils to x x x x x [*sic*] Oct 1815 [– Oct. 1835], NLM MS B 118. Ramsbotham's first advertisement for his course at the London appeared in 1815; *Times*, 26 Sept. 1815.

26 Theophilus Lobb, *A Compendium of the Practice of Physick: or the Heads of a System of Practical Physick, contained in twenty-four lectures* (London: James Buckland, 1747), vi.

27 *Gazetteer and London Daily Advertiser*, 22 Sept. 1756.

28 John Hall, "Experiments and Observations on the Contents of the Medullary Cells in Dropsy," *London Medical Journal* 7 (1786): 155.

Table 5.2.   *Institutional affiliations of lecturing physicians, surgeons, and chemists, 1750-1815*

	1750-1789	1790-1815	Total
Physicians			
General hospital	15(37%)	17(40%)	32
Dispensary or lying-in charity	8(19%)	9(21%)	17
Other	18(44%)	16(38%)	34
Total physicians	41	42	83
Surgeons			
General hospital	11(25%)	9(35%)	20
Dispensary or lying-in charity	2 (5%)	8(30%)	10
Other	31(70%)	9(35%)	40
Total surgeons	44	26	70
Non-MD Chemists:	--	3	3
Total	85	71	156

Sources: Appendix III.

in Table 5.2 extends this general point. It shows that physicians were just as active as surgeons in providing educational opportunities for London pupils and platforms for themselves as experts. In doing so, degree-bearing physicians used public mastery of certain kinds of knowledge subtly to undermine the university systems that gave them authority in the first place.[29] They taught potential competitors among surgeon–apothecaries the theories and practices central to the physician's medical status, revealing concepts and arguments that nonphysicians could adopt. So, too, did surgeon–anatomists supply apothecaries and physicians with the hands-on anatomy of dissection, and lecturers on midwifery enlarge the ranks of male practitioners educated about childbirth. How they did so, and the

29 George Tuthill, who noted he was "of Caius College, Cambridge," in his advertisement (*Times*, 13 Sept. 1810), is an obvious example of a physician who disseminated knowledge with a university pedigree. When Tuthill began lecturing in London in 1810, he had a Cambridge AB and AM. He received the license ad practicandum in 1812, and the MD in 1816. He was elected physician to the Westminster in 1813 and noted this in his later advertisements, too (*Times*, 24 Sept. 1814). Munk, *Roll*, 3: 171–2.

implications of their enterprises for changing medical knowledge, concern the rest of this chapter.

ENTREPRENEURS: ENTERTAINMENT AND EXPERTISE,
1700–1760

The men who began lecturing on medical subjects in eighteenth-century London shared both business models and audiences with scores of others tapping an urban market in education. From the late seventeenth century, Londoners had found amusement, enlightenment, and self-improvement in numerous lectures and courses offered across the metropolis. Tutors, lecturers, and modest schoolteachers competed with charity schools, grammar schools, craftmasters, and universities for malleable youths. Educational entrepreneurs sought adults who were ready to invest some time pursuing intriguing or socially advantageous subjects. Vocational or practical aims, such as acquiring skill in bookkeeping or composition, often overlapped with the more nebulous desires for the social ease and possible social mobility promised by learning to dance, to speak French, or to understand Latin.[30] As historians have recently emphasized, lectures on natural philosophy and chemistry especially piqued public curiosity.[31] In the early eighteenth century, lecturing men enlivened their talks with mechanical and electrical displays in order to attract diverse audiences. John Theophilus Desaguliers, for instance, became one of the best-known lecturers in natural philosophy in London for his staged experiments.[32]

Such instructors frequently promoted their work as rational knowledge and equally rational pastimes, suitable – by cost and implicit ideology – for the ubiquitous eighteenth-century "gentlemen" and – sometimes – "ladies."[33] Yet allusions to cultural advancement existed side by side with claims to impart pragmatic and utilitarian scientific knowledge for busi-

30 Nicholas Hans, *New Trends in Education in the Eighteenth-Century* (London: Routledge and Kegan Paul, 1961), 63–70, 99–116, 136–50, 185–9.
31 Considerable work on eighteenth-century lecturing has appeared in the last twelve years. See Roy Porter, *English Society in the Eighteenth Century* (Harmondsworth: Penguin Books, 1982), 63–112, 247–60; J. H. Plumb, "The Commercialization of Leisure in Eighteenth-Century England," in *The Birth of a Consumer Society*, 265–85; Simon Schaffer, "Natural Philosophy and Public Spectacle in the Eighteenth Century," *History of Science* 21 (1983): 1–43; J. N. Hays, "The London Lecturing Empire, 1800–1850," in *Metropolis and Province: Science in British Culture, 1780–1850*, ed. Ian Inkster and Jack Morrell (Philadelphia: University of Pennsylvania Press, 1983), 91–119; Stewart, *The Rise of Public Science*.
32 Hans, *New Trends*, 136–50, 152–60; A. E. Musson and E. Robinson, *Science and Technology in the Industrial Revolution* (Manchester: Manchester University Press, 1969), 37–43, 51–4, 57–8, 120–4, 129–31; Larry Stewart, "Public Lectures and Private Patronage in Newtonian England," *Isis* 77 (1986): 47–58.
33 Advertisements explicitly inviting women to attend courses are rare, but see Charles Lucas's chemistry course in 1753, directed at "curious persons of either sex." *Daily Advertiser*, 10 Oct. 1753.

ness, trade, or profession. Chemistry, for example, drew craftsmen, mechanics, manufacturers, and interested gentlemen, as well as aspiring physicians, surgeons, and apothecaries.[34] Anatomy lecturers, depending upon their course's style, appealed not only to surgeons eager to operate competently, but also to those who saw human and animal bodies as objects of natural history.[35] William Cheselden and Francis Hauksbee aimed their 1721 course in human and comparative anatomy, with its "Mechanical Experiments," at "Gentlemen." They promised that "such things only will be omitted as are neither instructive or entertaining, and Care will be taken to have Nothing offensive."[36] In 1772, William Hewson still directed his anatomy lectures "not only to the Students of Medicine and Surgery, but to such Philosophical Gentlemen as wish to acquire a Knowledge of the Animal Oeconomy."[37] That a practical apothecary or surgeon was also a devotée of chemistry for its nonmedical manufacturing applications or of anatomy for its insight into God's rationality challenges any attempts to demarcate strictly vocational from avocational interests in this period.[38] Indeed, eighteenth-century lecturers (and authors) on topics about nature constantly re-created and maintained the twin ideologies of practical and gentlemanly knowledge since neither sufficed alone to establish their technical expertise, cultural authority – or income.

The broader enthusiasm for private courses and the multiple motives that inspired London's inhabitants and visitors to pay for them do not

34 Musson and Robinson, *Science and Technology*, 119–22; Jan V. Golinski, "Peter Shaw: Chemistry and Communication in Augustan England," *Ambix* 30 (1983): 21–2; advertisement by Henry Pemberton for his chemistry lectures at Gresham College, *London Daily Post and General Advertiser*, 19 Jan. 1738. John Thornton, when advertising his lectures on botany at Guy's, explicitly noted, "Other Gentlemen than Medical are admitted to these Lectures," *Morning Chronicle*, 22 Sept. 1798.

35 Andrew C. Cunningham, "The Kinds of Anatomy," *Medical History* 19 (1975): 1–19; Christopher Lawrence, "Alexander Monro *Primus* and the Edinburgh Manner of Anatomy," *Bulletin of the History of Medicine* 62 (1988): 193–214; Porter, "William Hunter: A Surgeon and a Gentleman," 22. Anatomical displays also intrigued the simply curious, as in the 1719 show of waxwork figures that included a newly born child, eyes, the head, and a female torso. In contrast, John Douglas pointedly stated in his published *Syllabus of . . . a Course of Anatomy, Chirurgical Operations, and Bandages* in 1719, that *his* course was "of a different nature from those commonly given, and is entirely calculated for students of surgery being essentially practical." Quoted in Peachey, *Memoir*, 22; for the waxworks, see p. 26.

36 *Daily Courant*, 9 Nov. 1721; also quoted in Peachey, *Memoir*, 18; Sir Zachary Cope, *William Cheselden, 1688–1752)*, (London: E. & S. Livingstone, 1953), 4–5.

37 *Daily Advertiser*, 12 Sept. 1772.

38 Schaeffer, "Natural Philosophy and Public Spectacle in the Eighteenth Century," 5–6, 26–7; Musson and Robinson, *Science and Technology*; Robert E. Schofield, *The Lunar Society of Birmingham* (Oxford: Clarendon Press, 1963); Paul Weindling, "Science and Sedition: How Effective Were the Acts Licensing Lectures and Meetings?" *British Journal of the History of Science* 12 (1980): 139–53; John R. Millburn, "James Ferguson's Lecture Tour of the English Midlands, 1771," *Annals of Science* 42 (1985): 397–415; John Gascoigne, *Cambridge in the Age of the Enlightenment* (Cambridge: Cambridge University Press, 1989).

entirely account for the emergence of medical lecturing. Learning physic or anatomy, after all, differed from taking Latin lessons or admiring Newtonian mechanics. There were established institutions for obtaining professional instruction, in addition to apprenticeship to a surgeon or an apothecary. Physicians went to university for physic. Aspiring surgeons saw internal human anatomy at the Company of Barber–Surgeons. Most literate practitioners had texts to read for theoretical systems and advice. Private lecturers somehow had to make these routes seem inadequate or inaccessible for obtaining "good" knowledge. In general, these early entrepreneurs did so by presenting themselves as blending elite, textual knowledge with the wisdom and expertise of personal experience. Lecturers in physic, anatomy, and midwifery, however, placed rather different emphases on how students could learn to absorb and apply the theoretical and the empirical foundations of their subjects. Their arguments and strategies thus reveal how they established private instruction as the new venue for fashioning regular medical men in the English metropolis.

Physic

Lectures on physic most directly subverted the connection between the physician's knowledge and the university in early-eighteenth-century England. Before 1750, only six men advertised courses on physic in London, starting with an extremely mysterious "T.C." in 1710. None of them (except perhaps T.C.?) had a degree from Oxford or Cambridge; none appears to have lectured for more than a few years.[39] William Graeme and Theophilus Lobb, two of these physician–lecturers, addressed the lack of lectures on physic in the metropolis. Graeme's and Lobb's rather obvious hopes to be heard highlight the persuasive intent of their arguments: lecturing on physic needed advocates as well as advertisements during these decades.

Graeme, an upstart young man from Scotland, claimed to respond to criticism of his plan to lecture in *An Essay on the Method of Acquiring Knowledge in Physick,* published in 1729. Lobb, a dissenting minister who had practiced physic (with a Glasgow MD) for years in the provinces, started teaching after settling in London as a full-time physician in the late

39 Peachey, *Memoir,* 45, lists four lecturers on physic for 1710–1743, "T.C.," William Graeme, William Schaw, and Nicholas Robinson, presumably from newspaper advertisements he found. Unfortunately, I have not discovered any of their notices in the papers I used for this study, but certainly have no reason to doubt Peachey's information. The British Library copy [544e4(5)] of Nicholas Robinson's *A General Scheme for a Course of Medical Lectures Intended for the Improvement of Young Physicians and Gentlemen* [London, n.d.] was dated to ca. 1725. Other copies date from ca. 1742, perhaps giving rise to Peachey's placing Robinson's lectures in 1743. Robinson had a 1718 MD from Rheims and obtained the LRCP in 1727, so the 1725 date is possible. He published extensively on medical topics and died in 1775. Munk, *Roll,* 2: 108.

1730s.[40] He explained his modest mission in his 1747 *Compendium of the Practice of Physick: or the Heads of a System of Practical Physick contained in twenty-four lectures.* Graeme and Lobb wrote as entrepreneurs on the fringes of London medical circles. Indeed, Graeme made a point of his marginal status. He was not a member of the Royal College of Physicians of London, he told his readers, but the College had no jurisdiction over teaching.[41] Graeme forthrightly asserted that attending a university – at least an *English* university – did not suffice to make a good practitioner. According to Graeme, those "young Gentlemen, just come from Universities where a System of Physick is taught," were particularly inept. They "have believed themselves sufficiently qualified to practice in every Case," but, as "we know from daily Experience," soon discovered otherwise if they had any sense. Some universities abroad provided excellent training, of course, but Graeme invoked the specter of Continental competition to emphasize that young physicians should be spending their money at home.[42]

Neither Graeme nor Lobb even hinted that attending London lectures could replace a medical degree for a physician. They aimed, instead, to detach physic from universities and their lackeys, the physician-elites who kept medical knowledge difficult and unnecessarily obscure, but without then reducing it to quackery or easy self-care. Graeme noted that critics disliked his decision to lecture in English, not in Latin. He belittled those who feared that "the Mysteries of the Profession were liable to be laid too open, the Honor of it lessened, and the whole exposed to too many People."[43] Rather, he countered, serious lectures would show the "lazy" how difficult physic really was. So, unlike the few lectures on physic already given in the metropolis, such as those presented in Latin at the Royal College of Physicians, Graeme "exposed" physic in a course for any beginner, and welcomed surgeons to attend.[44] Similarly, Lobb lectured to bring his expertise not only to "Young Physicians," but also to "Apothecaries and Surgeons" and "other Gentlemen." He *published* his lectures,

40 Lobb took the LRCP in 1740, and soon started offering courses. He died in London in 1763; Munk, *Roll*, 2: 146–7.
41 William Graeme, *An Essay on the Method of Acquiring Knowledge in Physick* (London: Lawton Gulliver, 1729), 28.
42 Graeme, *An Essay*, 16, 22–5, 53.
43 Graeme, *An Essay*, 28–35, 47–9; quotation p. 47. Graeme never became a member of the London RCP, although he claimed that he would (p. 28), but he was a member of the Royal College of Physicians of Edinburgh. He had his "foreign degree" recognized by a "University in the Kingdom," but I have been unable to discover where he obtained his MD.
44 Graeme, *An Essay*, 3–10, 19–26. Graeme also mentioned the occasional lectures on physic given at Greshem College (p. 19). For Gresham College, see William Maitland, *The History of London from its foundation to the Present Time*, 2 vols. (London: T. Osborne and J. Shipton, 1756), 2: 805–13.

however, in order to help "Gentlemen and Others, who live remote from any Physician," to "escape the pernicious Effects of complying with mistaken Advices."[45] His text places a ghostly physician at the bedside as an assistant to, not as a substitute for, regular medical practitioners. Later physician–authors of domestic medical manuals, such as the well-known William Buchan, refined this voice of the friendly confidant who knew when to direct a reader to qualified practitioners.[46] In multiple senses, then, these lecturers could claim that they gave learned physic to audiences previously denied it.

If unmasking the "Mysteries of the Profession" were the primary goal, then writing plain books would do. Both Graeme and Lobb tried to establish the lecturer's unique role in disseminating good knowledge. For them, only a lecturer could adequately straddle the lines between books and bedsides. A lecturer could "render things plainer," Graeme argued, and provide a basis for the perceptions and judgment that the beginner then took to the patient. Graeme had a problem here, for he noted that critics claimed he was too young and too marginal to have much of his own to say. He carefully pointed out that he taught by combining the best information from well-respected texts, especially Boerhaave's, hence giving the neophyte a useful tour through competing ideas and therapies. Lobb, too, had "read different Systems." He had "daily prayed, that God would be pleased to direct, assist and succeed me [*sic*] in my Studies; and guide my Thoughts in them, and communicate to me that Wisdom, which was a necessary means for successful Practice."[47] Having had such help, Lobb confidently recommended his course "especially [to] those who have but little Time for the Reading Books [*sic*], [and] would be glad of such Assistance." No book could replace a lecturer, Lobb went on, "who has long practiced [medicine], and is capable of Answering questions, and solving Difficulties about it."[48]

Graeme and Lobb undermined the sufficiency of books for those either too ignorant or too learned to recognize the dangers of taking a "System"

45 Lobb, *Compendium*, ix–x. The knowledgeable patient, in his view, can deal with the misguided apothecary using the physician-in-the-book, but only in lieu of a practitioner as well informed as Lobb. Lobb gives explicit examples on how the lay person could respond to unwanted advice. A pregnant woman afraid of miscarrying might find her apothecary recommending bleeding. She was to answer, "I cannot approve of such Advice; I never want Blood so much as when I am in this Condition; and for me to have it diminished, will only render me, and the Child I go with weaker" (pp. x–xi).
46 Charles Rosenberg, "Medical Text and Social Context: Explaining William Buchan's *Domestic Medicine*," *Bulletin of the History of Medicine* 57 (1983): 22–42; Ginnie Smith, "Prescribing the Rules of Health: Self-Help and Advice in the Late-Eighteenth Century," in *Patients and Practitioners: Lay Perceptions of Medicine in Pre-Industrial Society*, ed. Roy Porter (Cambridge: Cambridge University Press, 1985), 249–82.
47 Lobb, *Compendium*, iii, v.
48 Lobb, *Compendium*, vi–vii, iii; and see his notice in *The General Advertiser*, 11 Aug. 1749.

too literally in practice. But what, then, of those who believed that physic was "only to be learned by attending the sick, and making Observations on the Course of their Diseases"? Both of these authors welcomed – even urged – apothecaries and surgeons who "undertake to advise for the cure of internal Diseases" to attend their lectures.[49] A student unacquainted with medical theory "cannot be the better for what he sees [at the bedside], but rather the worse," Graeme protested. He called upon physicians' common arguments against untutored empiricism, labeling the rational foundations of physic "a science" and stressing the efficiency of building upon what was already known in understanding illness.[50] Lobb similarly stressed the importance of knowing "Principles" and the abstract "Nature of Causes" to truly treat disease.[51] "The Patient's Bed-side is not a convenient place for such a System to be taught," Graeme observed.[52] Lectures were the best way to address these deficiencies.[53]

Graeme and Lobb needed to justify lectures on physic in London because such innovative ventures lacked conventional credibility. Their arguments – presuming that they were even read – did not convince many aspiring practitioners or lecturers to crowd immediately into London class-rooms, since so few physician–entrepreneurs advertised courses before the 1760s. What Graeme and Lobb envisioned, nevertheless, underlay physicians' continuing efforts to offer courses, and the later incorporation of lectures on physic as a regular part of the London curriculum. These London lecturers met head-on the continuing tension between understanding abstract principles and treating the individual sick person, especially if lecturers were open to interrogation about their own practice. Apothecaries and surgeons learned medical systems from those whose experience lay with books as well as patients, but without needing to matriculate at a university. Becoming a "good" medical practitioner demanded guidance through *both* theoretical and experiential realms of expertise; and paying pupils ultimately agreed that lecturers were indeed efficient synthesizers and critics of knowledge.

Anatomy

Learning anatomy, like learning physic, had a long textual and erudite lineage, as well as a perceptual and pragmatic one. For centuries in Europe

---

49 Lobb, *Compendium*, vi.
50 Graeme, *An Essay*, 3–10, 19.
51 Lobb, *Compendium*, iv.
52 Graeme, *An Essay*, 10.
53 For an argument that lectures were far too superficial, and led the "poor *mistaken Pupil*" to believe he actually knew something, see William Douglass, *A Letter to Dr Smelle* [sic]

and in Britain, university lecturers and authors had discoursed on the physical and philosophical attributes of the human body, describing the organs and systems relevant to medicine while enthusing over their divine designs and functions. Public dissections at universities (mostly on the Continent), carried out by anatomically inclined physicians or surgeons, displayed body parts through rituals that made specific corpses into medical objects.[54] Similarly, various surgeons' companies acquired social and legal sanction to dissect certain bodies in order to prepare apprentices for their craft. By the late seventeenth century in Britain, talking and reading about human anatomy did not upset the literate, if indeed armchair study of human parts had ever seemed offensive. Cutting up corpses, however, remained socially and medically contained. Those who believed that disease left meaningful organic signs accepted autopsies, especially those performed at the request of family and friends who hoped that investigating causes of death would prove useful to the living.[55] Dissecting a dead person simply to learn about normal anatomical structures, however, had strict boundaries.

As I explained in Chapter 3, anatomy teachers in early-eighteenth-century London encountered corporate rights and lay concerns over the access to the human corpses they needed to dismember and display. Only the Barber–Surgeons' Company, the Royal College of Physicians, and the Royal Society of London technically had any right to the bodies of executed criminals, although by the early 1700s the Royal College of Physicians and Royal Society rarely pressed for corpses.[56] While the Barber–Surgeons jealously guarded their near-monopoly over the bodies obtained at executions, the company had no mandate to police either general lectures that did not involve dissection or the private use of other (that is, illegal) human material.[57] Instead, they had the right to present public anatomies organized around the full dissection of a criminal's corpse, to authorize private anatomies on other felons' bodies if available, and to protect *those*

Shewing the Impropriety of his New invented Wooded Forceps; as also the Absurdity of his Method of Teaching and Practicing Midwifery (London: J. Roberts, 1748), 14–17 (quotation p. 15, original emphasis).

54 Jan C. C. Rupp, "Matters of Life and Death: The Social and Cultural Conditions of the Rise of Anatomical Theatres, with Special Reference to Seventeenth Century Holland," *History of Science* 28 (1990): 263–87.

55 Robert L. Martensen, " 'Habits of Reason': Anatomy and Anglicanism in Restoration England," *Bulletin of the History of Medicine* 66 (1992): 511–35.

56 For references to early anatomy teaching by physicians, see George Norman Clark, *A History of the Royal College of Physicians of London*, 3 vols. (Oxford: Clarendon Press for the Royal College of Physicians, 1962–1972), 1: 85, 256, 264.

57 See the minutes of the Court of Assistants, 25 Mar. 1714/15 in John Flint South, *Memorials of the Craft of Surgery in England*, ed. D'Arcy Power (London, New York: Cassell & Co., 1886), 233, n. 2.

privileges in London.[58] Anatomy instructors could offer extramural
courses, in short, only if they avoided compromising the Company's state-
sanctioned license to dissect human corpses. Whatever dissection occurred
in secret – always a tempting area of speculation – the ways anatomical
teaching became public through newspaper advertisements for courses reveal the social and corporate acceptance of human anatomy as an appropriate subject for lay curiosity and professional betterment.

The distinction between lecturing about the body and actually dissecting
fresh corpses strongly shaped the emergence of private anatomy teaching in
eighteenth-century London. This would be an easy and obvious historical
dichotomy except that lecturers promised to *demonstrate* anatomy during
their courses.[59] As already noted, several of the early anatomy instructors –
notably Cheselden and Hauksbee – promoted anatomy as an entertaining
and enlightening subject of natural philosophy. Just as natural philosophers
and chemists presented machines and experiments to embed their statements in material displays of "facts," so too did anatomists promise visual
confirmation of their verbal descriptions. Indeed, a few rather sensationalist
entrepreneurs advertised exhibits of "monsters" and wax models, such as
Chovet's "New figure of Anatomy, which represents a woman chained
down upon a table, suppos'd opened alive," in 1733.[60] While such sights
seemed aimed at a more popular audience than those paying for a series of
lectures, titillation probably had a place in creating a market even for
serious anatomists. In 1720, for instance, Nathaniel St. André vowed that
"all the modern discoveries will be shewn with the Doctrine of the Animal
Oeconomy demonstrated on a curious Collection of Preparations" in his
"Course of Human and Comparative Anatomy" without specifying
whether his "curious" pieces included human parts.[61] Throughout the later

58 From the start of the eighteenth century, but probably well before, the Barber–Surgeons'
   Company had sheltered "private" anatomies for members. George Rolfe, in 1701, and
   Nathaniel Smith, in 1708, for instance, were among those with early newspaper notices
   for private anatomy lectures, and they gave them *at* Surgeons' Hall. Peachey, *Memoir*, 12,
   14. A Dr. Connor appears to have been the first private anatomy teacher in London,
   giving a course in 1697. His notices have not been found in newspapers, however.
   Cunningham, "The Kinds of Anatomy," 14.
59 In 1703, George Rolfe advertised "a complete Course of Anatomy on Humane Bodies" to
   be given "at his house." His announcement is one of the earliest to appear in London's
   newspapers and mentioned neither dissection nor demonstrations. Peachey, *Memoir*, 12–
   19; *The Daily Courant*, 9 Sept. 1703; James Earle reported that "Mr. Nourse was one of
   the few who then gave anatomical lectures [ca. 1729]; his school was at London-house, in
   Aldersgate-street; and Mr. Pott was employed in preparing the subjects for demonstration." Presumably these were human subjects. James Earle, "A Short Account of the Life
   of the Author," in *Chirurgical Works of Percival Pott*, 3 vols. (London: J. Johnson, 1790),
   1: viii.
60 Quoted from the *London Evening Post*, 27 Dec. 1733, in Peachey, *Memoir*, 30.
61 *Daily Courant*, 21 Feb. 1719/20; Peachey, *Memoir*, 12, 14, 20, 28, 34; *Daily Courant*, 5 Oct.
   1721; see also *The Art of Dissecting the Human Body in a plain, easy and compendious Method*,
   translated from Lyserus by G. Thompson (London: Joseph Davidson, 1740) advertised in

1720s and 1730s, newspaper readers knew that inquisitive folk could see specimens of (human?) bones, organs, and flesh in lecturers' chambers as they heard about the human body's forms and functions.

As William Graeme noted matter-of-factly in his pamphlet on teaching physic, discussing and demonstrating anatomical information in lectures did not suffice to make an anatomist. *Really* learning anatomy was "best done by attending Dissections, and working with one's own Hands."[62] Graeme did not specify where, when, or upon what sorts of dead creatures the student could use his "own Hands." Vague references from the 1720s and 1730s show that, while anatomists limited their public advertisements to benign-sounding lectures, students could gain experience dissecting if they belonged to the right circles.[63] Nathaniel St. André came closest to revealing the existence of two sorts of anatomy courses available outside the Barber–Surgeons' Hall. In a 1721 advertisement, as in the one for 1720, St. André announced his "Course of Human and Comparative Anatomy" to all comers. He continued, however,

Mr. St. André will also give a Private Course of Anatomy in which he will demonstrate the Method of Dissection, Preparations, Mounting of Skeletons, &c. NB The Skeletons already bought will be ready to be delivered at the end of the Publick Course.[64]

Learning how to be a do-it-oneself anatomist clearly took place in "Private," demarcating such experience from the "Publick" display of anatomical knowledge that St. André provided on Northumberland Court, near Charing Cross. Once again, nevertheless, the notice refrained from promising practice on human parts.

With the apparent success and popularity of private teaching established in London during the 1700s to 1730s, anatomists became more explicit about access to dissecting experience. In 1740, William Hewitt advertised "a Course of Anatomy . . . at his house in Leicester-fields, where all pupils will have the advantage to dissect and prepare with directions and assis-

---

the *London Daily Post and Advertiser*, 4 Feb. 1739/40. In his notice for his course on anatomy and surgery in 1721, John Douglas proclaimed that he would demonstrate "the new method of cutting for stone" answering "all objections" to it. He promised to show "3 persons in whom I have already performed this operation, whose wounds are not only perfectly healed, but they themselves in as good a state of health, as if they had never had the stone." Quoted from a *Postboy* advertisement in Peachey, *Memoir*, 22–3.

62 Graeme, *An Essay*, 32–3. In this discussion, Graeme remarked that he included anatomy in his course on physic, but taught it from figures, drawings, and textual descriptions.

63 Peachey, *Memoir*, 14; Toby Gelfand, "The 'Paris Manner' of Dissection: Student Anatomical Dissection in Early Eighteenth-Century Paris," *Bulletin of the History of Medicine* 46 (1972): 101–2, nn. 11, 15. For contemporary comments on the importance of dissection to surgeons learning anatomy, see Peter Linebaugh, "The Tyburn Riot against the Surgeons," in *Albion's Fatal Tree*, ed. Douglas Hay, et al. (New York: Pantheon, 1975), 70–2.

64 *Daily Courant*, 5 Oct. 1721. Peachey described this advertisement in *Memoirs*, 20–21, but without noting the connection to a "publick" course.

tance in everything of a difficult nature in making their own preparations."
Mr. Vitrack "proposes to give courses on the method of dissecting the
human body" in which "beginners" would have "the opportunity to dissect
with their own hands."[65] In the autumn of 1746, William Hunter published
the well-known notice of his course, in which he promised that "Gentlemen may have the opportunity of learning the Art of Dissecting during the
whole winter season in the same manner as at Paris."[66] This euphemistic
phrase referred, as only contemporaries conscious of French practice knew,
to the ease with which students in the rival capital could practice dissection
on human corpses, not just see the parts demonstrated by a lecturer or
develop skills on animals. His advertisement, however, revealed no more
than Hewitt's or Vitrack's about what it meant to learn to dissect. It was
only through a letter from the anonymous "Publicus" to the *Westminster
Journal* a few months later that browsing readers discovered that a "gentleman," imitating the Parisians, "provid[ed] each of his pupils with one
entire body" to cut up during the course. According to Publicus, each of
London's anatomy teachers already needed to have "at least one fresh body
once a week."[67]

Hunter's and his competitors' apparent boldness in openly offering anatomy courses with dissection followed upon the separation of the Barbers
from the Surgeons in 1745. The new Surgeons' Company maintained its
rights over criminals' corpses, but omitted references to jurisdiction over
private anatomies. Whatever meager responsibility the previous Company
had had for extramural teaching evaporated. The private anatomy teachers'
use of corpses obtained illicitly thus could cast no shadows on the Company as a corporate entity. The Company, in turn, sustained the pleasing
public fiction that novice surgeons had sufficient exposure to dissected
humans in the Company's sanctioned space, with the traditional demonstrations of felons' bodies carried out in a few days of intense observation.
The company's laissez-faire stance nicely supported its members' entrepreneurial ventures, of course, especially during the absence of official anatomies between 1745 and 1752. While the Surgeons' Company built a new
theater, private courses were the only place where aspiring practitioners
could study dissected material.[68]

65 Quoted respectively from the *London Evening Post*, 18 Sept. 1740, and the *London Daily
Post*, 4 Nov. 1741, in Peachey, *Memoir*, 38, 40. Vitrack only advertised once, and Peachey
believed that "it seems likely that the intended teaching of practical dissection was forbidden by the Company" of Barber–Surgeons (p. 40). His conclusions, however, are noticeably underdetermined by the existing evidence.
66 Quoted from the *London Evening Post*, 16 Sept. 1746, in Peachey, *Memoir*, 80; Peachey
discusses Hunter's teaching at length. See also Gelfand, "The 'Paris Manner' "; Simmons
and Hunter, *Hunter*, 5, contrasts Hunter's course with those of his immediate rivals,
William Hewitt, William Bromfield, and Thomas Lawrence.
67 *Westminster Journal*, 20 Dec. 1746, quoted in Peachey, *Memoir*, 95–6. "Publicus" sounds
suspiciously like an anatomy lecturer championing such private teaching.
68 See Chapter 3.

By the 1750s private teachers had clearly developed a market for their lectures, as supplements and alternatives to the official anatomies seen at Surgeons' Hall or studied from anatomists' texts.[69] Newspapers carried advertisements for both "philosophical" and "practical" anatomy for the rest of the century. In the former, lecturers presented anatomy from the podium, using specimens to demonstrate the parts, interspersing more or less practical comments with their renditions of names, anatomical relationships, and nods to divine design. This was the genre that the Monros performed so well at the University of Edinburgh in the mid-eighteenth century, as Christopher Lawrence has discussed.[70] In the "practical" anatomy courses, London lecturers presided over dissection, directly or through assistants. Isaac Minors, in 1753, for example, promised that "those Gentlemen that enter for Dissection, &c. will be constantly attended by Mr. Minors, every morning during the whole Winter Season."[71] Such advertisements remained circumspect about precisely *what* students dissected, but it was probably not difficult to guess. While students could take either lectures or dissection, most instructors advertised these opportunities together. Intertwining academic presentation, visual demonstrations and hands-on experience gave the metropolis a reputation for anatomical instruction that neither British apprenticeship nor university courses could match. For all intents and purposes, moreover, neighbors and newspaper readers implicitly tolerated these business ventures. Whatever fears and revulsions beset Londoners at the thought of students' dissecting illicit corpses, the private system worked.[72]

Midwifery

A few lectures on midwifery, the third broad subject in London's de facto curriculum, appeared off and on during the first decades of the eighteenth century. Thomas Griffiths, for instance, announced that he would include "proper Lectures on the Art of Midwifery" in his 1739 anatomy course; Edmund Chapman, in an advertisement for his *A Treatise on the Improve-*

---

69 Peachey, *Memoir,* 12–13, 18, 47–8. Private courses could also last much longer than those at Surgeons' Hall. George Rolfe's lectures, for example, continued for about six weeks, meeting Mondays, Wednesdays, and Fridays. William Cheselden's, in the 1710s, took about two months. Lectures appealing directly to a lay audience could also last several weeks. Peter Macculloch's 1726 course, centered around John Sargeant's popular "wax figures," had three morning lectures a week for five weeks, while his 1727 class for "gentlemen" lasted six weeks (pp. 27–8). Dale Ingram, in contrast, in the course he claimed he started in 1743–4, sped through his "Anatomico-Chirurgical Lectures" in three weeks. *Lloyd's Evening Post and British Chronicle,* 29 Dec. 1758. At this time, Ingram noted that he limited his class to ten students.
70 C. Lawrence, "The Edinburgh Manner of Anatomy," 193–5.
71 *Public Advertiser,* 1 Sept. 1753.
72 Susan C. Lawrence, "Anatomy and Address: Creating Medical Gentlemen in Eighteenth Century London," in *The History of Medical Education in Britain,* ed. Vivian Nutton and Roy Porter (Amsterdam: Rodopi, 1995).

ment of Midwifery, noted that he "has undertaken the instruction of Gentlemen in the Art of Midwifery with good Success."[73] Historians have already produced an extensive literature on the emergence of men-midwives, their relationships with female practitioners, and their claims to improve the understanding and management of childbirth, but have rarely discussed how men learned the necessary skills.[74] Aspiring men-midwives had several texts to guide them, of course, as well as the potential instruction of raw experience, with or without masters and tutors.[75] In the early 1750s, however, courses on midwifery took off in London and became regular features of metropolitan medical training.

The timing is hardly coincidental. In the uprush of interest in the amelioration of social and economic conditions in the 1740s, philanthropists founded several lying-in charities to help deserving poor (married) women during childbirth. Medical men, such as Sir Richard Manningham (LRCP 1720 and knighted in 1721), who had made midwifery his specialty, championed such efforts. They blended arguments for saving women and infants through appropriate care with appeals to medical expertise, provided by female midwives with support from male practitioners in emergencies.[76] The apparent success of these charities, along with the growing reputations of male accoucheurs such as Manningham and William Smellie, enhanced the visibility of midwifery as a subject useful to those in general practice. Christopher Kelly, "one of the Men Midwives at the British Lying-in Hospital," for instance, encouraged "Gentlemen in the Practice of Physick or Surgery" to learn "this art" from him in 1757.[77] These lecturers thus competed with midwives not only by instructing men, but also by promoting the institutions that could reduce female practitioners' livelihoods among women of the lower orders.

Midcentury midwifery lecturers advertised demonstrations and clinical practice as key advantages in their courses. Indeed, in the newspapers of the 1750s and 1760s, midwifery lecturers drew the most explicit public connections between charitable service and teaching that appeared during

73 *London Daily Post and General Advertiser*, 1 Mar. 1739; 12 Aug. 1738; Peachey found earlier advertisements for John Maubray (1724) and Edmund Chapman (1736). *Memoirs*, 46.

74 For an introduction to this extensive subject, see Donnison, *Midwives and Medical Men*; Adrian Wilson, "William Hunter and the Varieties of Man-Midwifery," and Edward Shorter, "The Management of Normal Deliveries and the Generation of William Hunter," both in Bynum and Porter, *William Hunter*, 343–84; Judith Leavitt, *Brought to Bed: Childbearing in America, 1750–1950* (New York: Oxford University Press, 1986).

75 Many announcements for midwifery texts appear in the newspapers. See, for example, the *Daily Courant*, 4 Jan. 1704/5, for notice of an English version of Paul Portal's book, *The Compleat Practice of Men and Women Mid-wives, or the true manner of Assisting a Woman in Child-bearing: Illustrated with a considerable Number of Observations . . . Adorn'd with many Copper Plates* (London: S. Crouch, 1705).

76 Donna T. Andrew, *Philanthropy and Police: London Charity in the Eighteenth Century* (Princeton, NJ: Princeton University Press, 1989), 65–9; *General Advertiser*, 21 Nov. 1744.

77 *Daily Advertiser*, 1 Jan. 1757.

the entire century. Notices that announced "machinery, on which the various Cases that occur in Practice, are very naturally represented" became commonplace in the 1750s.[78] Christopher Kelly promised that he would demonstrate "the most respectful method" on the machine, which would then "be repeated by each Pupil, whereby the truest ideas thereof are imprinted on the memory." Yet Kelly's final enticement was that "opportunities of seeing and performing the real practices are plentifully provided."[79] Felix Macdonough claimed that he would "advance nothing but what may be indisputably demonstrated on the natural Subject by every individual Student . . . at the Lying-in Hospital, St. James."[80] Lecturing men without connections to the new hospitals exploited personal charity for suitable patients. William Smellie, for instance, let students practice on women who went to him for free care, although he does not seem to have advertised that opportunity.[81] In contrast, the surgeon John Martin announced, in conjunction with his midwifery course, that at his apartments "constant attendance is given, and where poor women are desired to apply, who may expect the greatest Humanity and Encouragement."[82] For the newspaper-reading public, these lecturers overtly intertwined learning the principles of childbirth from the lectern with pupils' practice of midwifery on the poor.

A new business established

The appearance and establishment of courses on physic, anatomy, and midwifery during the first five decades of the century illustrate some of the common strategies and practices of these market-driven enterprises. Similar stories could be outlined for lectures on medical chemistry, the materia medica, and surgery. At various points between the 1750s and 1770s, what had been innovations – lectures on physic, student dissection, pupils practicing midwifery on the poor – became conventions in London's ad hoc curriculum of private teaching. Throughout this process, lecturers made technical medical knowledge accessible to open audiences of aspiring

78 *Daily Advertiser*, 25 Aug. 1753; for other midwifery lecturers' advertisements promising "machines," see *Daily Advertiser*, 31 July, 19 Oct. 1754.
79 *Daily Advertiser*, 25 Aug. 1753.
80 *Daily Advertiser*, 9 July 1754.
81 Richard Kay, *Diary;* William Smellie, *A Treatise on the Theory and Practice of Midwifery*, 2nd ed., 2 vols. (London: D. Wilson and T. Durham, 1752), 1: i–vi. Smellie claimed that "one thousand one hundred and fifty poor women have been delivered in presence [sic] of those who attended me; and supported during their lying-in, by the stated collections of my pupils: over and above those difficult cases to which we were often called by midwives, for the relief of the indigent" (p. v). See, too, William Douglass's criticism in *A Letter to Dr Smelle*, esp. 14–15.
82 *Daily Advertiser*, 25 Aug. 1755; see also Hugh Crawford's advertisement in the *Daily Advertiser*, 19 Oct. 1754.

practitioners and curious laity – but not *too* accessible. Courses cost money and took time, usually lasting for weeks or months of daily or thrice-weekly meetings. Medical lecturers, moreover, simply did not advertise quick routes for the layperson to become his or her own physician, surgeon, or apothecary. They primarily sold occupational improvement, not self-help, even when they welcomed other gentlemen into their rooms to gain knowledge about nature or the complexities of disease and treatment.

Not only was private medical lecturing well established by 1760, it was also socially visible through the newspapers that carried course advertisements. Unlike the syllabi and books that lecturers published, newspaper notices clearly displayed medical courses as commodities – and opportunities – to the vast majority of Londoners with little interest in taking them. Private teaching clearly went on in the early eighteenth century, as it likely had for centuries before, when neophytes gathered for discussions, dissections, and consultations with those more experienced, whether masters or physician–patrons. Publicly advertised private teaching, however, informed the literate (and their circles of gossips) that practitioners, including *their* practitioners, could acquire medical knowledge from experts, several of whom promised "demonstrations," "machines," or "curious Preparations." Such notices, moreover, displayed Londoners' tacit toleration of human dissection and the use of charity patients for pupils' training, as they appeared season after season and year after year. The fundamental social and occupational acceptance of lecturing entrepreneurs and their marketing strategies enabled the London "system" to flourish for the rest of the century.

BODIES AND BUSINESSES: HOSPITAL LECTURING, 1760–1820

The number of private lecturers, the extent of their courses, and the organization of their businesses expanded and evolved in the later eighteenth century with few innovations – except for the fact that hospital staff men took private lecturing right onto the grounds of their charitable institutions. Lecturing medical men in London sought paying audiences to support their ventures. Giving lectures *at* a hospital where students walked the wards seems, in retrospect, such an obvious means to entice pupils and to promote "advancement" in medical education that the introduction and growth of on-site lecturing have inspired little curiosity over just how staff men managed this novel feat.

The introduction of lectures into the hospitals, like the introduction of ward-walking, depended upon a reconceptualization of the purposes of charity care. By the 1760s, the general hospitals' staff men and governors all more or less agreed that it was appropriate for short-term pupils to observe poor patients for their edification. Catering to pupils by allowing lectures on hospital grounds, however, was quite another matter. Staff men and governors across the metropolis responded differently to concerns about dissection and to local lecturing markets during the eighteenth century. Whatever motivated specific decisions about hospital lecturing, its uneven introduction suggests the range of social and occupational negotiations involved in grafting academic medical education onto these eighteenth-century institutions.

Tables 5.3 and 5.4 summarize the chronological and geographical distribution of medical lecturing at the general hospitals. Evidence for early hospital lectures is much more indirect than that for courses announced in the newspapers. Only Richard Kay's brief notes, taken when he was a pupil at Guy's in 1743–4, for example, reveal that Samuel Sharp, surgeon to Guy's, and John Girle, surgeon to St. Thomas's, gave lectures at these hospitals. John Harrison, surgeon to the London, received his fellow governors' permission to lecture at the hospital – subject unknown – in 1749, but he did not put notices in the newspapers for it.[83] Only one lecturer appears to have advertised a course at a hospital before the 1760s. In 1734, Edward Nourse, assistant surgeon to St. Bartholomew's, announced that his class on anatomy and surgery would take place at the hospital. The governors rescinded their approval the next summer, however, and Nourse returned to teaching off-site.[84]

Before midcentury, the only staff men who lectured either at the general hospitals or outside them were hospital surgeons. No hospital physicians in London, except the physician–accoucheurs of lying-in charities, deigned to give courses on physic, chemistry, or the materia medica until two Edinburgh graduates, Hugh Smith and Donald Monro, combined lecturing with hospital service in 1757–8.[85] Having hospital *physicians* willing to

---

83 Similarly, in 1768, the surgeon George Neale received permission to "make use of the room (formerly the Physicians' room) to read lectures to his pupils," and no advertisements have been found for his course. London Hospital, House Committee Minutes, 17 Oct. 1749, 30 Aug. 1768, LH/A/5/3,8, London Hospital Archives; Clark-Kennedy, *The London,* 1: 103, was incorrect in dating Harrison's permission to 1743.

84 Thornton, "The Medical College," 46; Peachey, *Memoir,* 34–5, discusses Nourse's advertisements; Moore, *St. Bartholomew's,* 2: 364.

85 For Hugh Smith at the Middlesex, see Middlesex Hospital, Minutes of the Weekly Board, Court of Governors, 28 June, 4 Aug. 1757; *Daily Advertiser,* 18 Sept. 1760. For Donald Monro, see his Lectures on the Practice of Physick, 2 vols., 1758, NLM MS B47. Monro does not appear to have advertised his lectures in the newspapers. Three physicians who lectured in London in the 1750s ceased advertising courses before they were elected to general hospital posts: Andrew Didier (MD Aberdeen) lectured on materia medica and physic from 1753 to 1755, the year he was elected physician to the Middlesex; James Greive (MD Edinburgh) advertised a chemistry course in 1753 but appears to have given up teaching years before his election to physician at St. Thomas's; Michael Morris (MD Rheims) offered chemistry courses from 1754 to 1757. He was elected physician to the Westminster in 1761.

Table 5.3. *Lectures at the London hospitals, 1760-1820*

Hospital	Known in/from	First advertised	Lecture theater/school
St. Thomas's			1765(?)
Surgery	1710s?	1765	"New theatre," 1775
Anatomy	1730s?	1765	New theater, 1813
Practical anatomy	1760s		
Guy's			1770(?)
[Anatomy (?)	1743]		"New theatre," 1777
Physic		1770	[Advertised
Materia Medica		1770	as "school"
Chemistry		1770	in 1807]
Midwifery		1785	
Physiology		1792	
The London			1782
Surgery	1749?	1782	[Joint advertisements
Anatomy		1782	1782-1807]
Practical anatomy		1802	
Physic		1782	
Materia Medica		1782	
Chemistry		1783	
Midwifery		1785	
St. Bartholomew's			1791
Surgery	1734/1767	1791	
Anatomy	1734/1767	1791	
Practical anatomy	1790s	1805	
Physic		1791	
Materia Medica		1791	
Chemistry		1791	
Midwifery		1791	
Comparative anatomy		1801	
The Middlesex			[A theater for pupils is
Physic	1757?	1809[a]	mentioned in the
Materia Medica		1817[a]	Governors' Minutes, 1796[b]]
Chemistry	1796?	1820[a]	["Middlesex Hospital
Midwifery		1812[a]	Medical School"
			established in 1835]

Table 5.3 (*cont.*)

Hospital	Known in/from	First advertised	Lecture theater/school
The Westminster			["Westminster
Surgery		1794[a]	Hospital Medical
Physic		1794[a]	School" established
Materia Medica		1794[a]	in 1840-1]
Chemistry		1794[a]	
St. George's			["Medical School"
No on-site lectures advertised			established in 1831]

[a] The dates for "first advertised" do not mark the start of continuous course offerings at the Westminster or the Middlesex.
[b] Middlesex Hospital, Minutes of the . . . Governors, 19 Jan. 1796.
Sources: See Appendix III; Richard Kay, *The Diary of Richard Kay, 1716-51, of Baldinstone, near Bury, A Lancaster Doctor*, eds. W. Brockbank and F. Kenworthy (Manchester: Chetham Society, 1968), 68-88; Norman Moore, *The History of St. Bartholomew's Hospital* (London: C. A. Pearson, 1918), 2: 364; J. Blomfield, *St. George's 1733-1933* (London: Medici Society, 1933), 31; R. R. James, *The School of Anatomy and Medicine Adjoining St. George's Hospital* (London: private printing, George Pullman & Sons, 1928); H. Campbell Thomson, *The Story of Middlesex Hospital Medical School* (London: John Murray, 1935), 1.

give courses enhanced the status of such ventures in the metropolis. The dates shown in Table 5.3 imply that physicians' involvement very likely influenced governors' and staffs' acceptance of newspaper advertisements for on-site lecturing. While the surgeons at St. Thomas's took the initiative to announce their courses in 1765, public notices for medical instruction at Guy's, the London, St. Bartholomew's, and, albeit briefly, the Westminster, all started when staff physicians, not just surgeons, wanted to teach on-site.

At the charities located in the City (St. Bartholomew's), in Southwark (St. Thomas's and Guy's), and in Whitechapel (the London), staff men established ongoing hospital lecturing between the 1760s and the 1790s (Table 5.4). These partnerships gradually dominated medical lecturing in the City and eastern parishes; relatively few entrepreneurs competed with them at separate premises between the 1790s and 1820, and none of these was a staff man. In contrast, at the three hospitals in the West End, St. George's, the Middlesex, and the Westminster, the staff rarely lectured on the premises, although at least one or more hospital physicians and surgeons gave courses, sometimes for years, off the hospital grounds. Non-hospital lecturers and lecturing flourished around the West End hospitals, attracting the pupils who walked their wards. Only in the 1830s did the

Table 5.4. *Geographical distribution of medical lectures in London: 1760, 1780, 1814, 1825*

	1760[a]		1780[a]		1814[a]		1825[b]	
	Hospital	Other	Hospital	Other	Hospital	Other	Hospital	Other
Central/Eastern London								
City	0	4	0	5	6	6	7	7
Southwark	0	1	3	1	7	0	14	8
Whitechapel	0	0	0	0	4	0	7	0
Central/Eastern subtotal	0	100% (5)	33% (3)	67% (6)	74% (17)	26% (6)	65% (28)	35% (15)
Western London	0	100% (5)	0	100% (6)	5% (1)	95% (20)	7% (3)	93% (42)
Total	0	100% (10)	20% (3)	80% (12)	40% (18)	60% (26)	35% (31)	65% (57)

Sources:
[a]Compiled from newspaper advertisements in London daily papers (autumn season only); see Appendix III.
[b]Compiled from the report on medical schools and lecturers in the *Lancet*, 1 October 1825.

governors and staff men of these eighteenth-century charities create schools
on (or close to) hospital property.[86]

Just why medical lecturing took hold in the City/East End hospitals in
the eighteenth century, but not in the West End ones until the nineteenth
century, remains only partially answered by hospital sources. In general,
the governors' minutes – more by what they do not say than by what
they do – suggest that disagreements and competition among the staff–
governors themselves undercut moves toward administrative consensus
about on-site lecturing in the West End charities during the few occasions
when hospital-based lectures were even broached in the boardrooms. The
market dynamics of entrepreneurial medical lecturing were as important as
staff rivalries, moreover, since lecturers outside a hospital's walls could
maintain a loyal following among pupils walking the wards at different
institutions. According to his friend Dr. Hawes, for example, Hugh
Smith – physician to the Middlesex – moved his lecturing location in 1760,
when "the pupils of St. George's Hospital, in conjunction with many
medical gentlemen, respectfully intreated the Doctor to deliver his course
at the West end of the town."[87]

From midcentury on, many lecturers probably sought to give courses in
the western parts of London to associate their enterprises with the more
genteel regions of the metropolis. William Hunter's lavish investment in
his home and anatomy theater on Great Windmill Street in 1768 illustrates
this conjunction of practice among the upper ranks, a reasonably up-scale
address, and medical lecturing to gentlemen pupils. Hospital men, notably
John Hunter and Dr. George Pearson of St. George's, and John Sheldon,
surgeon to the Middlesex, similarly invested in off-site premises in the
West End for their teaching. Their choices reveal that having their own
facilities in areas where other lecturers gave courses on diverse medical
subjects outweighed the purported advantages of linking their lectures to
hospital locations and hospital colleagues.

The interplay among the charities' governors, the staff men's businesses,
and the success of off-site lecturing underlies three aspects of London
hospital teaching explored in the rest of this section. First, while ward-
walking allowed pupils to study the living poor, access to their corpses was
much more problematic. Looking at anatomy teaching shows how the
connections between governors' moderate support of hospital instruction
and their concerns for charitable propriety worked in different ways across

86 S. Lawrence, "Entrepreneurs and Private Enterprise."
87 Hugh Smith, *Formulae Medicamentorum Concinnatae: or, Elegant Medical Prescriptions . . . to
which is prefix'd a sketch of his Life* (London: J. S. Barr, 1791), ii. In this account, Smith
moved to the Piazza Coffee-House in Covent Garden. If he had been lecturing at the
Middlesex in 1757 (see n. 85), then he moved from what was then a spot on the northwest-
ern edge of the metropolitan area to a more central location, although strictly speaking he
moved southeast toward the City.

the metropolis. Second, examining when and how governors allowed lecturing to proceed on-site, especially with the construction of purpose-built lecture theaters, shows how formal medical education was imbued with a charitable purpose and hence seen as appropriate to hospital interests. Third, while anatomical instruction and lecture courses entered the hospitals as fairly straightforward instances of private teaching in new places, once established there, hospital lecturing acquired institutional foundations and prestige. As hospital men began advertising collectively, with the hospital location headlined over the individual lecturers' names, they began to invest in institutional, rather than simply personal, reputations. By the 1820s, the hospital lecturer stepped to the podium with an authority increasingly built into the position he filled, whatever his background, demonstrable skills, or expertise in practice.

Anatomy at the hospitals

People died in hospitals. The newspaper-reading public for the most part overlooked how anatomy lecturers obtained the bodies they used for demonstration material and student practice in private theaters and dissecting rooms, but hospitals were an obvious source. The simple deduction that the corpses of the sick poor, separated from friends and relatives within institutional walls, might end up on anatomists' tables provoked an inestimable anxiety among the objects, observers, and patrons of charitable care.[88] Considering the extremely fragmentary evidence about how Londoners expressed such concerns, constructing the story of anatomy teaching *in* the hospitals demands extra caution. Hospital lecturers and pupils certainly dissected hospital corpses; hospital governors definitely passed rules about access to dead bodies. Yet how much the governors actually knew or cared about what students did, much less how much attention the staff and students routinely paid to the regulations, remains obscure. Many possible motives and conditions led governors to make rules but not necessarily to enforce them. Outright ignorance of hospital dissection, tacit tolerance in exchange for discretion, and accommodation to the claims of medical education instead of to patients' fears and outsiders' squeamishness allowed staff, pupils, and governors to work around their sometimes conflicting views on what to do with the dead.

The distinction between "philosophical" and "practical" anatomy that I have discussed is important for understanding references to anatomical instruction in the hospitals throughout the eighteenth century. Richard Kay, the note-taking Guy's pupil, wrote in his diary for 5 October 1743 that he had attended the "weekly Anatomical Lectures" at "the Hospitals."

88 Fissell, *Patients, Power and the Poor*, 14, 162–70; Ruth Richardson, *Death, Dissection and the Destitute* (London: Routledge and Kegan Paul, 1987), 75–99.

(He referred to St. Thomas's and Guy's together, a common locution for these neighboring institutions.) Throughout his visit, Kay jotted down the lecturers' topics: "Mr. Girle lectur'd to us upon the Eye," "Mr. Sharp lectur'd to us upon the Bones." On 9 November, however, Kay first noted, "Mr. Sharp lectur'd to us upon a dead Corpse." Two days later, he remarked, "Mr. Girle lectured to us upon a leg that he took off Yesterday."[89] Significantly, Kay did not refer to seeing corpses or parts in conjunction with the topical lectures, so Sharp and Girle may have talked about the body's parts without much (if any) demonstrating.[90] Similarly, Kay never specified that Sharp or Girle presented an anatomical *topic* when lecturing over corpses or limbs. Instead, these discourses appear to have occurred when material was available, suggesting that they were prompted in part by looking for the manifestations of disease involved in causes of death and disease, rather than being designed to display normal structures or to illustrate surgical procedures.

Surgeons probably first openly used dead patients for teaching purposes in conjunction with permission to perform autopsies.[91] From the beginning of the eighteenth century, the governors at St. Thomas's allowed staff physicians and surgeons to open corpses to look for the cause of death when the medical men had reasons and the patient's family, friends, or a hospital officer agreed. They established procedures that supposedly ensured that the surgeons and students did not take bodies for mere dissection. In 1702, for example, the Court of Governors ruled that "none of the surgeons' young men or apprentices shall presume to open, dissect or dismember any dead patient and no surgeon [is] to do so without the treasurer's consent."[92] In 1730, the St. Thomas's governors provided a room specifically for postmortems, separate from the dead-house where bodies were laid out to be claimed by their friends. The governors' decision to allocate a separate room for autopsies shows that they endorsed such inspections, if screened from public view. This room could well have been where Kay heard Girle lecture "upon a dead Body."[93]

Concern for proper authorization and discretion, rather than for ways to police patients' corpses on their journeys from ward to dead-house to friends or a pauper burial, marks the governors' regulations and actions at the other London hospitals. In 1731, for example, the Guy's governors suspended Richard Beal, an apprentice to the surgeon Baker, from the hospital because he "had dissected a body or Bodys of one or more of the

---

89 Kay, *Diary*, 72–5.
90 Kay, *Diary*, 79, has the one exception to these generalizations. Kay noted for 2 Feb. 1744 that "Mr. Sharp lectur'd to us upon a Heart and Lungs."
91 Fissell, *Patients, Power and the Poor*, 140–4.
92 Quoted in Parsons, *St. Thomas's*, 2: 149. The Court of Governors reiterated this rule in 1752 (p. 209).
93 Parsons, *St. Thomas's*, 2: 186–7; Kay, *Diary*, 79.

Patients dying in this House without leave of the Physicians or Surgeons."[94] Presumably those with leave could perform dissections, although whether "dissection" here meant the study of normal anatomy or referred more narrowly to opening the body only for autopsy is open to speculation. In 1750, the St. Bartholomew's governors, "being of Opinion, that this Practice might conduce greatly to the Benefit of the Publick in General, and also of the Poor Patients hereafter to be admitted into this Hospital," agreed to the staff physicians' and surgeons' formal request to open patients' bodies "to discover the Real Causes of their Death." They gave the hospital beadle responsibility to ensure that postmortems took place only in the presence of a staff man and that the body was then sewn up and placed in a coffin.[95] These last steps presumably deterred staff and students from taking away obviously large portions – the head, or a leg – for further dissection, but hardly precluded judicious removal of internal organs. If the body were completely shrouded or the coffin were to remain closed, of course, then hospital surgeon–anatomists (or others) could have taken more substantial portions of the corpse for student practice.

Some unusually explicit minutes from the Middlesex Hospital governors' meetings at midcentury show a further administrative reaction to the increasing popularity of anatomical studies. In 1758, the Middlesex governors ruled at a Weekly Board meeting that

no Pupil belonging to this Hospital, nor the Apothecary, House Pupil, or any other Person be permitted on pain of immediate Expulsion, to open the Body of any Patient dying in this Hospital, unless on very extraordinary Occassions & in the Presence of one of the [*1762 insert:* Physicians &] Surgeons, that they may see the same properly & decently performed, and that no part of the said deceased be taken away by any One on any Pretence whatsoever.[96]

Considering that two of the four staff surgeons, Isaac Minors and Henry Watson, were busy teaching anatomy at off-site locations, the governors probably had very good reason to suspect that hospital patients went to burial with parts missing. Henry Watson was present at the Weekly Board meeting, and if anyone knew what was going on, he did. Whether it was a warning *to* Watson and his colleagues, or Watson's own suggestion for appropriate control within the hospital, this statement shored up the distance between legitimate postmortem inspections and the possible use of bodies simply for student work.

Managing access to corpses remained an issue. At the 1758 meeting, the

94 Guy's Hospital, Court of Committees, 10 Mar. 1731, Greater London Record Office (GLRO) H9/GY/A3/1.
95 St. Bartholomew's Hospital, Journal of the Board of Governors, 19 Dec. 1750, Ha 1/12, St. Bartholomew's Hospital Archives, St. Bartholomew's Hospital.
96 Middlesex Hospital, Minutes of the . . . Governors, 22 Aug. 1758; the Quarterly General Court on 4 Feb. 1762 ruled that "the word Physicians be incerted [*sic*] immediately before the word surgeons."

governors entrusted the key to the "shell-house," where corpses were shrouded and held for removal by relatives, friends, or hospital burial attendants to the apothecary. The governors revised this practice early in 1762, placing the House Pupil in charge of the key. He then had orders "immediately on the decease of any Patient [to] inform the Physician or Surgeon to whom such Patient belong'd to know whether he thinks proper to Examine the Body." If so, the House Pupil had to tell the hospital Secretary, who would inform the patient's friends. "This & the former [1758] Order are to be understood & intended," the governors continued, "to take off any Odium that may be Thrown on the Hospital by the Younger part of the Faculty having any direction in these Affairs."[97] In 1771, the governors further ruled that when the patient's friends had agreed to a postmortem, "such Consent be given in Writing or before Witnesses."[98]

By the early 1760s, staff men in all the general hospitals had clear authority to request autopsies and to have pupils watch them. The governors' regulations may have circumscribed such procedures but did little more than ensure the patient's ultimate burial.[99] Any "odium" hospital governors feared rarely surfaced as a problem during the rest of the eighteenth century. At the Middlesex, St. George's, and the Westminster, the staff and governors basically avoided potential public awkwardness. Perhaps these hospital men had well-known but unwritten policies that forbade on-site teaching; at any rate, students found their anatomy lectures and dissection practice in the extramural theaters that flourished in the West End.[100] In the early nineteenth century, when the first printed notices for courses using body parts appeared in association with the Middlesex and St. George's, moreover, these distinctly centered on autopsy material. Richard Cartwright, for example, advertised a single course of "demon-

97 Middlesex Hospital, Minutes of the . . . Governors, 5 Jan., 4 Feb. 1762. What they meant by the "Younger part of the Faculty" is unclear, although they might have referred to James Moffat, elected surgeon on 1 Feb. 1759, who also taught anatomy off-site, or to the apothecary and house pupil.
98 Middlesex Hospital, Minutes of the . . . Governors, 29 Oct. 1771. For the similar regulations at the Westminster, see Westminster Hospital, Proceedings of the Trustees, 10 July 1782, 28 May 1788, 26 Dec. 1810, GLRO H2/WH/A1/19, 20, 24.
99 The various death registers that have survived for St. Bartholomew's, for example, record the patient's admission date, parish and ward, date of death, and place of burial. No reference to autopsies was included, although these registers were a likely place for such bureaucratic supervision to occur. Death Books, MR 5/1–3, 1762–9, 1807–16, 1826–34, St. Bartholomew's Hospital archives, St. Bartholomew's Hospital. For the 1781 regulation that pupils were to be notified of postmortems at St. George's, see St. George's, Laws and Regulations, p. 86, St. George's Hospital Medical School Library; St. George's Hospital, Board of Governors, 14 June 1793; Peachey, *Memoir*, 298.
100 In 1829, when St. George's staff pressed for space to give lectures at the hospital, the governors explicitly forbade them to have "practical anatomy" in the hospital. By this time, of course, dissection was clearly a volatile topic in the metropolis. St. George's Hospital, Board of Governors, v. 22, 11 Nov. 1829; see also R. R. James, *The School of Anatomy and Medicine Adjoining St. George's Hospital* (London: George Pullman, 1928), 10.

strations of morbid anatomy" at the Middlesex in the autumn of 1809, in the same notice that Dr. Satterly used to announce "Clinical instruction." In 1812 George Pearson, St. George's physician, similarly noted that Dr. Richard Harrison, "of St. John's College, Oxford," would "give the Pathological Demonstrations" on the cases that Pearson covered in his Saturday morning clinical lectures at the hospital.[101]

If those at the three western hospitals continued to worry that anatomy teaching might adversely affect their charities' reputations, those running the eastern hospitals contained their qualms. Staff surgeons started to advertise that they gave anatomy lectures at St. Thomas's in 1765, at the London in 1782, and at St. Bartholomew's in 1791. Like their more reticent off-site colleagues, hospital anatomists first opted for restrained announcements of anatomy lectures or courses, not the "practical" anatomy that other entrepreneurs promoted. William Blizard, the surgeon–anatomist at the London, actually had to promise the governors in 1781 that he would not "use any of the Patients out of this House."[102] What sources he then used for teaching material, of course, remained appropriately unmentioned. Eighteen years later the London's governors supported his enterprise – and discretion – enough for Blizard to be the first to advertise "Practical Anatomy during the Season" at a metropolitan hospital. The staff at St. Bartholomew's followed suit in 1805, including the announcement for William Lawrence's instruction in "Anatomical demonstrations and practical anatomy" in their notice in the *Times*.[103]

Well before these explicit items appeared in newspapers, "practical anatomy" at the London, St. Bartholomew's, and especially St. Thomas's had became an open secret: not advertised, but certainly not hidden from pupils and practitioners. In some of his articles for medical periodicals, for example, Joseph Else casually referred to patients' bodies or amputated parts being "conveyed to the anatomical theatre" at St. Thomas's in the 1760s, where "Mr. North, who . . . dissected for the lecturers," worked on them.[104] James Ware, a surgical pupil in 1775, noted in his diary that he attended Joseph Else's lectures on anatomy at the hospital and that his fees included a separate payment for "instruction in the dissecting room" and

101 *Times*, 22 Sept. 1809, 24 Sept. 1812, 30 Sept. 1814.
102 London Hospital, House Committee Minutes, 28 Aug. 1781; London Hospital, Court of Governors, 5 Sept. 1781; and see the House Committee Minutes, 20 Apr. 1782, for concern that "some unwarrantable means have been used in hastening the removal of Corpses of patients from this Hospital." The governors said that only the secretary, steward, or matron could call the undertaker: "The Credit of this Charity must suffer if the Friends of every deceas'd Patient have not due notice of every decease."
103 *Morning Chronicle*, 29 Sept. 1798; *Times*, 25 Sept. 1805. In 1802, the London hospital advertisement actually mentioned "dissection" under Armiger, the anatomical demonstrator; *Times*, 6 Sept. 1802.
104 Joseph Else, "Of tumors formed by ruptured veins sometimes mistaken for Aneurysms" (read 5 May 1766), *Medical Observations and Inquiries* 3 (1767): 169–77; idem, "An uncommon Case of a fatal Hernia" (read 15 Oct. 1770), *Medical Observations and Inquiries* 4 (1771): 355–7.

"1 guinea for a half share of a muscular subject to dissect."[105] Of course anatomy lecturers at the hospitals turned to "resurrectionists" to provide bodies for students' use, just as off-site teachers did.[106]

Patients' corpses nevertheless supplemented those from grave-robbing and the body trade for an ongoing supply of interesting observations and specimens used in teaching. As Hampton Weekes, a boarding apothecary's pupil at St. Thomas's in 1801–2, recounted with relish, Astley Cooper knew how to subvert mere hospital protocol. Weekes attended a clandestine postmortem on a woman who had just died in the hospital.

Mr. Cooper . . . laughd with us and said that Mr. Pohill, a great Tobaconist at St. Margaret's Hill, (with Whom this woman had been living), had sent word that she shd. not be inspected, (Mr. P is also a governor of this Hospital) But ye answer shd. be to him that she had been open'd before his message had arrived, but wh. was not ye. case, (This shd. not be told to your country Neddy's, neither to any one.) so we were very merry about it.[107]

While the connivance of students and staff may have concealed such goings-on from "country Neddys," it is hard to imagine from Hampton's account of his studies that hospital patients and attending governors were unaware of dissection within the charity's walls. Hampton spent long hours dissecting body parts that he purchased to learn normal anatomy. He described his work in enthusiastic detail in his letters home to Sussex, and sent his brother and father some of his preparations for their edification. He reported with great pleasure when he finally obtained a key to one of the private dissecting rooms, where privileged students helped the anatomy demonstrators to prepare material for lectures and for the surgeons' collections of pathological specimens.[108]

Throughout this period – from 1765 to the 1820s – the St. Thomas's

---

105 Quoted from James Ware's diary in Parsons, *St. Thomas's*, 2: 229. A few years later, another St. Thomas's pupil recorded in his notes Else's statement: "There is another division [of anatomical studies] called Comparative Anatomy, but this is almost extinct, owing to a good and constant supply of human subjects – This renders it therefore of little consequence." Joseph Else, "Introductory Lecture," Lectures on Anatomy delivered at St. Thomas's Hospital, ca. 1779–80, taken down by John Williams, n.p. MS. St. Thomas's Hospital Medical School Library.

106 Henry Cline, Surgical Operations by Henry Cline, delivered 1788, taken down by Richard Whitfield of Southwark, 43, WIHM MS 1672: "Mr Cline relates the following laughable story . . . The man who supplied the dissecting room with subjects happened to pass at the time of the accident . . . and claimed him [a beggar who suffocated on a cabbage] as his brother, he called a coach immediately and carried him to the theatre"; and see the letter from John Jeffrey, a governor, to the hospital treasurer, dated 5 Dec. [1831], complaining about the sale of bodies at the hospital in GLRO H1/ST/A76/5. Richardson, *Death Dissection and the Destitute*, discusses the resurrectionists' trade in some detail.

107 Hampton Weekes to his father, 17 Feb. 1802, in Ford, ed., *A Medical Student*, 130.

108 Weekes to his father, 24 Sept., 1 Nov., 15 Nov., 7 Dec. 1801; Weekes to his brother, 13 Dec. 1801, 30 Mar. 1802, in Ford, ed., *A Medical Student*, 43, 59–61, 90–4, 147–9. For further details on dissection at Guy's and St. Thomas's, see B. B. Cooper, *Cooper*, 1: 26, 268–72, 2 :11–18, 23–5.

men never advertised "practical anatomy" in the London newspapers. This ongoing decision may well reflect the hospital administrators' hopes for public discretion. Weekes's letters, however, unmistakably show how little such silence deterred staff and students from finding and using what they could to pursue their own goals. Like observing patients on the wards, watching postmortem inspections, and dissecting pilfered body parts appealed to pupils convinced that such experience would make them better practitioners at the bedside, in the marketplace, and among their peers.

Hospital theaters

Toleration of dissection implies lay acknowledgment that medical men did indeed need a "good" education, one which demanded experiences that many people found abhorrent. From this perspective, the relative success of "practical anatomy" on and off hospital grounds in eighteenth-century London shows how practitioners set standards for medical training quite apart from corporate regulations, university degree requirements, or overt social approval. Similarly, the emergence of entrepreneurial medical lecturing on other subjects during the first half of the eighteenth century entailed pupils' agreement that taking courses added to their medical expertise. When lecturers moved onto hospitals' grounds after midcentury, they taught just as they had, and others did, in off-site businesses, offering courses for which pupils paid fees only to the instructors, not to the hospitals. Yet when staff men obtained permission to lecture on-site, apparent approval to advertise their courses, and support for constructing purpose-built theaters, they acquired more than convenient facilities. Medical lecturing itself gained a basic mark of legitimation. Lay governors, from local tradesmen to peers of the realm, appeared to endorse such enterprises. Lecturing became associated with what took place *at* hospitals, with what prestigious staff men did, and with what hospital pupils wanted. On-site lecturing, even when as administratively distinct from hospital business as it was, linked the provision of academic knowledge to students with the provision of medical care to the poor.

At various moments in the 1700s, the governors at all of the general hospitals allowed staff men to lecture on-site; by the end of the century, those at St. Thomas's, Guy's, the London, and St. Bartholomew's had supported the construction of purpose-built theaters (Table 5.3). In most cases, hospital surgeons and physicians had to ask the governors for permission to lecture. And such innovations were debatable points. At the London in January of 1755, for example, the House Committee governors decided that Henry Thompson could lecture on surgery in the hospital. Two weeks later they changed their minds: "The Committee apprehending that Some Inconveniencys might arise from Reading such Lectures agreed

that Mr. Thomson [*sic*] be desired to find another place for that purpose."
He and Gabriel Risoliere, his surgical colleague at the hospital, continued
with the lectures they had begun off-site in 1754. In 1768, however, the
House Committee agreed that George Neale, staff surgeon, could "make
use of the room (formerly the Physicians room) to read lectures to his
pupils."[109] In contrast, when Dr. Hugh Smith wrote to the Middlesex
governors in 1757 to "beg the favour to be allowed the Liberty of giving
Lectures upon some of the particular Cases that may offer amongst the
patients," the Quarterly General Court passed the much more general
motion "that the Physicians & Surgeons of this Hospital have Liberty to
read Lectures on Physic and Surgery in the Hospital."[110] Yet this privilege
may well have been understood as referring only to occasional clinical
lectures, as neither Smith nor his surgical colleagues advertised that any
courses took place at the Middlesex in these years.

As Neale's request to use the former "Physicians room" at the London
indicates, staff men found a variety of areas within the hospitals for their
courses. In the 1720s to 1750s, when the general hospitals were being
renovated or built, several included separate "theaters" where the surgeons
could perform operations off the wards.[111] Not surprisingly, hospital men
used them for their courses from at least the 1760s. At St. Bartholomew's
in 1767, for example, the "Physicians and Surgeons desired that they may
have leave to make use of the Theatre for operations and also of the room
adjoyning thereto in the pyle of Building lately finished to read lectures in
to their pupils," and the governors agreed.[112] The first newspaper advertisements for lectures at "the theatre" at St. Thomas's in 1765, and at
Guy's in 1770, almost certainly refer to these hospitals' operating rooms.
Not until 1775 at St. Thomas's, 1777 at Guy's, 1783 at the London, and
1791 at St. Bartholomew's did notices for a "new theatre" at each institution mean that these hospitals had spaces devoted specifically to lecturing.[113]

109 London Hospital, House Committee Minutes, 21, 25 Jan., 4 Feb. 1755, 30 Aug. 1768;
   Clark-Kennedy, *The London*, 1: 103–4; *Public Advertiser*, 26 Sept. 1754; *Daily Advertiser*,
   7 Oct. 1755; *Gazetteer and London Daily Advertiser*, 30 Sept. 1756.
110 Middlesex Hospital, Minutes of the . . . Governors, 28 June, 4 Aug. 1757; Wilson,
   Middlesex, 193.
111 At Guy's, for instance, the Court of Governors thanked Moses Raper "for his Generosity
   in building a theatre at this Hospital" in 1738; Guy's Hospital, Court of Governors, 16
   Jan. 1738.
112 Quoted from the governors' Journal Books in Thornton, "The Medical College," 46–7;
   only the surgeon Percival Pott seems to have given lectures, however.
113 For Guy's, see n. 117; Parsons, *St. Thomas's*, 2: 184; 3: 39–40; Thornton, "The Medical
   College," 48. In 1796 the Middlesex hospital seems to have had a lecture theater (a
   modified operating theater?) and a room for chemistry teaching. The only references I
   have found to these facilities, however, are in the governors' minutes, not in newspaper
   advertisements or course notes. In January 1796, "it was moved and seconded that leave
   be granted for fitting up the Laboratory, in order that Chymical Lectures may be given

The first two of these, at St. Thomas's and Guy's, appeared less than ten years after the governors strengthened hospital ward-walking in 1768. That autumn, after committee reports and negotiations, the St. Thomas's and Guy's governors reestablished the agreement that ward-walking pupils at one hospital could attend the other's practice. While the governors did not discuss on-site lecturing, they clearly approved of it, since the St. Thomas's surgeons had advertised their courses at the hospital since 1765. William Saunders, with a 1765 MD from Edinburgh, had already lectured on chemistry, physic, and materia medica at various places in London. After his election as physician to Guy's in 1770, Saunders promptly advertised that he would give courses on these subjects, along with clinical lectures, at the hospital. Then, without any mention of plans or permissions in the governors' minutes, Joseph Else announced his course of "Anatomical Lectures" in the "new Theatre" at St. Thomas's in 1775; two years later Saunders advertised his lectures at the "new Theatre" at Guy's.[114] Whether or not these rooms doubled as operating theaters, the notices for "new" facilities suggest they were designed with lecturing in mind. From the 1770s to the 1820s, lecturers at St. Thomas's and Guy's maintained an understanding that courses on anatomy and surgery took place at St. Thomas's, while those on physic, chemistry, and materia medica occurred at Guy's. That a physician's subjects were obviously less associated with anatomy than a surgeon's surely helped the Guy's governors to enjoy being patrons of medical teaching.

St. Thomas's and Guy's staff men had advertised their "new theaters" for only a few years when the London elected William Blizard surgeon in September 1780. Blizard had had experience lecturing in the City and went to the London determined to introduce lectures to the hospital in Whitechapel. He got permission to use "the demonstrating Theatre" for courses in August of 1781. A year later, he and three of his colleagues (one surgeon and two physicians) submitted a letter to the House Committee requesting authorization to construct "a proper building" for lectures. The

therein, and that the Physician's Room be used for that purpose until the Laboratory be put into a proper state" (19 Jan.). In June of that year, the minutes note "that leave be granted to enlarge the room adjoining the theatre, also to alter the seats of the Theatre for the further accomodation of the Pupils, the above alterations to be done without putting the hospital to any expense" (7 June 1796). These latter changes may have been done primarily to allow more students to observe operations, while the former clearly served for lectures. That these were not advertised, however, suggests that the chemistry course was a particularly private one.
114 *Morning Chronicle and London Advertiser*, 26 Sept. 1775; *Daily Advertiser*, 19 Sept. 1777. Cameron, *Guy's*, 89–90, dates the lecture theater at Guy's to 1770, when William Saunders began at the hospital. Yet neither the governors' minutes nor cash books have any reference to a building project remotely resembling a place to lecture until 1781, when work was done on a new "laboratory" at the hospital, so Saunders's reference in 1777 is still obscure. Guy's Hospital, Court of Committees, 16 Feb. 1781; Cash Book, 1765–94, 6 Nov. 1781, GLRO H9/GY/D11/4.

governors eventually called a special meeting to consider this idea, and a "great Majority" of the fifty men present decided the staff could build "a Theater at the East End . . . provided no additionall Expense be brought upon this Hospital."[115] The hospital agreed to provide the land, but the staff had to pay for the building. Blizard and James Maddocks, a staff physician, prepared two fulsome pamphlets to attract subscribers' donations to a building fund. *Of the Expedience and Utility of Teaching the Several Branches of Physic and Surgery, By Lectures at the London Hospital,* and *An Address to the Friends of the London Hospital and of Medical Learning* laid out all the arguments they could come up with for why lecturing – not just bedside observations – belonged in hospitals.[116]

"Governors of Hospitals of the highest reputation justly consider *teaching* as naturally connected with *curing,* and of the greatest importance to the interests of mankind," Blizard and Maddocks proclaimed. They quoted from one of the Bishop of Litchfield's sermons celebrating an anniversary of the London Hospital. The Bishop had publicly endorsed ward-walking, picturing the hospital as "a nursery for the useful science of medicine . . . its [benefits] extended over the whole of mankind. . . . Thus the treasures of knowledge are increased . . . by the exercise of our charity."[117] Yet, while ward-walking offered students experience, such work had little meaning "without a proper knowledge of principles." They pressed on: "But the principles of Medicine and Surgery cannot be taught but by means of lectures publicly read [as] the experience of learned men from the beginning of science to the present time has proved."[118] Lectures by staff men at the hospital, moreover, provided a valuable synthesis. "The instruction conveyed will be more efficacious, as the teacher will have continual opportunities of exemplifying and confirming by practice the principles he teaches." And students presumably knew this. Blizard and Maddocks claimed – with considerable exaggeration – that "few [students] chuse to attend any hospital where Lectures are not given."[119]

These staff men knew that such pedagogical insights were not enough to

---

115 London Hospital, House Committee Minutes, 5 Oct. 1782; Court of Governors Minutes, 4 Dec. 1782 (Quarterly General Court), 5 Feb. 1783 (Extraordinary General Court). A notice for the Extraordinary General Court appeared in the *Daily Advertiser*, 11 Jan. 1783. It announced that the topic would be the "new Theatre for Lectures upon the Practice of Physick, Chemistry and Surgery." The start of the "medical school" at the London is discussed (with some inaccuracies) in Morris, *The London,* 171–5; Clark-Kennedy, *The London,* 164–8; and John Ellis, *The Story of the London Hospital Medical College: England's First Medical School* (London: London Hospital Medical Club, 1986).

116 *Of the Expedience and Utility of Teaching* is internally dated 23 May 1783. It listed the names of the men who accepted subscriptions to the theater fund; *An Address to the Friends of the London Hospital and of Medical Learning,* a revised version of the former pamphlet, has an internal date of 12 Aug. 1783.

117 Blizard and Maddocks, *Expedience and Utility of Teaching,* 6, note on p. 5.

118 Blizard and Maddocks, *Address to the Friends,* 6–7.

119 Blizard and Maddocks, *Expedience and Utility of Teaching,* 6; *Address to the Friends,* 7.

persuade governors (or others) to part with cash to build a theater when it could be spent directly on charitable care. So they appealed to utility and to collective vanity. Patients in the hospital suffered from the London's place in the medical education market, since pupils had to travel a good way to hear the lectures they wanted.[120] With lectures on site, students would be "much more in the house" and hence more likely "to give the necessary attention to their patients," a not-so-subtle reminder of the free labor that pupils provided. Pupils educated at the hospital who formed "an attachment to it, may be a means of greatly promoting its interests" by becoming governors and encouraging others to do so.[121] The lecturers, of course, would get direct financial rewards, but the hospital would benefit from their "truest zeal for the interest and credit of the institution." Staff lecturers, they claimed, would "devote the greatest part of their time to the service of the charity." All of these elements converged, Blizard and Maddocks argued, to enhance the "reputation of an hospital."[122] They predicted that

if Public Lectures on the various branches of Medicine are delivered at this Hospital, its reputation will be raised, its fame generally extended, and it will become an object more generally noted.[123]

Men of "good sense and liberality" would of course "encourage them in the undertaking."[124] Governors like Thomas Wellings, a "plaisterer and painter," did, too. Wellings, an active governor and a theater subscriber, received £2.6s. from the hospital's accounts in August 1783 for painting the "Letters marked over the Theatre Door."[125] Some governors' interests were very close to home.

The fund-raising scheme worked. In the autumn of 1783, newspapers carried notices for the "new medical theatre" at the London, with courses on anatomy and surgery, chemistry, the materia medica, and medicine.[126]

120 London Hospital, House Committee Minutes, 2 Dec. 1778, 12 Jan. 1780. In 1780, a subcommittee reported, "It appears on Investigation, that the Pupils of the Surgeons absent themselves under pretence [of] attending lectures."
121 Blizard and Maddocks, *Address to the Friends*, 8–9.
122 Blizard and Maddocks, *Expedience and Utility of Teaching*, 8 (note by Maddocks), 7.
123 Blizard and Maddocks, *Address to the Friends*, 8.
124 Blizard and Maddocks, *Expedience and Utility of Teaching*, 8.
125 Two "Thomas Wellings" (probably senior and junior) were governors of the London. Both attended the Court of Governors' meeting that approved the lecture theatre. Both subscribed to it. For the payments to Thomas Wellings for work on the theater, see London Hospital, Tradesmens Ledgers (1782–85), 24 July, 7 Aug., 12 Aug. 1783, LH/F/ 8/7, London Hospital Archives.
126 Blizard taught anatomy, physiology, and surgery; Maddocks lectured on the theory and practice of medicine; Dr. Thomas Healde offered materia medica and pharmacy; and Dr. John Cooke, who was not yet on staff, gave a course on chemistry. *Daily Advertiser*, 10 Sept. 1783. The governors announced the new theater in their printed report for 1785, noting proudly that "every Part of Medical Science is encouraged and promoted for the

Blizard's and Maddocks's appeals managed to make a hospital founded to care for the sick poor seem an obvious place for medical lectures. In this case, indeed, they did far more. They succeeded in making the construction of a lecture theater itself into a worthy project for lay patrons.[127] They transformed what was, and remained, an independent business into a mark of medical enlightenment and charitable care.

Lecturers' publicly advertised courses at St. Thomas's, Guy's, the London, and, in 1791, St. Bartholomew's reveal the fruits of cooperation between staff men and governors. Events at St. George's in the 1790s aptly illustrate the effects of conflict and competition. Since at least the early 1770s, the absence of lectures at St. George's arose from staff reluctance, not from lay governors' resistance to medical teaching.[128] As I explained in Chapter 4, John Hunter's decision to keep all of his ward-walking pupils' fees for himself inspired a full-fledged inquiry into teaching at St. George's in 1793. Most of the investigation concerned ward-walking, but the final report from the subcommittee (one actually written by all the hospital surgeons except Hunter) urged St. George's to catch up to "the improved state of other hospitals."[129] They should have a "Medical School" like those "allowed and provided by the Governors of other hospitals." St. Thomas's and Guy's, the London, and St. Bartholomew's, they noted, each had a "complete school" with courses in the full range of medical subjects.[130] In

common Good." *An Account of the Rise, Progress and State of the London Hospital* (London, 1785), advertisement to the list of governors in 1785. Clark-Kennedy, *The London*, 1: 167, dates the opening of "the new school" to October 1785, when a celebratory dinner took place at the building's completion.

127 *An Address to the Friends* (12 Aug. 1783) included a list of the first fifty-two subscribers, who had given a total of £457 (pp. 11–14). Blizard gave £31.10s. and Richard Grindall, another staff surgeon, donated £21. At least eighteen of the subscribers were hospital governors who had attended meetings where teaching at the hospital had been discussed, including Thomas Wellings [I] (£10.10s.) and Thomas Wellings [II] (£2.2s.). Other subscribers included Robert Maclaurin, Blizard's former lecturing partner, who gave £3.3s. and Jonas Hanway, the noted Quaker philanthropist (see *Dictionary of National Biography* [DNB]), who gave £5.5s.

The London was the only medical theater in the eighteenth century built with money raised by public subscription. The theaters at St. Thomas's, Guy's, and St. Bartholomew's were built from the charities' funds, but these were endowed institutions. In 1813, Henry Cline and Astley Cooper each contributed £1,000 to the new teaching facilities at St. Thomas's, while the hospital provided £3,000. Cline and Cooper had a significant stake in the profits of their enterprise that clearly made their investments worthwhile. Parsons, *St. Thomas's*, 3: 39.

128 Peachey, *Memoir*, 200–4, 277–9, 288–92.

129 "Surgeons' Letter to the Committee (27 May 1793)," printed in Peachey, *Memoir*, 300; a nearly identical version was transcribed into the Board of Governors Minutes, 29 May 1793. For the governors' committee, see the Minutes for 17 Apr. 1793. The committee consisted of the two hospital Treasurers, three physicians retired from staff positions, Drs. Gisborne, Warren, and Burges; and the Hon. Mr. Pusey; Sir Joseph Andrews, Bt.; William Drake, Jr.; and James Gladill Vernon, Esq.

130 They noted, for example, that St. Thomas's and Guy's together offered "Midwifery, Surgery, the Materia Medica, with the practice of Physick, Chymistry and Anatomy."

both Hunter's letters and his colleagues' replies and report, St. George's reputation (not patient welfare) figured as a chief rallying cry to rouse their fellow governors' attention.

In contrast to the arrangements at St. Thomas's, Guy's, St. Bartholomew's, and the London, at St. George's staff physicians and surgeons served as regular governors as long as they paid subscription fees. They recommended patients, attended meetings, and voted. They undoubtedly needed to lobby lay governors to get their views accepted, just as staff men elsewhere did, but clearly had on-the-spot influence at crucial moments. And all of the staff practitioners except John Hunter and Dr. John Robertson Barclay attended the Special General Court called to consider the subcommittee's report on 14 June 1793. Including the staff, twenty of the fifty-nine governors there that day were medical men; it is safe to suppose that the Court heard from medical interests during the discussion. Most of the surgeons' ideas for ward-walking passed verbatim as resolutions, but when it came to lecturing the Court decided "that Professors of Surgery and Midwifery shall be permitted to give lectures at this Hospital . . . having first been approved of by the Governors of the Weekly Board."[131] Without courses in anatomy, medicine, chemistry, and materia medica, this was nowhere near a "complete" curriculum. At that time, of course, John Hunter taught surgery and anatomy off-site – a point that Gunning, Walker, and Keate had raised to demonstrate how "the gentleman . . . [regarded] the hospital as a second consideration" in his life.[132] Everard Home, assistant surgeon and Hunter's teaching partner, was there, however. Also present were two lecturing staff physicians. Dr. Matthew Baillie was then in charge of the well-known anatomy theater on Great Windmill Street. Dr. George Pearson had recently started giving courses on medicine, chemistry, and materia medica at his own off-site "Laboratory." Surgery and midwifery were the only lecturing subjects that did not step on any staff man's toes – except John Hunter's.

Why Matthew Baillie and George Pearson did not want to move their courses to St. George's remains unknown, but with such high tensions among the surgeons at the hospital it is not surprising that they avoided it. Nor would they have been thrilled to support other staff men's teaching the same subjects there, even if the other physicians and surgeons had seemed willing to do so. Considering that Gunning, Walker, and Keate did not take advantage of permission to lecture on surgery, even after John Hunter's death that autumn, and that lectures on midwifery alone would

"Surgeons' Report," in Peachey, *Memoir*, 300–1; St. George's, Board of Governors Minutes, 29 May 1793.

131 St. George's Hospital, Board of Governors, 14 June 1793; compare with the surgeons' report printed in Peachey, *Memoir*, 302–3.

132 "Surgeons' Reply to Hunter's Address (1793)," in Peachey, *Memoir*, 289.

be embarrassing, it seems to me quite probable that the governors *really* unswayed by appeals to enhance St. George's metropolitan reputation were the medical lecturers themselves. The hospital's physicians and surgeons continued to give courses off-site, among the other entrepreneurs in London's West End, until new rivalries established St. George's medical school in the 1830s.

Making institutions

Implicit partnerships among the lecturers at St. Thomas's, Guy's, the London, and St. Bartholomew's began the process of embedding ongoing medical courses into the London hospitals. The hosptials' physicians and surgeons developed the shared locations, customary lecturing times, relationships with their hospitals' governors, and collective reputations that gradually made their hospital-based courses the foundations for formal educational institutions. Lecture theaters provided concrete sites for continuing enterprises. From the 1780s, staff men started advertising together, heading the notice with the hospital's name instead of using separate announcements under each individual's name or his course's subject. While sometimes inconsistent and irregular, such joint announcements displayed a group identity that transcended the names of specific lecturers.[133] Staff names appeared and disappeared from the lists, but for the most part the courses were always there.[134]

As I have stressed throughout this discussion, the hospital governors generally left the staff alone to run their businesses and to reap the profits. If hospital physicians and surgeons met to negotiate who was to lecture, when, on what subjects, and for what fees, or even to thrash out how much everyone needed to pay for candles and lamps, they did not meet formally enough to keep minute books with records of their ad hoc policies. Certainly they did not have to make official reports to the governors, as the paucity of references to lecturing in administrative records demonstrates. Such a laissez-faire attitude seems to have been most governors' choice, not an expression of staff men's power. St. Thomas's was the exception that supports this generalization, for in 1781 a General Court confirmed "that no person be allowed the use of the Theatre belonging to this Hospital without leave from the Grand Committee or the Treasurer

---

133 See, for example, *Daily Advertiser*, 13 Jan. 1780; 10 Sept. 1783; 10, 21 Sept. 1790; 29 Sept. 1791; Thornton, "The Medical College," 48.
134 Three St. George's lecturers attempted to construct a hospital identity in 1806, when Pearson, Gunning, and Home advertised together under the heading "St. George's Hospital." They placed this notice, moreover, in the *Edinburgh Medical and Surgical Journal* [2 (1806): 508], for a medical audience. But the description of the courses made it clear that this cooperation was only on paper: they all lectured at different locations off the hospital's grounds.

when the Committee is not sitting," and the Grand Committee actually used their authority to "appoint" hospital lecturers.[135]

Even without hospital rules, staff men shared an understanding that only hospital physicians and surgeons could offer courses on site. Exceptions were made for midwifery lecturers, anatomy demonstrators, and, in a few cases, lecturers in chemistry. Presumably no staff physician or surgeon wanted to teach midwifery, as it compromised their status as "pure" practitioners. Young surgeon–assistants took on the tedious job of supervising students doing dissection. Staff men probably turned to outsiders for chemistry when none of them wished to teach it. These exceptions show that by the late eighteenth century it was more important for hospital collaborators to have these subjects covered than it was for them to maintain closed ranks.[136]

These quasi-institutions managed fairly well until the 1820s. With the success of hospital schools, however, came a spate of internal conflicts that undermined the gentlemen's agreements sustaining them. These disputes centered, not surprisingly, on questions of staff authority and governors' control. Events at the united "school" at St. Thomas's and Guy's provide the best early example of the shift from complete staff autonomy to governors' intervention in "school" affairs. The united school dissolved in 1825 when the St. Thomas's governors refused to let Bransby Cooper, Astley Cooper's nephew and surgeon at Guy's, succeed his uncle in the coveted post of lecturer on anatomy and surgery at St. Thomas's. The issue was simple: Astley Cooper felt that he should have the power to appoint his successor, and the St. Thomas's governors disagreed. Instead of acquiescing to the long-standing tradition of dividing the lectures between the two hospitals, much less bowing to the 1781 rule giving St. Thomas's governors the authority to appoint lecturers, Astley Cooper declared that anatomy and surgery would henceforth be taught at Guy's. With the support of the influential Treasurer at Guy's, he proceeded to install his nephew in that position.[137] In the 1820s, such nepotism raised reformers' criticism

135 The Grand Committee had appointed "Mr. Cline to read the Lectures in Anatomy and Surgery at this Hospital." The governors paid attention to their regulation, moreover. They approved Henry Cline, Jr.'s, and Astley Cooper's (surgeon to Guy's) petition to take over the senior Cline's lectures in 1813 and refused Dr. George Currey's (staff physician with an Oxford MD) request for permission to lecture on medicine in the hospital in 1815; St. Thomas's, Board of Governors, 8 Aug. 1781, GLRO H1/ST/A1/7; Grand Committee Minutes, 8 Aug. 1781, 8 Nov. 1815, 7 June 1820; GLRO H1/ST/A6/7, 8.

136 In Appendix III, see Richard Dennison, Andrew Thynne, and Robert Gooch, midwifery lecturers at the hospitals; and William Allen, Richard Edwards, and Clement Hue, nonstaff chemistry lecturers.

137 Cameron, *Guy's,* 145–6, 162–74. See Guy's Hospital, Court of Committees, 12 May 1824; 23 Feb., 13 Apr. 1825; 21 June 1826, for the Cooper affair; 30 Aug., 8 Nov. 1826 for a new dispute with the staff physician, Dr. Cholmely, who claimed a right to give lectures. For the governors' view from St. Thomas's, see its Grand Committee Minutes, 26 Jan., 2 Mar., 29 June, 28, 30 Sept. 1825.

and, in Bransby's case, entailed public humiliation. In 1828, Bransby sued Thomas Wakley, editor of *The Lancet,* for libel, when Wakley published a description of Bransby's hesitancy and ignorance during an operation (seen, of course, by the hospital pupil public) at Guy's. To uphold his dignity, Bransby had to hear accounts of his presumed surgical incompetence aired in court, along with his uncle's staunch defense of his knowledge and skills on the witness stand. Bransby technically won the case, but, as the jury awarded him only token damages, in effect he lost it.[138]

Bransby Cooper, by all accounts a pleasant man yet a diffident lecturer and awkward surgeon – quite unlike his popular and talented uncle – both stood for, and suffered from, the successful institutionalization of hospital knowledge. According to Wakley's well-publicized statements, Bransby Cooper was not supposed to be just an adequate practitioner but, as surgeon to Guy's, a great one. Whether great or not, however, he continued to instruct pupils on the wards and to lecture to students in Guy's Theatre, precisely because he was already ensconced as surgeon and lecturer to Guy's Hospital. And students went to Guy's – because it was *Guy's.*

Throughout the eighteenth century, London lecturers prospered because they offered convincing prizes for the attentive student. Reading dozens of course notes has convinced me that men paid for lectures because they promised not only practical information but also an entrée into professional learnedness. Lecturers with hospital posts may have had an advantage when claiming that what they taught was drawn from experience and based on up-to-date practice, since they had (for whatever reasons) been entrusted with care of large numbers of patients. But men without such positions flourished as well, because they had an equally valuable commodity. Students' notes show that much of what they heard and recorded concerned the more abstract aspects of medical knowledge. Lecturers gave them the appropriate language for being a well-informed practitioner, conversant with the systems that provided explanations for disease, trauma, and death.[139]

The acquisition of suitably sophisticated ways to express medical theories and therapies, to converse on natural philosophy, and to join discussions of natural history had long marked the physician. Advice given to young gentleman–practitioners – indeed advocates of university studies generally – underscored the multiple intellectual and social benefits that followed from a liberal education. Londoners, I have argued in this chapter, wanted similar advantages, aptly expressed to the Guy's Court of Committees in 1785:

---

138 S. Squire Sprigge, *The Life and Times of Thomas Wakley* (New York: Robert E. Krieger, 1974; originally published 1897), 135–55.

139 Susan C. Lawrence, "Educating the Senses: Students, Teachers and Medical Rhetoric in Eighteenth-Century London," in *Medicine and the Five Senses,* ed. W. F. Bynum and Roy Porter (Cambridge: Cambridge University Press, 1993), 154–78.

Mr. Treasurer acquainted the Court that it was the opinion of the Medical Gentlemen belonging to the Hospital and also of several Governors that it would render the Hospital a more complete school of instruction to the Students who attend this Hospital to finish their education . . . if a course of Lectures in experimental philosophy could be established to be read in the Hospital. And that the Students have express'd an earnest desire of . . . acquiring such knowledge equally replete with entertainment and utility.[140]

Seeing natural philosophy as a way "to finish their education" with "entertainment and utility" encapsulates the dual appeal of natural knowledge for medical men and their lay associates. In this scheme, social ease and useful knowledge were inseparable. As the content of useful knowledge changed during the eighteenth century, the concepts and practices that neophyte medical men learned to value changed right along with it.

Chemistry, for instance, underwent a considerable reconceptualization between the 1760s and 1820s, for all sorts of reasons that had little to do with the mundane concerns of medical practitioners. But chemistry belonged to the subjects "replete with entertainment and utility," and chemistry lecturers – most of them physicians with Edinburgh MDs – did well in London. Many of these enthusiasts championed the image of progress in chemistry, taking up Lavoisier's system in the 1790s and introducing new experimental techniques in their demonstrations.[141] In 1802, William Babington told his students at Guy's that he taught them "a new science expressed in a new language." And Hampton Weekes delighted in reporting "a very good Lecture on Chemistry" when he saw "Oxygen Gas & Hydrogen" united "by ye. Electric spark" to make water.[142] Modernlooking "science," in short, entered London medical education of rank-and-file practitioners in the wake of the protracted commercial and cultural changes underlying the emergence of private lecturing in the metropolis.

I pointed out in Chapter 4 that pupils walked hospital wards under either the physicians or the surgeons or the apothecary, a custom that maintained the traditional corporate divisions among elite medical practitioners. Students preparing to practice physic and surgery, and to make up their own prescriptions, treated these divisions as different subjects, but not as distinct *occupations*. Private medical lecturing in London explicitly dispensed with the boundaries that kept certain areas of knowledge and expertise within the older tripartite categories. Surgeons and apothecaries could learn the physicians' erudite vocabulary for physiological processes and convoluted

140 Guy's, Court of Committees, 4 Feb. 1785. Also quoted in Cameron, *Guy's*, 160–1.
141 Jan Golinski, *Science as Public Culture: Chemistry and Enlightenment in Britain, 1760–1820* (Cambridge: Cambridge University Press, 1992), 129–52, 249–52.
142 William Babington and William Allen, *A Syllabus of a Course of Chemical Lectures read at Guy's Hospital* (London, 1802), iv; Hampton Weekes to his father, 3 Dec. 1801, in Ford, ed., *A Medical Student*, 88.

regimens if attentive during class. Physicians and apothecaries could acquire the surgeons' technical terms if they paid to spend hours dissecting and listening to lectures about surgical diseases, traumas, and operations. Physicians and surgeons could master the apothecaries' lexicons for the materia medica and chemical procedures if they studied their course notes.

During the eighteenth century, practitioners educated in this seemingly ad hoc way became adept at discussing – *not* necessarily at applying or practicing – a range of subjects and skills previously separated by the different kinds of work they did. This common familiarity with professional languages allowed London's alumni to read the medical journals and to join medical societies that emerged from the 1750s. This shared understanding and experience allowed all sorts of regular practitioners gradually to constitute a medical community with knowledge, expectations, and interests distinct from those of their patients, patrons, neighbors, and families. In a very pragmatic, day-to-day sense, London's private lecturers created this community. And hospital lecturers, with their auras of public authority over patients, pupils, up-to-date theories, and acceptable therapies, made themselves a central part of the new community's elite.

PART II

Community and knowledge

6

Gentlemen scholars and clinical cases, 1700–1760

On 1 May 1740, the Fellows of the Royal Society elected James Hawley, MD, to join them as an FRS. His nomination letter, exhibited at the society from 31 January to 24 April for his potential colleagues to examine, described Dr. Hawley as a

Member [FRCP 1739] of the College of Physicians & Fellow of Oriel College in Oxford. Now residing in Bow Street Covent Garden.
A Gentleman well skilled in Mathematicks, Natural Philosophy, & other parts of Polite Literature, is desirous of becoming a Fellow of the Royal Society, and is recommended as a person who is likely to become a Usefull Member thereof by us.[1]

Signed by four relatively undistinguished members, Hawley's certificate followed a pattern already familiar to the Fellows: this man would fit in. In contrast, those had who nominated John Andrée the previous October had stated that he was a

Doctor of Physick residing in London; who among other ingenious Performances, has publish'd an account of the Tilbury Mineral Waters, and translated from the french [sic] a Treatise on the Venereal Disease, with a Dissertation on the Hydrophobia, and another on Consumptions, written by Dr. Pierre Desault, and being well Qualified, & desirous of the honour of becoming a Member of this Society, is recommended by us.[2]

Andrée's supporters included Sir Hans Sloane, President of the Society, and Cromwell Mortimer, MD, its Secretary. Yet it was unusual to detail publications in nomination letters: perhaps this man did not fit in. The Fellows rejected him on 24 January 1740. Andrée never got his FRS, however desirous.

The way that the anonymously balloting Fellows reacted to Hawley and Andrée provides a launching point for this chapter. In the convoluted

---

1 Nomination certificate I.150, Royal Society of London Library. William Sloane, J. Hamilton, Henry Rowe, and R. Graham signed the certificate.
2 Certificate I.144, Royal Society.

social and intellectual worlds of early- to mid-eighteenth-century London medicine, natural philosophy, and "other parts of Polite Literature," the Fellows of the Royal Society marked a mainstream elite among those pursuing natural knowledge. Hospital physicians and surgeons sought acceptance there, likely for a wide range of motives. For James Hawley, recently elected physician to the Westminster Hospital, requesting the FRS followed upon getting the FRCP and perhaps, like the hospital post, helped him establish his London practice. For John Andrée, who had just received his MD from Rheims at age forty-two, the FRS could well have seemed a major coup for beginning his career as a physician. Denied it, however, Andrée still went on to be a cofounder and first physician of the London Hospital (October 1740) and, when he got around to it, to obtain his Licentiate from the Royal College of Physicians (in December 1741).[3]

Having the FRS or a hospital post was only one part of a practitioner's identity for social approbation or occupational authority in any particular instance.[4] Yet Royal Society meetings and hospital wards were not simply symbols: they were concrete places where people generated, accepted, criticized, and disseminated particular kinds of knowledge, along with all the values, expectations, and rituals associated with what made "good" knowledge and practice. The standards at work in the Royal Society, from choosing Fellows to publishing the *Philosophical Transactions,* depicted what mattered for many educated gentlemen – a group including potential patients and hospital governors, as well as practitioners. What hospital men did, in turn, in seeking the FRS and, more generally, in what they published reveals how they intersected with the cultural elite in the Royal Society and presented themselves as producers of textual knowledge. In the end, James Hawley's only foray into print was his Harveian oration to the Royal College of Physicians in 1747, in suitably ornate Latin.[5] John Andrée, in contrast, wrote another medical book, discussed later, in which he presented hospital cases as specific elements in his arguments against using hemlock to treat cancers. Andrée may have exploited his hospital post in a way that Hawley did not, but his use of evidence was well grounded in the criteria for good knowledge already displayed by Hawley's colleagues at the Royal Society. Medical men, indeed several hospital men,

3 William Munk, *Roll of the Royal College of Physicians of London,* 2nd. ed., 4 vols. (London: Royal College of Physicians, 1878), 2: 144, 148. No biographical information on Andrée's early life, other than that he descended from Swiss who immigrated to England in the sixteenth century, exists in the standard sources. See E. W. Morris, *A History of the London Hospital,* 3rd ed. (London: Arnold, 1926), 236.

4 For an extended discussion of how medical practitioners sought social success, see Dorothy Porter and Roy Porter, *Patient's Progress: Doctors and Doctoring in Eighteenth-Century England* (Stanford, CA: Stanford University Press, 1989), 16–29, 53–69, 117–32.

5 James Hawley, *Oratio anniversaria in theatro collegii Regalis Medicorum Londinensis ex Harveii instituto habita postridie D. Lucae, 1747* (London: J. Whiston, 1747).

had used the Society's meetings and the *Philosophical Transactions* as a place
to reaffirm the significance of individual case histories to establish medical
"matters of fact," however they were then used to support or contest
various theories and practices.[6]

In the pages that follow, I look at hospital physicians and surgeons as
particular subsets of London practitioners. I discuss the range of ways that
they presented themselves as knowledgeable men and illustrate their criteria for "good" knowledge. Examining all the staff men to the seven general
hospitals underscores the diversity of their approaches to medical knowledge and hence highlights the implications of the work they chose to do.[7]
Clustering the ways they attempted to achieve medical authority, such as
appealing to classical authors, adapting medical theories to prevailing
trends in natural philosophy, or calling on personal experience, establishes
what these men believed would convince other practitioners, their patients,
and, for some, their pupils to accept their ideas.

As diverse as their work was, one very basic characteristic unites them.
At least in print hospital men were epistemological imitators, not innova-
tors. However new their theoretical suggestions or potentially risky their
therapeutics, in this period hospital practitioners, like their university colleagues or fellow master-surgeons, followed the paths to natural knowledge already well trod by respectable gentlemen. (Even when they hurled
rude epithets at one another, elite practitioners followed coffee-shop wits
who cultivated polemics and satire.) This chapter thus illustrates and deep-
ens the concept of "safe" science introduced in Chapter 1: elite practitioners
conformed to cultural sensibilities about both the style and the substance of
scientific inquiries. Their compliance simultaneously enhanced their personal credibility and reinforced for other medical men the acceptable ways
to make "good" professional knowledge. Innovations that elite physicians
and surgeons adopted – publishing case histories in the *Philosophical Transactions,* for instance, which, I argue later, was a transformative event for
medical knowledge – introduced new methods and ideas into medicine.
Safe, because they originated under gentlemanly purview, such new no-

---

6 Steven Shapin and Simon Schaffer, *Leviathan and the Air-Pump: Hobbes, Boyle and the
  Experimental Life* (Princeton: Princeton University Press, 1985), discuss the important epistemological arguments about the creation of "matters of fact" as a category of natural
  philosophical knowledge within the Royal Society. See also Peter Dear, "Narratives, Anecdotes and Experiments: Turning Experience into Science in the Seventeenth Century," in
  The Literary Structure of Scientific Argument, ed. Peter Dear (Philadelphia: University of
  Pennsylvania Press, 1991).
7 Historians looking for "progress" in eighteenth-century medicine have frequently decried
  this century's practitioners for their "confusion" over methods and the multitude of systems
  and therapies they produced. See, for example, Lester King, *The Medical World of the
  Eighteenth Century* [1958] (Chicago: University of Chicago Press, 1971), chapters 7, 9, and
  10; Richard H. Shyrock, *The Development of Modern Medicine* [1936] (Madison: University
  of Wisconsin Press, 1974), chapters 2–4.

tions then gradually modified medical culture while keeping the medical elite firmly ensconsced as its polite and well-behaved masters.

PUBLIC PERSONA: PUBLISHING

Before embarking upon just what hospital men did to make "good" knowledge, I offer four approximate measures of the number of physicians and surgeons who participated in the creation and dissemination of medical information in some public way: (1) The number of hospital men who published medical work provides a rough index to how they appeared before a literate public; (2) the number whom the Royal Society chose to include as Fellows suggests their connections to the broader metropolitan community of intellectuals; (3) the number of those who lectured on medical topics shows the proportion of hospital men who sold their expert knowledge to students (and others); and (4) the percentage of men who published among all of those who joined the Royal College of Physicians, divided between those with general hospital posts and those without, reveals the relative visibility of hospital physicians as "contributors" to knowledge compared with their professional peers.

Table 6.1 summarizes the data from my investigations into (1), (2), and (3). It includes all of the physicians and surgeons who joined one of the general hospitals between 1700 and 1759.[8] From the most general perspective, over half of the hospital men in these six decades had some investment in offering their expertise or erudition beyond their practices and personal collaborations. Of course there was an overlap among those who published, obtained the FRS, and lectured, although only five hospital men (one physician and four surgeons) did all three. Table 6.2 shows the results of my analysis of (4). Seen as a subset of RCP men, hospital physicians as a group were not a great deal more likely to produce publications than nonhospital men. Overall, 46 percent of hospital physicians chose to write for the press, while 31 percent of physicians without posts at the general hospitals did so. Indeed, the most "marginal" group – nonhospital physicians with the LRCP – published most frequently, a fact which underscores the way that writing for the press probably revealed their hopes of appearing suitably learned.

In contrast, the publishing rate among hospital surgeons (29 percent) compared to that of a sample of other London surgeons clearly shows that

---

8 As Londoners founded five of these hospitals in this period, the Westminster (1719), Guy's (1725), St. George's (1733), the London (1740), and the Middlesex (1745), moreover, the number of opportunities for charity service multiplied considerably. In 1700–9, six men joined St. Thomas's and St. Bartholomew's, out of a total of twelve places for physicians and surgeons. In 1750–9, forty-two new men were elected to the seven hospitals, a sign of the high turnover among some of the forty-four existing staff positions. See Chapter 2.

Table 6.1. *Physicians and surgeons elected to St. Bartholomew's, St. Thomas's, the Westminster, Guy's, St. George's, the London, and the Middlesex hospitals, 1700-1759*

Position	Elected	Published	FRS	Lectured	Did only one	Did all three
Physicians	75	48% (36)	43% (32)	4% (3)	65% (49)	1% (1)
Surgeons	80	29% (23)	26% (21)	8% (6)	45% (36)	5% (4)
Total	155	38% (59)	34% (53)	6 % (9)	55% (85)	3% (5)

these staff men were already part of a literate occupational elite. Among the fifty surgeons licensed by the Bishop of London from 1700 to 1725 to practice in or near the metropolis, only three (6 percent) appear to have published during their lives, and two of them, William Cheselden and Ambrose Dickens, were hospital surgeons who had obtained the Bishop's license before climbing to prominence and publishing. The remaining forty-seven were thus more typical of surgeons, in the sense that the vast majority of ordinary practitioners did not publish.[9] As noted in Chapter 3, when the surgeons separated from the Barber–Surgeons' Company in 1745–6 the new company declared that its ruling officers had to "be of no trade but that of the profession of Surgery only."[10] The "pure" surgeons at the top of the occupational – and social – hierarchy included an increasing number of hospital men. From the perspective of "contributions" to knowledge, as a group hospital surgeons more closely resembled their physician counterparts than ordinary practitioners.

Tables 6.1 and 6.2 provide a vital sense of who I mean when I refer to the hospital elite in the rest of this chapter. While such data can serve only to sketch in the contours of medical men's ambitions to appear publicly knowledgeable, they provide important curbs on overgeneralization. Since only a third of hospital surgeons published *anything*, the two-thirds who

9 James Harvey Bloom and Robert Rutson James, *Medical Practitioners in the Diocese of London, Licensed under the Act of 3 Henry VIII, c.II; An Annotated List, 1529–1725* (Cambridge: At the University Press, 1935), 36–74. The third surgeon who published was the prolific author Daniel Turner, who later turned physician; see Munk, *Roll*, 2: 35–7, and recent work by Phillip Wilson, especially his "Surgeon 'Turned' Physician: The Career and Writings of Daniel Turner (1667–1741)," Ph.D. Dissertation, University of London, 1992. I was unable to consult Wilson's dissertation while writing this book.

10 Bernice Hamilton, "The Medical Professions in the Eighteenth Century," *Economic History Review*, 2nd ser., 4 (1951): 150. Quoted from "Problems Presented to Counsel" by the Surgeons' Company, 1746.

Table 6.2.   *Physicians and publishing, 1700-1759*
            By year of entry into the Royal College of Physicians

	Hospital	Other	Total
Fellows	41	75	116
Published	20 (49%)	24 (32%)	44 (40%)
Licentiates	12	76	88
Published	4 (33%)	40 (53%)	44 (50%)
Extralicentiates	0	101	101
Published		15 (15%)	15 (15%)
Non-RCP	8		8
Published	4 (50%)		4 (50%)
Total	61	256	313
Published	28 (46%)	79 (31%)	107 (34%)

Note: The data include all physicians who entered the Royal College of Physicians between 1700 and 1759, as Fellows, Licentiates, or Extralicentiates. The eight hospital physicians who did not become FRCP or LRCP obtained their posts during this period. The hospital category includes physicians to St. Bartholomew's, St. Thomas's, the Westminster, Guy's, St. George's, the London, and the Middlesex hospitals, but omits physician-accoucheurs to the Middlesex.

did not have an imposing, if inarticulate, presence. Similarly, as learned as they likely were, fifty-four percent of the hospital physicians abstained from writing out their thoughts for the press. Publishing, in short, simply was not necessary for establishing a professional identity among the elite before the late eighteenth and early nineteenth centuries. Making a published contribution to knowledge gradually became a required mark of medical status only after the formation of a large medical community in which, as I argue in Chapter 7, ordinary medical men could add their own articles to the common stock of "good" knowledge.

While most of the hospital men who did not publish remain quite obscure, the stories of a few of those who acheived fame and fortune without such trappings of learned lives illustrate the other paths to success in eighteenth-century London. For them, public notice primarily arrived through patronage and political activity. Caesar Hawkins, surgeon to St. George's from 1735 to 1774, provides an apt – although rare – example of a surgeon's social advancement unmarked by publications or election to the Royal Society. Hawkins gained prominence through patronage. While he lectured on anatomy during his first year or so as a hospital surgeon, he stopped before his appointment as surgeon to the Prince of Wales in 1737. Serjeant-surgeon to George II and George III, Hawkins was created baronet in 1778. He was the first hospital surgeon to get a "Sir," and this clearly rewarded his royal practice, not his intellectual or scholarly attainments. Hawkins followed a path familiar to physicians like Dr. Edward Wilmot, who received his MD from Cambridge, served as physician to St. Thomas's from 1729 to 1740, held various royal appointments, and was created baronet in 1759. Wilmot was elected to the Royal Society in 1729, and, like Hawley, gave the Harveian oration at the College of Physicians, yet died unpublished at age ninety-three.[11] Positions at Court, in short, could bestow prestige, aristocratic patients, and healthy fortunes on favored practitioners quite apart from any public displays of medical knowledge in print.[12]

Royal patronage hardly excluded the learned, of course. Several hospital physicians and surgeons combined their charity work and time spent writing with attendance on the monarch, royal family, or other Court luminaries. Dr. Richard Mead (St. Thomas's, 1703–15) and William Cheselden (surgeon and lithotomist to St. Thomas's, 1718–38; the Westminster, 1724–33, St. George's, 1733–8), for example, both obtained royal positions well after being elected to a hospital position, getting the FRS, and publishing. In Cheselden's case especially, becoming surgeon to Queen Caroline in 1727 literally embellished his reputation, as he printed the royal arms in his major work, the *Osteographia* of 1733.[13] This elegant display, just as the fulsome praise regularly offered to patrons in dedications and prefaces throughout the literary – including medical – world, presented knowledge as a gift to the great. In turn, such "presence" of the powerful cast a penumbra of social, if not also intellectual, authority over the contents.

Hospital physicians and surgeons participated in such subtle exchanges marking status, learning, and authority throughout the eighteenth century. During the first six decades, in particular, patronage helped. So also did the style of presentation, combined with content, serve in shaping hospital men's work for particular audiences and purposes. Four interrelated approaches stand out in early to midcentury publications, each carrying im-

11 For Hawkins, see George Peachey, *A Memoir of William and John Hunter* (Plymouth: William Brendon & Son), 8, 35–6 and the *Dictionary of National Biography* [*DNB*]; for Wilmot, see Munk, *Roll*, 2: 106–7.
12 William F. Bynum, "Medicine at the English Court, 1688–1837," in *Medicine at the Courts of Europe, 1500–1837*, ed. Vivian Nutton (London and New York: Routledge, 1990), 262–9, esp. 282–4; see also Vivian Nutton, "Introduction," in *Medicine at the Courts of Europe*, 4–6, 8–12.
13 William Cheselden, *Osteographia* (London, 1733); Sir Zachary Cope, *William Cheselden, 1688–1752* (Edinburgh and London: E. & S. Livingstone, 1953), 31–2.

plications for what constituted good medical knowledge. First, like other practitioners, hospital men wrote for the medical marketplace. They published to call attention to their practice and to associate themselves with particular conditions or therapies. Several embroiled themselves in the excitement of polemical literature, producing tracts, pamphlets, and cutting remarks about others' work. By midcentury, priority disputes especially called forth such vituperative stabs, as eighteenth-century medical men claimed discoveries and personal fame. Second, a scholarly style characterized many elite practitioners, particularly physicians who maintained the Latin of their university training and would not write without allusions, references, or direct appeal to classical authorities. Third, medical men had a complex relationship with the "new" science of the seventeenth century as it spilled over, with an aging Newton, into their modern era. Among the publishing hospital practitioners, natural philosophy and natural history furthered both cultural and medical ends, and hence they interwove the new styles of science with their own concerns about theory and practice. Fourth, hospital men presented clinical cases within a new genre of public medical writing centered on the short account of a particular person's story of illness. Only here did access to charity patients begin to demarcate the hospital practitioner from his peers, as hospital cases were drawn into the stock of clinical knowledge already bestowed by experience with the "private" ill.

PUBLICITY AND POLEMICS

No hospital men (as far as I have discovered) used the broadsheets, newspaper advertisements, and catchy pamphlets that empirics and other more entrepreneurial practitioners did to attract attention to their cures in early-eighteenth-century London.[14] Yet some of their works seem to have been more market-oriented than others: publications on mineral waters, gout, smallpox, venereal disease, "pestilential contagion," or "the Art of Healing" all had great potential interest for lay readers, whether seeking self-help or – as the authors implicitly hoped – wondering whether they needed professional advice.[15] At least from the amount of paper generated, however, displays of intense competition and rivalry, not just popular

14 Roy Porter, *Health for Sale: Quackery in England 1660–1850* (Manchester: Manchester University Press, 1989); Andrew Wear, "Medical Practice in Late Seventeenth- and Early Eighteenth-Century England: Continuity and Union," in *The Medical Revolution of the Seventeenth Century*, ed. Roger French and Andrew Wear (Cambridge: Cambridge University Press, 1989), 394–420.
15 John Andrée, *An Account of the Tilbury Water* (London: M. Jenour, 1737); Donald Monro, MD, *A Treatise on Mineral Waters*, 2 vols. (London: D. Wilson & G. Nicol, 1770); Thomas Reeve, [MD], *A cure for the epidemical madness of drinking tar-water* (London: J. & P. Knapton, 1744); Richard Mead, MD, *A Short Discourse Concerning Pestilential Contagion, and the Methods to prevent it* (London: S. Buckley, 1720); Thomas Dawson, MD, *Cases in the Acute Rheumatism and the Gout* (London: J. Johnson, 1774); Thomas Gataker [surgeon],

topics, brought gratifying notice and presumably some occupational benefit. Hospital men, like those jousting over political positions, battling religious doctrines, or otherwise embroiled in controversies in the wider world, turned to print to trade insults, condemnations, and self-justifications. Late-seventeenth- and eighteenth-century authors honed their satirical styles and proclaimed their biting individualism in a rich pamphlet and monographic literature. Lay wits enjoyed ridiculing medical practitioners from learned physicians to quacks, playing with medical language, and creating stock figures and phrases for public amusement.[16] Such language decorated collegial abuse, as when the pseudonymous Dod Pierce mocked Dr. Pierce Dod (St. Bartholomew's, 1725–54) in 1746: "This delirious Scribbler was violently infected with the Itch of Authorism." The Grub-Street disease was the only possible reason Dr. Dod could have written his appalling book.[17] Many intramedical attacks, some directly

Observations on venereal complaints and on the methods recommended for their cure (London: R. and J. Dodsley, 1754); John Freke [surgeon], *An essay on the art of Healing. In which Pus laudable or matter, as also incarning or cicatrizing, and the causes of various diseases, are endeavored to be accounted for from both nature and reason* (London: W. Innys, 1748). Among the hospital physicians writing on smallpox and inoculation were William Wagstaffe and Pierce Dodd from St. Bartholomew's, and Daniel Cox and William Douglass of the Middlesex: Daniel Cox, *A Letter to a Friend on Inoculation* (London, 1757); Pierce Dodd, *Several Cases in Physic, Small-pox, and Fever* (London, 1746); William Douglass, *Practical Essays Concerning Smallpox* (London, 1730); and William Wagstaffe, *A Letter Showing the Danger and Uncertainty of Inoculating the Smallpox* (London, 1722). For the considerable literature on, and context of, smallpox and the inoculation controversy, see Andrea Alice Rusnock, "The Quantification of Things Human: Medicine and Political Arithmetic in Enlightenment England and France," Ph.D. dissertation, Princeton University, 1990; Noel G. Coley, "Physicians and the Chemical Analysis of Mineral Waters in Eighteenth-Century England," *Medical History* 26 (1982): 170–87; Roy Porter, "The Early Royal Society and the Spread of Medical Knowledge," in French and Wear, *The Medical Revolution of the Seventeenth Century*, 280–1.

16 David Harley, "Honour and Property: The Structure of Professional Disputes in Eighteenth-Century English Medicine," in *The Medical Enlightenment of the Eighteenth Century*, ed. Andrew Cunningham and Roger French (Cambridge: Cambridge University Press, 1990). See, for example, Edward Ravenscraft, *The Anatomist; or the Sham Doctor* (London: R. Baldwin, 1697); this play went through many editions and performances throughout eighteenth century. S. H. Misodolus [pseud.], *The young-man's Counsellor, or The Way of the World Display'd; in several profitable essays, serious and comical*, 2nd ed. (London: Robert Gifford, 1713), 109–17; Porter and Porter, *Patient's Progress*, 124–6.

17 Dod Pierce, *A Letter to the Real and Genuine Pierce Dod, MD, actual Physician of St. Bartholomew's Hospital* (London: M. Cooper, 1746), 2–3; Pierce Dodd, *Several Cases in Physick* (London: C. Davies, 1746); In 1750, John Starr, MD, introduced his letter to Cromwell Mortimer at the Royal Society by claiming, "It is not, I'll assure you, an Itch for Scribbling, but the Concern I feel . . . for the . . . Well-being of my Fellow-Creatures" that induced him to send in his case. "An Account of the *Morbus Strangulatorius*," *Philosophical Transactions* 46 (1749–50), 435. The public stir around Mary Toft, who claimed to give birth to rabbits, led to the downfall of a hospital surgeon, Nathaniel St. Andrée. He was anatomist to the household under George I and surgeon to the Westminster Infirmary around 1723. In 1727, he published *A Short Narrative of an Extraordinary Delivery of Rabbits* (London, 1727), which showed that he was taken in by Mary Toft and her unnatural brood. When Toft was exposed and the butt of much ridicule, St. Andrée lost much of his practice (*DNB*).

involving hospital physicians and surgeons, were less amusing and equally public. Notable nastiness between Dr. John Woodward and Dr. Richard Mead (St. Thomas's, 1703–15); John Douglass, (lithotomist, Westminster, 1721–42) and William Cheselden; William Hunter and his rivals, Alexander Monro, Jr., and Percival Pott (surgeon, St. Bartholomew's, 1745–87); and Dr. Donald Monro (St. George's, 1758–86) and Dr. John Millar, for example, marks how significant claims for particular discoveries and practices were for personal reputations, and how far medical men would go to revile one another in print.[18] Even titles could convey contempt. William Douglas, briefly physician and physician-accoucheur to the Middlesex (1750–52), broadcast his opinions on a rival in *A letter to Dr. Smelle* [sic] *Shewing the impropriety of his new-invented wooden forceps; and also, the absurdity of his method of teaching and practicing midwifery* (1748).

Such displays and disputes reveal not only the intense competitiveness among practitioners, but also some of the grounds that London men used to critique or justify claims for good medical knowledge. Yet the very polemicism of their language sometimes points to love of controversy and the apt phrase, not necessarily to serious epistemological commitments that authors (on either side) adhered to. Sir John Colbatch (LRCP 1696; knighted 1716), for example, who had a tenuous relationship with the Westminster Hospital from 1716 to 1723, exchanged heated declarations of knowledge based on personal experience, on "true" observations and "experiments," with his critics. The authority of personal experience was undoubtedly crucial for eighteenth-century medical men. That Colbatch went on to assert, however, that he had been "publickly threatened to be murder'd" and "afterwards my self, with two of my Friends were secretly poison'd" indicates the more exciting ways he used personal experience to demonstrate the threatening truth of *his* facts.[19]

18 Joseph M. Levine, *Dr. Woodward's Shield: History, Science and Satire in Augustan England* (Berkeley: University of California Press, 1977), 11–17; Peachey, *Memoir*, 104, 111, 115–6; Ulrich Tröhler, "Quantification in British Medicine and Surgery, 1750–1830, with Special Reference to its Introduction into Therapeutics," Ph.D. dissertation, University of London, 1978, 58–9; Cope, *William Cheselden*, 68–9; see also, Thomas Thomson, MD, *The Case of the Rt. Hon. Thomas Winnington, Esq.* (London: T. Gardner, 1746); William Douglas, MD, *A Letter to Dr. Thomson in answer to the Case of the Rt. Honorable Thomas Winnington, Esq.* (London: J. Roberts, 1746); Porter, *Health for Sale*, provides an overview of public controversy in the marketplace.
19 John Colbatch, *A Collection of Tracts, Chirurgical and Medical* (London: D. Brown, 1704), 11; Colbatch, *Novum Chirurgicum Vindicatum: or, The New Light of Chirurgery Vindicated. From the many unjust Aspersions of some unknown Calumniators* (London: D. Brown, 1695); W. W., *Novum Lumen Chirurgicum Extinctum* (London: Andrew Bell, 1695); John Langdon-Davies, *Westminster Hospital: Two Centuries of Voluntary Service 1719–1948* (London: J. Murray, 1952), 18–19; Harold J. Cook details Colbatch's polemics and their implications in his "Sir John Colbatch and Augustan Medicine: Experimentalism, Character and Entre-preneurialism," *Annals of Science* 47 (1990): 475–505.

ANCIENTS AND MODERNS

Compared with Drs. Douglas and Colbatch, those caught up in the disagreements between "ancients" and "moderns" in medicine were, for the most part, rather modest. By the early eighteenth century in Britain, the debate over the relative stature of the ancients and the moderns had been going on for decades. Recent analysts of these discussions have probed the cultural and scholarly meanings embodied in this contest, which superficially concerned the "greatness" of Greco-Roman philosophers, artists, and authors versus the "greatness" of recent knowledge, usually referring to contributions since the Renaissance. While nearly all polemicists in this fray conceded that the moderns excelled the ancients in certain sciences, such as mathematics and astronomy, and some practical arts, such as weaving and navigation, defining the "sciences and the arts" in the eighteenth century had a contentious aspect all its own. The ancients' achievements in the polite arts of literature, drama, and rhetoric, nevertheless, had staunch defenders – and imitators – in Augustan England.[20]

Disputes over medicine's character as both art and science, both ancient and modern, had similarly exercised scholars for centuries.[21] Eighteenth-century appeals to classical authors, then, had multiple functions. For physician graduates of Oxford and Cambridge, and hence for the Fellows of the Royal College of Physicians, Latin – and sometimes Greek – ostensibly remained the active languages of medical scholarship. At a rhetorical level, reading, writing, and speaking Latin denoted the academic gentleman; similarly, reading, writing, and speaking English grounded in familiarity with great classical literature suited some circles of polite learning. Practitioners aspiring to touch these audiences, whether lay or medical, knew these basics well.[22] Dr. James Greive (St. Thomas's, 1762–73) re-

20 David Spadafora, *The Idea of Progress in Eighteenth Century Britain* (New Haven, CT, and London: Yale University Press, 1990), 21–84; Joseph M. Levine, *The Battle of the Books: History and Literature in the Augustan Age* (Ithaca, NY, and London: Cornell University Press), 1–9, ff. For a sweeping account of Continental issues, see Anthony Grafton, *Defenders of the Text: The Traditions of Scholarship in an Age of Science, 1450–1800* (Cambridge, MA: Harvard University Press, 1991).

21 John Freind, *The history of physick: from the time of Galen, to the beginning of the sixteenth century. Chiefly with regard to practice*, 2 vols. (London: J. Walthoe, 1725–7); Levine, *Dr. Woodward's Shield*, 2, 9–10, passim; see also: Laurence Brockliss, *French Higher Education in the Seventeenth and Eighteenth Centuries: A Cultural History* (Oxford: Clarendon Press, 1987); Nancy G. Siraisi, *Taddeo Alderotti and His Pupils: Two Generations of Italian Medical Learning* (Princeton, NJ: Princeton University Press, 1981).

22 For the general popularity of classical authors and style, see Dorothy Marshall, *Dr. Johnson's London* (New York: Wiley, 1968), 195–7. The status associated with classical expertise is emphasized in William Machmicael's anecdotal reminiscences of major eighteenth-century physicians, *The Gold-Headed Cane (1827)*, ed. George C. Peachey (London: H. Kimpton, 1923). See especially the descriptions of Mead, Askew, and Pitcairne, 39–169.

marked in dedicating his translation of Celsus' *Of Medicine* (1756) to Samuel Sharp (surgeon to Guy's, 1733–57), that no one but Sharp, who "esteeme[d] Celsus," had "imitated his [Celsus'] conciseness and elegance with so much success."[23] Favorable comparison to an ancient's prose was praise indeed.

For some hospital authors, such conventions were merely stylistic ones, ways to embellish their writing with appropriate quotations and rhythms. Throughout the century, in fact, practitioners dropped Latin or Greek tags into their medical work as flags waving for educated readers' appreciation.[24] For others, however, ancient knowledge was a serious matter, still offering vital knowledge in theory and practice for contemporary practitioners. While acknowledging gaps and errors in classical authors, both physicians and surgeons used them as ahistorical authorities even when aware of their historical provenance. Dr. John Brisbane (Middlesex, 1758–73), for example, presented Aretaeus' clinical description of diabetes as a timeless standard.[25] In this sense, the medical scholars who produced new editions of classical texts, as Dr. John Wigan (Westminster, 1733–7) did in his edition of *Aretai Cappadocis, De Causis* (1723), contributed to the advancement of knowledge.[26] So too did practitioners like Greive, who, by publishing English translations of classical authors, made their work more accessible to those not so comfortable with Latin or Greek.[27]

Intense attention to what the ancients had to say, on the other hand, also comforted the moderns with the evident progress of the recent past, particularly by the mid-eighteenth century. Presenting detailed commentaries on classical authors simultaneously served to display familiarity with the learned sources and to elaborate on their defects. Dr. Thomas Dickson (London, 1759–84) began a project to "review . . . the Materia Medica" with a short treatise on bloodletting that concentrated on Hippocrates and Galen. Hippocrates, for whom Dickson had "due respect," had been

---

23 Cornelius Celsus, *Of Medicine. In Eight Books,* trans. James Greive, MD (London: D. Wilson and T. Durham, 1756), dedication, see also v–vi. Greive added "notes critical and explanatory."

24 See, for example, Joseph Warner, *An Account of the Testicles, Their Common Coverings and Coats and the Diseases to which They are Liable* (London: L. Davis, 1774), 26–7. On the general characteristic of physicians to be especially liberal with their classical allusions, see also Coley, "Physicians and the Chemical Analysis of Mineral Waters," 127.

25 John Brisbane, *Select Cases in the Practice of Medicine* (London: G. Scott, 1772), 1–3.

26 John Wigan, ed., *Aretai Cappadocis, De Causis* (Oxford: Clarendon Press, 1723); Munk, *Roll,* 2: 121–3.

27 See also, for example, Hippocrates, *Upon air, water, and situation; Upon epidemical diseases; and Upon prognosticks, in acute cases especially,* trans. Francis Clifton (London: J. Watts, 1734). Hospital men also made "modern" works available to an English-reading audience. Thomas Gataker (surgeon, Westminster, 1754–60 and St. George's, 1760–9), for example, translated Le Dran's *Traité des operations de chirurgie;* Dr. Benjamin Alexander (London, 1765–8) translated Morgagni's *De Sedibus et causis morborum* from the Latin; it was published posthumously in 1769.

swayed by his "crude notions of the animal economy." Hippocrates' work, in short, contained therapeutic advice that could not have been "the fruit of genuine observation."[28] In his *History of Medicine and Surgery* (1782), the outspoken physician William Black encapsulated the Enlightenment shift away from ancient authority when noting that "a perusal of a great part of their works might, *at this day,* be dispensed with by students and physicians, except as objects of curiosity."[29] Black's own concern with such "objects of curiosity" nevertheless underscores their importance for eighteenth-century medicine, as authors positioned themselves around how the ancients defined health, disease, and therapies, whether in praise or criticism.[30] In both writing and lecturing among London hospital men, the "ancients" were at once markers of cultural authority, connecting medicine with a venerable past of remarkable philosophers, practitioners, and stylists, and foils for contemporary improvements.[31] In sum, "good" medical knowledge for many learned physicians in the first decades of the century needed to be embedded in a classical base; "good" knowledge for the moderns, in contrast, demanded a careful distancing from aged authorities in content and method, if not in literary style. In between lay the way authors of both persuasions used classical figures – especially Hippocrates – as archetypes not for specific knowledge, but for methodology and the proper character for the investigative practitioner.

GENTLEMANLY KNOWLEDGE: NATURE, MEDICINE, AND THE
ROYAL SOCIETY

As other historians of science have recently stressed, one of the central themes underlying both the formation of the Royal Society in the late seventeenth century and its continuing attempts to disassociate certain kinds of natural knowledge produced by "gentlemen" from religious and political controversy lay precisely in strategies to reach consensus over "matters of fact" and to avoid the polarizations of rhetorical excess.[32] Part

28 Thomas Dickson, *A Treatise on Blood-Letting; with an introduction recommending a Review of the Materia Medica, Part I* (London: D. Wilson, 1765), 15, 13, 11. Dickson published no further parts.
29 William Black, *A Historical Sketch of Medicine and Surgery* (London: J. Johnson, 1782), 302, emphasis in original.
30 See, for example, Donald Monro, *An Essay on the Dropsy and its different Species,* 3rd ed. (London: D. Wilson and T. Durham, 1765), 3–8. Monro was physician to St. George's 1758–86; the first edition of this work appeared in 1755. John Barker, *An Essay on the Agreement between Ancient and Modern Physicians: or, a Comparison between the Practice of Hippocrates, Galen, Sydenham and Boerhaave* (London: G. Hawkins, 1747). Barker, MD Oxford 1743, became physician to the Westminster in 1746, and died in 1749.
31 Henry Banyer, *Micro-techne: or A Methodical Introduction to the Art of Chirurgery; translated from the Latin of Johannes van Horne, Professor of Anatomy and Chirurgery in Leyden* (London: J. Darby, 1717), i–xiv.
32 The early Royal Society and changes in late-seventeenth- and-early-eighteenth century arguments about natural knowledge, not to mention the broader debates over epistemol-

of the strength of this analysis rests on how much, indeed, natural history and natural philosophy were gentlemanly avocations in seventeenth- and eighteenth-century society. The notion of "gentleman" here has several connotations that are often inadequately developed in discussions of gentlemenly science. Two of these are important for my argument. First, natural knowledge, like intimacy with classical authors and modern philosophers, demarcated gentlemen and gentlewomen from the lower social orders, and continued to do so throughout the eighteenth century. Second, gentlemen (rarely gentlewomen) bestowed the authority of their status and, more importantly, of their idealized character as impartial participants, on the creation of "true" science when they made statements about natural knowledge.

In the first sense, knowledge of natural philosophy and natural history were among the attributes that distinguished a cultivated person. James Hawley's election notice for the Royal Society, as noted, played into this widespread social convention. Like an appreciation of music, modern literature, classical texts, art, or antiquities, natural knowledge ornamented its bearer. It signaled an appropriate education and leisure time spent in "improving" activities. (Hence the once-prevalent characterization of pre-nineteenth-century British science as "amateur," compared to the "professional" science of an industrializing world.)[33] Those contemplating an elite medical career included natural philosophy and natural history as parts of a liberal education, not a premedical requirement. Sir John Floyer, for example, recommended in 1720 that the medical student first acquire Latin, Greek, and natural philosophy and "for his diversion study botany."[34]

ogy in the "Scientific Revolution," have had decades of attention. Discussion in this chapter relies most centrally on: Shapin and Schaffer, *Leviathan and the Air-Pump*; Dear, "Narratives, Anecdotes and Experiments"; Peter Dear, "*Totius in verba*: Rhetoric and Authority in the Early Royal Society," *Isis* 76 (1985): 145–61; Steven Shapin, "The House of Experiment in Seventeenth Century England," *Isis* 79 (1988): 373–404; Simon Schaffer, "Natural Philosophy and Public Spectacle in the Eighteenth Century," *History of Science* 21 (1983): 1–43; Michael C. W. Hunter, *Establishing the New Science: The Experience of the Early Royal Society* (Woodbridge, Suffolk, UK: The Boydell Press, 1989).

33 James E. McClellan III, *Science Reorganized: Scientific Societies in the Eighteenth Century* (New York: Columbia University Press, 1985), xxiii–xxvi; Robert H. Kargon, *Science in Victorian Manchester: Enterprise and Expertise* (Baltimore: Johns Hopkins University Press, 1977), ch. 1; Morris Berman, " 'Hegemony' and the Amateur Tradition in British Science," *Journal of Social History* 8 (1975): 34; William R. Le Fanu, "The Lost Half Century of English Medicine, 1700–1750," *Bulletin of the History of Medicine* 46 (1972): 319–48.

34 D. D. Gibbs, "Recommendations of Sir John Floyer on the Education of a Physician," *Proceedings of the XXIII International Congress on the History of Medicine* (London, 1974), 368. Quoted from Floyer's "Advice to a Young Student of Physic," a manuscript in Oxford. At the universities, anatomy and medical botany were treated far more as branches of natural philosophy and history than as knowledge for practical application. Andrew R. Cunningham, "Aspects of Medical Education in Britain in Seventeenth and Early Eighteenth Century England," Ph.D. dissertation, University of London, 1974, 155–9, 163, 169, 180–3, 210, 224.

Several prominent hospital men heartily pursued nonmedical parts of natural knowledge for their "diversions." James Jurin (Guy's physician, 1725–31), for example, Secretary to the Royal Society from 1721 to 1737, was a skilled Newtonian and worked intensely in mathematics and mechanics, as well as publishing on medical subjects.[35] With study of nature merely one of many gentlemanly pursuits, hospital practitioners – mostly physicians – chose other avocations, from writing poetry to standing for Parliament, that had little academic relevance to their success in practice.[36]

The second sense of "gentlemanly" evokes the rituals of personal and consensual knowledge that had emerged as grounds for epistemological authority to supplement (or replace) those of church, state, and university eroded over the previous two centuries. Considerable historical work on the intellectual implications of the political, social, and religious upheavals of seventeenth-century Britain has established how deeply intertwined beliefs about nature were with ideas of God, secular power, and social order, and how such interconnections persisted throughout the ostensibly calmer eighteenth century. As Steven Shapin and Simon Schaffer have persuasively insisted, the Royal Society in the 1660s to 1690s literally demonstrated a place where gentlemen, and invited others, met to discuss nature as though the matters before them, whether reported or performed, could be separated from their religious or political implications. Within the Royal Society's rooms, gentlemen did not raise socially tendentious topics.[37]

In the late seventeenth and early eighteenth centuries, "gentleman" de-

35 Munk, *Roll*, 2: 65–7; Lyons, *Royal Society*, 148. He published extensively in the *Philosophical Transactions* from 1717–19 to 1744–5.
36 Dr. Mark Akenside (St. Thomas's, 1759–1770) tried (yet failed) to maintain his youthful stature as a poet. He consorted with literary figures and collected rare manuscripts. Munk, *Roll*, 2: 196–7, Samuel Johnson, "Akenside" in *Lives of the English Poets*, ed. George Birkbeck Hill (Oxford, 1905; rptd. New York, 1967), 3: 411–20; Horace Walpole, *The Letters of Horace Walpole, Fourth Earl of Orford*, ed. Mrs. Paget Toynbee, 16 vols. (Oxford: Clarendon Press, 1903–5), 2: 82; 4: 88; Dr. Charles Coates (Westminster, 1733–9) served as a Member of Parliament while hospital physician. Munk, *Roll*, 2: 137. John Baillie (physician to St. George's, 1735–44, and not a member of the RCP), as far as I have discovered, only wrote essays and plays, including *An Essay on the Sublime* (1747), *A Married Coquet: A Comedy* (1746), and *The Patriot* (1736), about William of Orange. See Bernard Mandeville, *A Treatise of the Hypochondriack and Hysterick Diseases* (London: 1709, 1730), 39–40, for excellent satirical advice for the physician to "shew your self a Scholar, write a Poem, either a good one, or a long one." I am grateful to Dennis Smith for this reference.
37 In addition to the references cited previously in n. 32, see Charles Webster, *The Great Instauration: Science, Medicine and Reform, 1626–1660* (New York: Holmes & Meier, 1975); Harold J. Cook, *The Decline of the Old Medical Regime in Stuart London* (Ithaca, NY: Cornell University Press, 1986); John Redwood, *Reason, Ridicule and Religion: The Age of Enlightenment in England* (Cambridge, MA: Harvard University Press, 1976); C.B. Wilde, "Hutchisonianism, Natural Philosophy and Religious Controversy in Eighteenth Century Britain," *History of Science* 18 (1980): 1–24; John Gascoigne, *Cambridge in the Age of Enlightenment: Science, Religion and Politics from the Restoration to the French Revolution* (Cambridge: Cambridge University Press, 1989).

noted an educated, morally sound, landed man free from the narrow economic and material interests besetting those in commerce, professions, trades, and wage-driven occupations. He was free to have the "comprehensive view" necessary for political participation in the Crown-and-Commons state ideologically dear to Englishmen during the Restoration, the Glorious Revolution, and the Hanoverian succession. Such a gentleman was, by definition, "disinterested," an objective, independent observer.[38] At root, in short, the Royal Society's own claims for knowledge worked because the *character* of the ideal gentleman sanctioned them. Unswayed by self-interested biases, a (landed) gentleman told the truth, eschewed enthusiasm and radicalism, and respected other gentlemen's testimony.[39] Hospital medical men in early-eighteenth-century London, whether of the learned profession of physic or the manual trade of surgery had problems being gentlemen of this sort. Unless made so by virtue of birth, family, marriage, or landed income, they were immediately implicated in occupational interests. Indeed, after the 1730s "gentlemen" had problems being gentlemen. Various commentators discovered the "landed" interest and exposed the fallacy of a really "comprehensive" – not to mention detached – view of anything.[40] In the process of separating the landed from their innate republican virtues, however, those discussing the "gentleman" retained the sense of honorable conduct and attempts at disinterested judgment that had sustained the early Royal Society. As more and more people claimed to be gentlemen, the title continued to denote character, whether inborn or acquired, displayed through manners, style, and other nuances recognized by polite society, even when watered down to include merchants, tradesmen – and surgeons.[41]

It was the subtle implication that a "gentleman" was a man of worthy character, in conjunction with its hints of social acceptance and appropriate income, that induced medical practitioners to crave this standing.[42] It was, moreover, the continuing role of the Royal Society as a group of gentlemen exchanging, advancing, and validating natural knowledge – its boundaries, methods and acceptable forms – that helped to define "good" *medical*

---

38 John Barrell, *English Literature in History 1730–1780* (London: St. Martin's Press, 1983), 31–6.
39 Shapin, "House of Experiment," 395–9.
40 Barrell, *English Literature*, 36–49.
41 Porter, *English Society in the Eighteenth Century* 1st ed. (Harmondsworth, UK: Penguin Books, 1982), 87–8, 320; Barrell, *English Literature*, 44.
42 A university education had, at least before the late seventeenth century, implied that Oxbridge physicians had acquired the moral character required for a wise counselor, as well as a scholarly medical training. This pastoral aura had significantly diminished with the growth of marketplace medicine. Harold J. Cook, "Good Advice and Little Medicine: The Professional Authority of Early Modern English Physicians," *Journal of British Studies* 33 (1994): 1–31; I am extremely grateful to Hal Cook for sharing this article with me before its publication.

knowledge in early- to mid-eighteenth century London. I have only begun to explore the intellectual and cultural dynamics of the Royal Society in the eighteenth century, particularly from the 1710s to the 1780s.[43] Yet enough is at hand to present a plausible view that the Royal Society authenticated *kinds* of medical theories, styles, and evidence for practitioners, their learned colleagues, and their gentleman patients.[44] Likely through discussions within Royal Society meetings, but certainly through the printed *Philosophical Transactions,* the authoritative stance of its "gentlemanly" knowledge persisted, however much the concept of "gentleman" changed from the Society's early days of philosophical insecurity.

The heyday of mechanical natural philosophy, particularly the Newtonian version(s), amply illustrates the acceptance and propagation of a theoretical and methodological stance into medicine supported by the learned culture of the Royal Society. Multiple Newtons, Newtonians, and Newtonianisms existed in the 1680s to 1730s, including the "experimental" Newton of prisms, the mathematical Newton of the *Principia Mathematicae,* and the speculative Newton of subtle matter, the aether, and God's sensorium. However much English Whig and latitudinarian apologists invoked a Newtonian universe for their political and religious purposes and hence, when in power, helped to make Newtonian styles the sine qua non of early-eighteenth-century natural philosophy, the Royal Society ostensibly embraced Newtonianism(s) as good science without explicitly concentrating on its social implications.[45] With Newton himself President of the Society from 1703 to 1727, its later leanings were hardly surprising.

The shift to corpuscular and mechanistic models to explain anatomical structures and physiological processes among learned physicians, as Brown and Guerrini have shown, reflected neither necessarily better explanations nor Whig political leanings, but the outright replacement of old-fashioned

43 David P. Miller, "Into the Valley of Darkness: Reflections on the Royal Society in the Eighteenth Century," *History of Science* 27 (1989): 155–66; David P. Miller, "The Royal Society of London: 1800–1835: A Study in the Cultural Politics of Scientific Organization," Ph.D. dissertation, University of Pennsylvania, 1981, 1–7. The most comprehensive – and quite inadequate – published source on the eighteenth-century Royal Society is still Charles Richard Weld, *A History of the Royal Society,* 2 vols. (London: John W. Parker, 1848), 1: 320–527, 2: 1–299.
44 Porter, "The Early Royal Society," 272–5.
45 For an introduction to the extensive literature on Newtonianism, latitudinarianism, and Whig political positions, see Colin Russell, *Science and Social Change, 1700–1900* (London: Macmillan Press, 1983), 16–21, 48–68. James Jacob and Margaret Jacob, *The Newtonians and the English Revolution, 1689–1720* (Ithaca, NY: Cornell University Press, 1976); James Jacob and Margaret Jacob, "Anglican Origins of Modern Science: The Metaphysical Foundations of the Whig Constitution," *Isis* 71 (1980): 251–67; Larry Stewart, "Samuel Clarke, Newtonianism and the Factions of Post-Revolutionary England," *Journal of the History of Ideas* 42 (1981): 53–72; Steven Shapin, "Of Gods and Kings: Natural philosophy and Politics in the Leibniz–Clarke Disputes," *Isis* 72 (1981): 187–215; Gascoigne, *Cambridge in the Age of Enlightenment,* esp. 142–84; see also Richard Westfall, *Never at Rest: A Biography of Isaac Newton* (Cambridge: Cambridge University Press, 1980).

Galenic and Aristotelian concepts with "modern" frameworks.[46] Such changes had been hotly criticized in the 1660s and 1670s, but by the turn of the century seeing the body at the minute level as a collection of particles and at the gross level as a hydraulic machine had begun to reinscribe traditional practice and definitions of disease (hence maintaining the ancients) on to the new strands of gentlemanly culture.[47] Several hospital physicians, such as James Jurin (Guy's, 1725–31, FRS 1717) and Alexander Stuart (Westminster, 1719–33; St. George's, 1733–6; FRS 1714) used explicitly Newtonian mechanisms in their physiological and clinical discussions. James Jurin, Richard Mead (physician, St. Thomas's, 1703–14), Joseph Tanner (surgeon, St. Thomas's, 1719–?), and Dr. Henry Pemberton, "who is no less skill'd in Mathematics and Philosophy, than in Anatomy and whatever relates to the Animal Economy," for example, collaborated on the revised 1724 edition of William Cowper's *MYOTOMIA REFORMATA: Or An Anatomical Treatise on the Muscles of the Human Body*. In this elaborately artistic text, a Newtonian language of mechanics and mathematics dominates the whole approach to muscular motion, especially in Jurin's sophisticated geometrical analysis of movement in joints.[48] Attentive readers of the *Philosophical Transactions* were already familiar with Jurin's approach, as he had several short essays on muscular power already in print.[49]

Fascination with muscles and muscular motion, both the gross anatomical object and the philosophical niceties of living powers, of course existed well before Newton's own speculations on subtle matters and forces. The transition to a mechanistic anatomy and physiology and its further mutation into various shades of midcentury vitalism had several other roots and other outlets in London circles besides the Royal Society. In the 1710s and 1720s, Boerhaave integrated broadly Newtonian styles into his physiology

---

46 Theodore M. Brown, "The Mechanical Philosophy and the 'Animal Oeconomy'," Ph.D. dissertation, Princeton University, 1968; Theodore M. Brown, "The College of Physicians and the Acceptance of Iatro-Mechanism in England, 1665–1695," *Bulletin of the History of Medicine* 44 (1970): 12–30; Anita Guerrini, "The Tory Newtonians: Gregory, Pitcairn, and Their Circle," *Journal of British Studies* 25 (1986): 288–311; Anita Guerrini, "Archibald Pitcairne and Newtonian Medicine," *Medical History* 31 (1987): 70–83; Robert E. Schofield, *Mechanism and Materialism: British Natural Philosophy in an Age of Reason* (Princeton, NJ: Princeton University Press, 1970), 3–4, 50–8, 192–4.

47 Harold J. Cook, "Physicians and the New Philosophy: Henry Stubbe and the Virtuosi–Physicians," in French and Wear, *The Medical Revolution of the Seventeenth Century*, 246–69. Wear, "Medical Practice," 294–320 has an excellent discussion of how medical practitioners (physicians and "empirics") blended traditional "rational" medicine and practices with the rhetoric of the new philosophy.

48 William Cowper, *MYOTOMIA REFORMATA: Or An Anatomical Treatise on the Muscles of the Human Body* (London: R. Knaplock and William and John Innys, 1724); see the "Advertisement" by Richard Mead, the preface (n.p.), and pp. ii–xxxiii, lxiii–lxvi, lxxvii, by James Jurin.

49 See, for example, James Jurin, "A Discourse on the Power of the Heart [in Latin]" *Philosophical Transactions* 30 (1717–19): 863–72, 929–38.

and chemistry, using the language of mechanics, particle attractions, and repulsions. Boerhaave's influence through his Leiden pupils, their diaspora, and his texts heavily shaped medical doctrines in this period. Concepts of fibers and minute powers had as much room for interpretation, debate, and dissension as had Galenic or Aristotelian qualities, and these terms became commonplace in medical lecturers' repertoires as well as in published works.[50] The Royal Society nevertheless provided an ongoing, semipublic place to display in person and in print these intersections of natural philosophy, natural history, and medical concerns.

When the bequest endowing the Croonian lecture on "the Nature and Property of Local Motion" finally became available to the Society in the late 1730s, for example, it was devoted to "muscular motion," according to the interests of its namesake, William Croone (d. 1684).[51] As Dr. Alexander Stuart (Westminster, 1719–33; St. George's, 1733–6) prepared to give the first Croonian lecture, he requested through the physician–secretary Charles Mortimer that the Society get executed "Bodies" from the Sheriffs, one of their "Right[s] by their Charter." The Society's Council – for unknown reasons – did not press this privilege, to Stuart's evident disappointment.[52] He fulfilled the Society's "constitution and custom" to have work "founded upon some one or more experiments, observations, or histories of facts," however, by providing his own experimental material (frogs, calf veins) and anatomical preparations (dissected muscles of the arm).[53] Stuart's lectures, and those that followed in the next fifteen years by other physicians, neatly combined the presence of a learned physician, some demonstrations of dissected parts, resonances of "new" science, and medically interesting topics for the Society's members. In his 1740 lectures, which remained unpublished, for instance, Stuart declaimed on "the peristaltic motion of the Gutts," and later showed the Society "anatomical Preparations of the Coats of the Intestines," perhaps indulging his well-fed audience in some personal enlightenment.[54]

Muscular motion was but one medical subject among the scores the Society printed in its *Philosophical Transactions* that entertained and in-

---

50 Brown, "Mechanical Philosophy," 344–53; Schofield, *Mechanism and Materialism*; James Parsons, MD, "The Crounian [*sic*] Lectures on Muscular Motion for the Years MDCCXLIV and MDCCXLV," *Philosophical Transactions,* supplement, 43 (1744–5): 2–43, summarizes various published theories on muscular motion; William Hunter, *Hunter's Lectures of Anatomy* (1752), facsimile edition (Amsterdam: Elsevier Publishing, 1972), 1–47.
51 Parsons, "Crounian Lectures [1744–5]," 5–12.
52 Royal Society, Council Minutes, 15 Jan. 1738/9, vol. 3 (1727–47). Royal Society of London Library; Alexander Stuart, "Three Lectures on Muscular Motion," *Philosophical Transactions,* supplement, 40 (1737–8), Lecture I, i.
53 Stuart, "Three Lectures," iii–xi, xxxvii–xl.
54 Royal Society, Journal Book, 19 Mar. and 26 Mar. 1740/1, vol. 18. Royal Society of London Library.

structed eighteenth-century readers. Their diversity has occasioned some historians' contempt, appearing as the products of amateurs flitting from one curiosity to another and only rarely producing "serious" science. As Roy Porter has noted for medicine in the Royal Society of the 1660s to 1680s, such dismissals miss the point of how this experimental enterprise worked as a center for the exchange of information and ideas. The Society's members, but particularly its Secretaries, such as the prolific correspondent Henry Oldenburg, struggled to decide what to accept as "good" knowledge, especially for accounts of nonexperimental experience reported to them. Hence, once again, the reliance on reliable witnesses – gentlemen – who could either provide firsthand observations with enough detail to be convincing or, rather less welcomed, character assessments of those telling their stories.[55]

In the process of absorbing, transmitting, reporting on, discussing, and printing "new" knowledge, from muscular motion to possible cures, the Royal Society created and promoted the appropriate forms for experiential accounts. These styles, as they appeared in the *Philosophical Transactions,* shaped medical journalism throughout the eighteenth century. Not merely because it was the first – and only – English scientific and medical periodical between the 1660s and 1730s, but also because it retained the sanction of gentlemen-approved arguments and content, the *Philosophical Transactions* provided an initial model for the later medical press.[56] Several of the emerging genres, such as the book review, the report of experiments in chemistry and physiology, and the essay on items of natural history, await further analysis. For London hospital men, other practitioners, and medical pupils, looking at that peculiarly medical story – the case history – affords insight into what it could mean to "advance" medical knowledge in the first half of the eighteenth century.

CLINICAL KNOWLEDGE: PUBLIC AND PRIVATE

In the welter of accounts of human disorders and reports of possible therapies published in the *Philosophical Transactions* between 1700 and 1760, I found two interconnected articles by hospital practitioners that encapsulate the multiple meanings of case histories within the Royal Society. In May of 1733, a Mr. La Grange "died of an Abscess in the *Vesica Fellis.*" Claudius Amyand, "Serjeant Surgeon to His Majesty, and F.R.S.," and also surgeon to St. George's Hospital, participated in treating Mr. La

55 Porter, "The Early Royal Society," 275–92.
56 Thomas H. Broman, "J. C. Reil and the 'Journalization' of Physiology," in Dear, *The Literary Structure of Scientific Argument,* 13–42. Broman has insightfully adopted the concept of "genre" for medical publishing in Germany in the late eighteenth and early nineteenth centuries.

Grange and wrote an account of his unusual case. Alexander Stuart, "M.D. F.R.S., &c.," Amyand's physician–colleague at St. George's, had also observed parts of Mr. La Grange and followed the surgeon's paper with a discourse on "the mechanical and necessary Connection between these apparent Causes and their Effects, in this uncommon Case."[57]

Amyand, as an elite surgeon, was consulted in this case by Dr. Vatas, La Grange's "Physician in Ordinary," and Mr. Fiquel, his surgeon. In his account, Amyand focused on his own observations, but supplemented these with Dr. Vatas's information on La Grange's previous life story, reaching at least fourteen years back to an episode of "a Tertian Ague." Already Amyand had established the well-to-do social context of this patient, and, as important, his own status as the surgeon called in to consult, to open Mr. La Grange's abscess, and to participate in his care until his death, when Amyand "attended the Dissection." The surgeon detailed the specific care from the operation to death, describing the amount and qualities of the material discharged from "the Orifice of the Bursted Bag," using a first-person narration. After the operation, Mr. La Grange became "the Patient" who recovered slowly until he could walk, when he "went to air himself in another Room, and caught Cold: This is presum'd to have occasion'd a Fever follow'd with a Lethargy" and his death. At the dissection, Amyand performed as an expert witness, describing the appearances in both common and Latinate anatomical language ("the *Cystis,* or grand Bag") and participating in the investigation of the relationship between the abscess and the internal organs. He concluded with some general remarks on how, for example, Mr. La Grange could have continued to digest his food well, despite the great quantity of bilious fluid discharged daily. Amyand also noted the constraints on the investigation, politely mentioning that they would have continued the anatomical study, "but the Time allow'd for Dissection did not permit us to pursue this Inquiry" and the accompanying figures "were done by Memory, we not being permitted to take the Liver out of the Body."

In this presentation, Amyand was simultaneously the expert practicing surgeon, the polished consultant, the experienced anatomist, the learned man, and the trusted narrator. When detailing La Grange's treatment after he lanced the abscess, Amyand offered practical points that seemed to help, such as placing "a short and thick *Cannula*" into the wound for constant drainage. La Grange's death, in turn, resulted from the patient's own behavior, which, although not directly ascribed to ignoring his physician's

---

57 Claudius Amyand, "Of an Obstruction of the Biliary Ducts, and an Impostumation of the Gall-Bladder, discharging upwards of 18 Quarts of bilious Matter in 25 Days, without any apparent Defect in the Animal Functions," *Philosophical Transactions* 40 (1737–8): 317–25; Alexander Stuart, "Some Observations on the Case of Mr. Le [*sic*] Grange," *Philosophical Transactions* 40 (1737–8): 325–31.

advice, relieved Amyand of responsibility. The dissection emphasized anatomical names and relationships, to identify the normal and the diseased parts. The conclusion drew physiological implications from the connections between the morbid appearances and La Grange's symptoms and recovery. In short, Amyand's case history gave the gruesome technicalities of a curious case, but shaped these around both pragmatic and philosophical concerns.

Alexander Stuart's following "observations" transformed Amyand's case into a mechanical physician's learned interpretation of symptoms and anatomical relationships within a hydraulic animal economy. Stuart (soon to be the first Croonian lecturer) appealed to gravity and to "the known Laws of Hydrostaticks and Mechanicks" to explain how La Grange's body could manage to digest food fairly well while producing and discharging large amounts of bile. Stuart also relied on the properties of bile in his disquisition, but for him the challenge was to propose a causal account somehow more fundamental than Amyand's anatomical one. He preferred an abstract analysis intelligible within the Royal Society's familiarity with quasi-mechanical views of human physiology. Stuart did state, in the very first sentence, that he "was Witness to" the dissection that Amyand had "fully narrated," thus both confirming Amyand's work and placing himself as participant, not just commentator. Yet none of his "observations" was in fact a *literal* observation, distinguished from Amyand's previous statement of the "facts" that had appeared before them.

As a paired set, the articles on Mr. La Grange nicely illustrate rather different concerns of the elite London surgeon and the physician. There is no simple dichotomy between empiric and theoretician, rather a satisfaction with different kinds of causal explanations, with the former anatomical and symptomatic and the latter, in this case, broadly "mechanical," evoking forces and laws of motion. Both centered their short discussions on the particular case at hand, drawing from it the grounds – at least rhetorically – for generalizations about physiological implications. In the end, nevertheless, the surgeon accomplished the manual acts in treatment and in the subsequent anatomical investigation, while the physician remained remote. As textual performances these articles maintained the practitioners' distinct areas of expertise and the subtle hierarchy that placed the physician as learned commentator on the surgeon's empirical report.

Although Stuart's paper relied on the details Amyand provided, both exemplify one of the *Philosophical Transactions'* standard styles, familiar by the 1730s, but already emerging in the 1680s and early 1700s.[58] More

<hr />

58 Porter, "The Early Royal Society," 277, describes a provincial letter writer as likely following the "house style" of the *Philosophical Transactions* in his passion for measuring an anatomical "wonder." For an example of an earlier case essay, see "An Account of an Extraordinary Aneurisma of the Arteria Aorta near to the Basis of the Heart, with the

formal than extracts from a letter, which were a common means for printing submitted information, these case commentaries appeared as complete narratives within self-contained essays, not as reports of immediate experience or observations.[59] In contrast to the "list" article, where the author primarily gave lists of observations, items, or experiments, or to the lengthy treatise sometimes printed in more than one number of the periodical, these essays stand out as pieces designed to be included in a journal and read through in one sitting, not consulted (like lists) or studied (like a treatise). In creating the *Philosophical Transactions,* the Royal Society provided a place where such stories (case histories, accounts of experiments) were publicly detached from a learned text, other more extensive printed work, or manuscript notes. As such, although obviously embedded in presumed systems of knowledge and practice, the case history surfaces as a distinct contribution to the "advancement" of medicine in and of itself.

Case histories – accounts of particular people with illnesses, with or without interpretive commentary – have of course an ancient pedigree and a history of their own that has yet to be written. There were scores of models for "the" case history available in various medical texts, displaying its basic form: a description of the patient; an account of his or her past experiences and current symptoms; the discovery of her or his individual patterns in sleep, diet, and exercise; and then the description of therapies, their effects, the ongoing state of the patient, and, usually, how the connection between practitioner and patient ended, in dismissal, relief, cure, or death.[60] Manuscript notebooks from the seventeenth century indicate that practitioners, at least fairly elite ones, more or less followed this style as they recorded – or rewrote – their own notes.[61] As much as the details of style varied, as in the differences between the way physicians and surgeons

Symptoms thereof; Dissected by Mr. Lasage, Surgeon, on the 10th of April, 1700," *Philosophical Transactions* 22 (1700–1): 666–8.

59 Some contributions, sent in as "letters," were certainly cast more like essays than simple communications. How the "article" arose from "letters" remains to be studied. See, for example, "Epistola D. Johannis Friend as Editorem missa, de Spasmi Rarioris Historia," *Philosophical Transactions* 22 (1700–1): 799–806.

60 See Christopher Lawrence, "Early Edinburgh Medicine: Theory and Practice," in *The Early Years of the Edinburgh Medical School*, ed. R. G. W. Anderson and A. D. C. Simpson (Edinburgh: The Royal Scottish Museum, 1976), 81, 86–90; Christopher Lawrence and Michael Neve, "Taxonomy and Practice: Medical Classifications in the Eighteenth Century," typescript in the conference papers of the meeting "New Perspectives in the History and Sociology of Knowledge," 28 Mar. 1980, Bath, England; for an example of an early publication of case histories, see John Hall, *Select Observations on English Bodies*, ed. and trans. James Cooke (London: John Sherley, 1657; facsimile edition in Harriet Joseph, ed., *John Hall Man and Physician* [1976]).

61 See, for example, Kenneth Dewhurst, ed., *Willis's Oxford Casebook (1650–52)* (Oxford: Sandford Publications, 1981); Lucinda McCray Beier, *Sufferers & Healers: The Experience of Illness in Seventeenth-Century England* (London and New York: Routledge & Kegan Paul), 51–3, 61–4; Michael MacDonald, *Mystical Bedlam: Madness, Anxiety and Healing in Seventeenth-Century England* (Cambridge: Cambridge University Press, 1981).

used language and described treatments, of more concern here is the purported *purpose* of recording particular cases for publication, not just for private use.

At one level, as noted for Amyand and Stuart, publishing cases served to display the practitioner's expertise. They replicated relationships between the medical man and his patients, informing both on how to act, to talk, to observe, and to accept. Such cultural and educational roles, however, certainly were not the overt ones declaimed by their authors. Case accounts, in multiple forms, explicitly offered the experience central to medical theory, as the physician Francis Clifton put it in 1732: "For what signifies *reasoning* or *philosophizing* without matters of fact to go upon?"[62] In early-eighteenth-century London (and beyond), Hippocrates and Thomas Sydenham were the outstanding heroes of clinical knowledge obtained through direct observation at the bedside.[63] They stood as the antagonists to those who spun theories of physiology and disease out of speculative flax. As champions of an educated empiricism, moreover, this "ancient" and this "modern" could return both the classical scholar and the "new science" aficionado back to the serious study of the patient, to recover or reinvent the primacy of "pure" observation.

The midseventeenth- to early-eighteenth-century Hippocratic revival, and the creation of the "English Hippocrates" in Thomas Sydenham, played into and reinforced the Royal Society's own adherence to a Baconian epistemology of plain observation, the collection of "facts."[64] The authors of most of the letters and essays published in the *Philosophical Transactions* between 1700 and 1760, at least on cases or other medically related topics, felt no need to justify in any way the submission of their accounts – or the secretaries removed such irrelevant excuses. Despite concern over the deluded empiricism of irregular practitioners and country folk, occasionally derided in reports to the Royal Society, gentlemen's empirical stories were significant items for the general store of knowledge.[65] At times a learned physician noted, as Nicholas Munckley (Guy's, 1748–70; FRCP 1754) did in 1758, that of course he could not draw a

---

62 Francis Clifton, *The State of Physic, Ancient and Modern* (London: W. Bowyer for John Nourse, 1732), 162.
63 Clifton, *The State of Physic*, 158–65; Black, *A Historical Sketch*, 236–8; Shyrock, *Modern Medicine*, 33, 69–70; Brown, "Mechanical Philosophy," 360–2; Othmar Keel, "Cabanis et la Généalogie Epistemologique de la Medicine Clinique," Ph.D. dissertation, McGill University, 1977, esp. chs. 1, 7, 8.
64 For a thorough discussion of the philosophical connections among Hippocrates, Sydenham, Bacon, and Locke, see Keel, "Cabanis," ii, viii, 5–9, 259–69, 272–9; Cook, "Physicians and the New Philosophy," 251–3, 265–7.
65 Richard Grindall, "A Remarkable Case of the Efficacy of the Bark in a Mortification," *Philosophical Transactions* 50 (1757): 379–80; Rev. James Bones, "Extract of a second letter . . . relating the case of a Mortification of Limbs in a Family," *Philosophical Transactions* 52 (1762): 531.

conclusion from "one single instance only" of the use of bark in a fever. Yet he went on to detail the case as important "both on its own account, and for the analogy, which being found by experience to subsist between diseases, affords the surest method of reasoning in practical subjects."[66] Once again, *claims* for rational reasoning embellished such clinical observations and upheld the elite practitioner's separation from others who might witness the same illness.

Examining case reports in the *Philosophical Transactions* during these decades strongly suggests that the very process of producing medical knowledge for the Royal Society legitimized practitioners' focus on clinical experience as valid "matters of fact." This style of article was particularly serviceable for surgeons, who concentrated on the details of a condition and its treatment as practical information in itself, with or without drawing more general conclusions. Surgeons, like others seeking to support mere testimony with visual evidence, sometimes took a diseased part or anatomical specimen to the Society meeting. John Belchier (surgeon, Guy's, 1736–68; FRS 1732), for example, introduced "the Man himself, and likewise the Arm" when presenting his account of this case in 1737, where "the Man" had had his arm and shoulder torn off in an accident.[67] Such displays quite literally identified the clinical "object" with interesting microscopes, rare plants, and curious antiquities. Discussion of new surgical treatments, such as Samuel Sharp's (Guy's, 1733–57, FRS 1749) enthusiasm for "Agaric of Oak" as a styptic for bleeding, pointedly relied upon case reports for sufficient substantiation, not on theoretical explanations or justifications.[68]

Amyand, Belchier, Sharp, Munckley, and several other hospital men laid cases before the Royal Society as "matters of fact" for discussion, publication, and distribution. As with case histories embedded within texts, or mimicked in testimonial advertisements in the daily press by midcentury, the authors frequently included the names of their patients, and other personal details, that emphasized the unassailability of direct experience. Such references also made the patient "public" and in ac-

---

66 Nicholas Munckley, "An Account of an Extraordinary Case of the Efficacy of Bark in the Delirium of a Fever," *Philosophical Transactions* 50 (1758): 611.

67 John Belchier, "An Account of a Man whose arm with the Shoulder Blade was torn off by a Mill, 15th of August 1737," *Philosophical Transactions* 40 (1737–8): 313–16.

68 Samuel Sharp, "Experiments concerning the Use of Agaric of Oak in Stopping Hemorrhages," *Philosophical Transactions* 48 (1754): 588–9; Joseph Warner, "The History of a case relating to the Effects of the Agaric of Oak," *Philosophical Transactions* 48 (1754): 590–2; Joseph Warner, "A Short History of the Effect of the Agaric of Oak," *Philosophical Transactions* 48 (1754): 593–8. Several other surgeons contributed to the debate over the use of agaric, both in the *Philosophical Transactions* and elsewhere. See William Thornhill, "Account of the success of agaric in amputations," *Philosophical Transactions* 49 (1755): 264–5 in which Thornhill gave the details of its use in four amputations; George Neale, surgeon to the London from 1753 to 1797, described his own case reports in his *Observations on the Use of the Agaric and its Insufficiency in Stopping Hemorrhages after Capital Operations* (London: J. Robinson, 1757).

counts – like Belchier's – of recent and successful treatments made his or her existence part of the truth of the story.[69] The case of Mr. La Grange, furthermore, shows how the conditions and care of ostensibly private, well-to-do patients could become public knowledge through a connection with a practitioner already aware of an audience for the unusual or instructive. Contemporaries certainly noticed this public display, at least in some of the pamphlet battles over disputed treatment. Dr. J. Campbell criticized Dr. Thomas Thomson's defensive account of *The Case of the Rt. Hon. Thomas Winnington, Esq.* (1746) with an acerbic remark:

I judg'd that learned Gentleman had more prudence than to encourage this newly-introduced Method of exposing Patients to publick View, after they are rotten in their Graves; and plaguing the Publick with Cases wherein they have not the least Concern. . . . All that can be learned from such publick Enquires, is, that the Science of Medicine is governed by no fix'd Principle.[70]

Dr. Campbell was undoubtedly correct. He voiced, yet again, the regular practitioner's fears of displaying too much that "the Publick" might not understand. Yet such worries did not seem to arise in the *Philosophical Transactions,* where "exposing Patients" ranked as unproblematic natural knowledge among disinterested gentlemen.

Part of the ease that medical men felt when discussing individuals at the Society and in print probably stemmed from the ways that the "private" also made themselves "public." One of the most notable examples of such personal exposure was "An Account of the Right Honorable Horace Walpole, Esq.; drawn up by himself," read to the Royal Society in 1751. Walpole suffered intensely from bladder stones. He discussed his symptoms; his advice from physicians, surgeons, and apothecaries; and his decision to treat himself with "soap and lime-water," which he eventually drank daily, a few months after reading Dr. Whytt's account of it in the "*Scots Medical Essays.*" The Earl of Morton's testimony that soap and lime-water had worked for Mr. Summers seems to have clinched its possible value for Walpole.[71] Not only did Walpole's essays confirm the significance

69 For an early-eighteenth-century example, see Christopher Birbeck, "An Account of a Woman, who voided the greatest part of a Foetus by the Navel," *Philosophical Transactions* 22 (1700–1): 1000–2: "The Woman laboured all this Season at Hay and Harvest" (1002). Other contributors took care to provide witnesses, especially of unusual circumstances. See, in the same volume, "An Account of a person who took a great quantity of Opium, without causing Sleep" (999–1000): "This is attested under the hands of her 3 Physicians, and the Apothecary."

70 J. Campbell, MD, *A Letter from J. Campbell M.D. to his Friend in Town, Occasion'd by the case of the Rt. Hon. Thomas Winington* [sic] *Esq.* (London: L. Raymond, 1746), 7–8; see also Douglas, *A Letter to Dr. Thomson.*

71 Horace Walpole, "An Account of the Right Honourable Horace Walpole Esq.; drawn up by himself," *Philosophical Transactions* 47 (1751–52): 43–8, quotation p. 44; Horace Walpole, "A Sequel of the Case of the Right Honourable Horace Walpole, Esq.; relating to

of empirical observation appropriately told by educated witnesses, but they also demonstrated how patients could delight in intimate details (e.g., "the irritation at the end of my yard"). Walpole's dedication to self-examination seems to have extended to permission for his autopsy. An account of his bladder (with stones) and other abdominal viscera, as observed by John Ranby and Caesar Hawkins and told to Dr. John Pringle, with Dr. Whytt's comments on soap and lime-water, appeared in 1757.[72]

HOSPITAL KNOWLEDGE

Throughout the preceding discussion, I have used "private" and "public" in referring both to the practitioner's relationship with a patient and to the audience privy to the details of a person's illness and corpse. For the former, "private" carried its modern sense of a fee-seeking practitioner whom the patient could choose as freely as money, time, status, and beliefs permitted; "public" has remained a shadowy opposite. In the latter, "private" suggested that the case remained within a domestic sphere, however much that extended to neighbors and friends in eighteenth-century London; "public" more obviously meant printed, spreading details to the unknown reader, or revealed at a meeting of the Royal Society. Just as private patients – La Grange, Walpole – became public through their case histories, so too did many "public" patients' stories remain essentially private, in the confines of the hospital ward or at home visited by a charity's practitioner. With the introduction of pupils into the hospitals, the ward patient's case became quasi-public, as I argued in Chapter 4, when his or her condition could be observed and discussed among groups of short-term students in ways that a private patient's could not. Making hospital cases public in the printed sense, however, did not demand a shift in attitudes toward the institutionalized poor. Indeed, looking for the "use" of charity patients as resources for clinical knowledge in the early to mid-eighteenth century reveals that many of the hospital men who published cases found them at best as useful as private ones and, more typically, just as easily ignored as sources for medical observations.

Because a few seventeenth- and early-eighteenth-century social commentators, particularly William Petty (in 1648) and John Bellers (in 1714),

the Stone, since his first Account in April 1750," *Philosophical Transactions* 47 (1751–2): 472–3; "An Account of the Case of the late Right Honourable Horace Lord Walpole; being a Sequel to his own Account," *Philosophical Transactions* 50 (1757): 205–20; this article is a collection of letters by John Pringle and Robert Whytt on Walpole's case.

72 Walpole, "An Account," 44; Pringle and Whytt, "An Account," 207–8. Two surgeons, Mr. Ranby (Serjeant-surgeon) and Caesar Hawkins, performed the autopsy, in which they only examined the abdomen, discovering stones in the urinary bladder and, to the surprise of all, stones in the gallbladder as well. Walpole had a notably antiphysician attitude in other contexts: see Porter and Porter, *Patient's Progress*, 38.

saw hospitals as places for the collection of empirical data on clinical medicine, historians have noted that hospital practitioners *could* have used them as research sites long before the early nineteenth century.[73] With Francis Clifton's scheme for the improvement of physic (1732), surely medical men realized the potential benefit if

three or four persons of proper qualifications shou'd be employ'd in the *Hospitals*. . . . to set down the cases of the Patients there from day to day, *candidly* and *judiciously*, without regard to private opinions or publick systems, and at the year's end publish these facts just as they are, leaving every one to make the best use of 'em he can for himself.[74]

Like the early Royal Society's plans for massive collections of information to bring Bacon's Solomon's house into being, Clifton's suggestions display the grandiosity of the new science and the rhetorical dream that, with the right conditions, regular medical practitioners would gain true knowledge and respect, while "*pretenders* of every kind wou'd . . . dwindle away to nothing."[75] No one embarked upon Clifton's project – not even Clifton; probably no one really took it seriously. The significant message for his contemporaries, I suggest, lies not in a possibly protoquantitative approach to hospital medicine, but in Clifton's appeal to appropriate character: the candid and judicious observer. "There is, it must be own'd a good deal of difficulty in following *Nature* close. The *Attention*, the *sagacity*, the *disinterestedness*, and the *diligence*, that is necessary, fall to the share of but few."[76] To display these gentlemanly qualities, it mattered little whether the patient were seen inside or outside a hospital ward. Instead, the way that the practitioner made his experience public, at the Royal Society or in print, could reveal his sagacity, disinterestedness, and diligence in the details of his case account.

Publishing hospital men thus used their charitable patients as they did their private ones, as potential stories of individual disorders. William Cheselden, to note just one example, dotted the pages of his *The Anatomy of the Human Body* with such indiscriminate observations.[77] Descriptions of patients – and the practitioners' attention to them – varied more according

73 William Petty, "The Advice of W. P. to Mr. Samuel Hartlib for the Advancement of Particular Parts of Learning (1648)," in *The Harleian Miscellany*, 6 (1810): 149–50; John Bellers, *An Essay Towards the Improvement of Physick in Twelve Proposals* (London: J. Sowle, 1714).

74 Clifton, *The State of Physic*, 171–2; see Tröhler, "Quantification," 94–7; this passage is also quoted and discussed in Max Neuburger, "Francis Clifton and William Black: Eighteenth Century Critical Historians of Medicine," *Journal of the History of Medicine* 5 (1950): 47.

75 Clifton, *The State of Physic*, 173.

76 Clifton, *The State of Physic*, 158.

77 William Cheselden, *The Anatomy of the Human Body*, 3rd ed. (London: W. Bowyer, 1726), 6–12, 54–5, 172–4; see also Richard Mead (briefly physician to St. Thomas's), *Medical Precepts and Cautions* (1751), in *The Medical Works* (London: J. Brindley, 1756), 385, 393; Percivall Pott, *The Chirurgical Works of Percivall Pott*, ed. James Earle, 3 vols. (London: J. Johnson, 1790), 1: 255–70, esp. p. 264.

to the sick person's status than to his or her location, with the poor at home or in wards sometimes given fewer visits and depicted more brusquely than the well-to-do.[78] Yet charitable kindness, whether or not sincere, also led some hospital men to personalize their hospital patients in the style suited to Mr. La Grange. Thomas Wilbraham, physician to the Westminster from 1739 to 1761, presented the case of Isaac Cranefield, "a waterman," to the Royal Society in 1752 with a tone of remarkable courtesy. Cranefield entered the Westminster with hydrophobia: "We desir'd him to give us the opportunity to see how he could bear an attempt to get down some liquid. He readily consented." He later died, as Wilbraham told his audience, after having "express'd much concern for the loss, which his wife and children would have of him."[79] Including the noble sentiments, compliance, or religiosity of the lower orders faced with illness and death allowed the case history to serve as an exemplary moral tale, just as the sad end to Mr. La Grange's careless airing offered a cautionary one. Comments on the patient's character and behavior let the practitioner invest his story with a whole range of social and medical meanings, whether the sick person appeared to him at hospital or at home.

Wilbraham ended Cranefield's case history at his death, noting casually that "that day we had him open'd" and duly providing a few sentences on the postmortem appearances of his lungs, esophagus, and stomach. The physician's perfunctory account in this case simultaneously suggests his aloofness from the procedure itself and the apparent routineness of a hospital autopsy. As I have explained in detailing anatomical teaching, postmortems to investigate particular causes of death had far more public acceptance than complete dissections merely to learn the parts of the body. Published autopsies, from *An Account of the dissection of His Highness William, Duke of Gloucester* (1700), to reports in medical texts and the *Philosophical Transactions*, reveal that this procedure had social and cultural approbation for seeking material evidence of the cause of death (however much or little it was actually performed) as long as the investigation was limited to the appropriate parts and these remained with the body for burial.[80] In this context, hospital patients, despite their removal from family and friends, seem to have been no more likely targets for postmortem study than private ones during this period. No evidence has appeared, at least, that

78 Claudius Amyand, "Of a Bubonocele or Rupture in the Groin, and the Operation made upon it," *Philosophical Transactions* 40 (1737–8): 361–7; Amyand's private patient was "my Lord Thomond's Coachman's Wife, Mrs. Bennet," whom he later called "this Old Woman."
79 Thomas Wilbraham, "An Account of an Hydrophobia," *Philosophical Transactions* 47 (1751–2): 412–14.
80 Bellers, *An Essay*, 7. See Royal College of Physicians (RCP) MS 101 for the manuscript accounts of postmortems of several prominent figures, including that of William, Duke of Gloucester, in which Charles Bernard and Edward Green (surgeons to St. Bartholomew's) took part, that was then published.

shows hospital surgeons or physicians in the early to mid-eighteenth century deliberately recounting a charity case *because* the body could be opened by virtue of a hospital demise.

Understanding the blurry boundaries between public and private helps considerably in explaining why hospital practitioners, despite perhaps seeing their charities as clinical resources as Clifton did, "used" them so little. With the single case history coming into its own as an exemplar of both venerable Hippocratic methodology and modern narration of matters of fact, closeness to the details of the well-to-do patient's life offered as many advantages to the observing practitioner as did the emotional and financial distance from the ward patient's opinions. Some social anxiety about the misuse of the poor for the benefit of their betters – and a likely more deeply felt fear that any patient might be the object of untried practice – did indeed arise during these decades, hinting that hospital cases might be treated differently than private ones. Yet such comments drew their strength more from the implications of "experiment" than from concern for the institutionalized as vulnerable objects of medical tinkering.

In the world of wits and social commentators, vivisectional experiments on animals performed in and around the Royal Society during the late seventeenth and early eighteenth centuries had been ridiculed for their purposelessness and, in some circles, deplored for their cruelty, even when some critics acknowledged their utility. Here the disinterested gentleman–observer met the eighteenth-century "man of feeling," in whom compassion and sensibility tempered the extremes of detachment that led, on the one hand, to the advancement of knowledge through "experiments" and, on the other, to brutality.[81] In the late 1720s, William Cheselden, for example, suggested that he perforate the eardrum of a convicted felon (who would then be pardoned) to see whether that might lead to insights on Queen Caroline's deafness. His notion attracted enough public notice, including satirical jibes about the "experiment," that Cheselden remarked that it was then "thought fit to be forbid."[82] In 1737, the Earl of Burlington withdrew his subscription from St. George's because he felt "that this once noble design will soon change from an hospital for relief into a school for experiments" when the senior surgeons, Ambrose Dickens and Claudius Amyand, resigned over an internal dispute involving surgical treatment.[83]

81 Andreas-Holger Maehle, "Literary Responses to Animal Experimentation in Seventeenth- and Eighteenth-Century Britain," *Medical History* 34 (1990): 27–51; Keith Thomas, *Man and the Natural World: Changing Attitudes in England, 1500–1800* (Harmondsworth, UK: Penguin Books, 1983), provides an extensive account of the complexities of cruelty and sensibility toward the animal world.

82 Cope, *Cheselden*, 32–4, includes the quotations from the *Grub-Street Journal* of 7 January 1731/2 and Cheselden's *Anatomy of the Human Body* (edition not cited).

83 George Peachey, in his *The History of St. George's Hospital (1733–1753)* (London, 1910), quoting from a 1737 letter to the governors, 276; I have not yet found the original of this letter.

"Mankind," observed Dr. Campbell in 1746, "naturally abhors the Thoughts of trying new Experiments in Physick; an honest physician is cautious of introducing a new Practice, however well he may be convinc'd of its Rectitude in Theory."[84]

For the most part, trying new treatments and therapies did not really pose a moral dilemma for early to mid-eighteenth-century practitioners or their patients. Doing "experiments" continued to display a progressive approach to clinical experience *and* to evoke the unscrupulous, unfeeling practitioner, depending on the polemical context. Hospital physicians and surgeons described trials of suggested techniques among their charity patients, the noninstitutionalized poor, the middling ranks, and the well-to-do during the first part of the eighteenth century with little sense that the hospital, much less the homes of the poor, distinguished a set of patients more easily observed or controlled than others.[85] Claudius Amyand, for example, told the Royal Society about a fairly elaborate surgical procedure attempted on the arm of a shepherd admitted to St. George's in August 1739, who died, and a similar operation on a private patient of his, begun in November of the same year, who was cured. The shepherd – according to Amyand – urged the search for an alternate treatment as he "was determined to forgo any thing, rather than submit to the Amputation that was propos'd."[86] Whether or not the shepherd actually requested the heroic effort, which ended in amputation and death anyway, Amyand depicted him as doing so; like Dr. Wilbraham's credibility, that of Amyand rested on the nuances of such personal observation and individualism.

John Andrée's midcentury work on hemlock offers a concluding example of the way that hospital practitioners combined "public" and private patients as they tested claims for a new treatment. Andrée's account, moreover, shows him using personal or "reliable" case histories for vital "matters of fact" while trying to undermine another's "matters of fact" through criticizing the author's narration of them. In 1760, Dr. Störck of Vienna published his treatise on hemlock, which was translated into English that year as *An Essay on the Medicinal Nature of Hemlock . . . in the Cure of Cancers.* Not surprisingly, a proclaimed cure for cancer by a Continental

---

84 Campbell, *A letter . . . [on] the case of the Rt. Hon. Thomas Winington,* 13–14.
85 The controversy over smallpox inoculation provides ample material for this point. See Rusnock, "The Quantification of Things Human"; John Douglas, *A Short Account of Mortifications, and of the Surprising Effect of the Bark, in putting a Stop to their Progress, &c.* (London: John Norse, 1732). See also the trials of agaric of oak reported in the *Philosophical Transactions* in the 1750s. London surgeons read a report from Paris that agaric of oak was used as a styptic to stop hemorrhages in operations. Both Samuel Sharp and Joseph Warner of Guy's submitted it to "experiment" at the request of the Royal Society in 1752. While the first case, successful, was indeed a Guy's patient, others soon followed from trials in private practice (see n. 68).
86 Claudius Amyand, "Some observations on the *spina ventosa,*" *Philosophical Transactions* 44 (1746–7): 193. This paper was read and published posthumously.

professor attracted attention, and even newspapers carried extracts of the English text (in part to advertise the publication), giving vivid details of some of the cases Störck presented.[87] In 1761 Andrée, noted as "senior physician to the London Hospital" (although *not* FRS), published his *Observations upon a Treatise of the Virtues of Hemlock . . . written by Dr. Störck, an eminent Physician in the Imperial City of Vienna.* From Störck's account, and the apparent sanction of other Continental physicians, Andrée stated that he, among others, was "induced . . . to try the Success of this important Discovery." Andrée thus neatly ascribed the initial experiments not just to another practitioner, but to an "eminent" one, clearly believed to be a learned gentleman. Having justified his reasonable faith in a way familiar, at least, to Fellows of the Royal Society, Andrée proceeded to describe the failure of hemlock in the internal treatment of cancers.[88]

Andrée began his exposé with the story of a hospital patient, Elizabeth Webb, who experienced dizziness, loss of sight, and numbness upon taking a preparation of hemlock (*Circuta vulgaris*). For a "lady" with breast cancer, seen in his private practice, hemlock "brought on paralysis." Reports from other London practitioners, including an "eminent surgeon," confirmed this disappointment. To bolster his account, however, Andrée then turned to textual authorities, from antiquity to the eighteenth century, who had associated the symptoms he saw with hemlock poisoning. In his search to be fair, Andrée sent for plant samples from Vienna, to see whether the English product differed from what Störck used. He even testified to his own belief that specifics for cancer likely existed in nature, underscoring his theoretical kinship with Dr. Störck.[89] In the end, however, his own experience triumphed and he dashed the hopes of those looking to hemlock for a nonsurgical treatment for cancer.

In supporting his claims, Andrée confronted the problem of using case histories as the primary sources of evidence and argumentation for medical practice. After his explicit efforts to procure samples of hemlock from Vienna, and his implicit attempts to show the results of the drug in a variety of "cancers" and among patients across the social spectrum, Andrée

87 See, for example, *London Chronicle: or Universal Evening Post*, 4–6 Sept. 1760. The original work appeared in Latin: Anton von Störck, *Libellus . . . quo demonstratur cicutam . . . non solum usu interno putissime exhiberi, sed et esse simul remedium valde utile in multis morbis, qui hueusque curatu impossibiles dicebantur*, in 2 parts (Vindoboae, 1760–1).
88 John Andrée, *Observations upon a Treatise on the Virtues of Hemlock, in the Cure of Cancers, written by Dr. Störck, an eminent Physician in the Imperial City of Vienna* (London: J. Meres, 1761), iii–iv. Andrée compared his investigation to that of the hospital surgeons Gataker (Westminster, 1754–60; St. George's, 1760–69) and Bromfield (St. George's, 1744–80) on claims for nightshade as a cure for cancer, a practice recommended in a French publication in 1756 (pp. 1–3). See Thomas Gataker, *Observations on the Internal Use of the Solanum or Nightshade* (London: R. and J. Dodsley, 1757), and William Bromfield, *An Account of the English Nightshades and their Effects* (London: R. Baldwin, 1757).
89 Andrée, *Observations*, 5–18, 54–8.

notably did not appeal to individual constitutions, local conditions, or national temperament to account for the discrepancy between his results compared to Störck's; nor could he dismiss the eminent Dr. Störck as a mere empiric or outright charlatan. He turned, instead, to the more subtle rhetorical strategy of questioning Störck's experiences as he had described them. "A material Criterion of the Veracity of the Cases produced is wanting, viz. the Names or Places of Abode of the Patients; that but a few of them were shewn to Dr. Van Swietan, the Empress's Head Physician, and some conjectured to be cured, tho' they were dismissed before the Event was determined."[90] Andrée had set up the implications of his suspicions with his own prefatory declaration:

Those who would be satisfied concerning the Cases introduced by me, may, if it is desired, be informed of the Patients, whose initial Letters are only mentioned; or of any other Particulars relating to the Veracity of the Facts, or the rest of the Matters submitted to the Consideration of the Public; not doubting but that they will bear the strictest Scrutiny.[91]

In this statement, John Andrée drew on decades of conventional language that sustained the empirical verification of "facts" through an appeal to personal "Scrutiny." By giving the full names of hospital patients and the initials and status of private ones, Andrée countered Störck's suffering but nameless cases, in an attempt to make his victims more "real" than those seen in Vienna. This tactic, along with appealing to gentlemen–witnesses, producing an anatomical part, or demonstrating an experiment, had become, at least in London's circles around the Royal Society, in popular and medical lectures, and in much medical writing, the way to cast "true" knowledge grounded in particular experience. These methods were, as Andrée's comments on Störck suggest, regularly contested and yet repeatedly confirmed among eighteenth-century practitioners, on and off hospital wards.

Andrée used his hospital position on the title page of his short work and presented ward cases within his text. For him, it seems that being a hospital physician gave him some status in the metropolis, but not necessarily privileged access to certain kinds of knowledge. During the middle decades of the century, other hospital physicians and surgeons began to refer to their charity posts as giving them the implicit authority of long "experience" rather than favored entry to unique realms of the sick. John Freke, for example, introduced his *An Essay on the Art of Healing* of 1748 by saying that he would not only dispense with the opinions of "learned Authors"

90 Andrée, *Observations*, 19; Andrée also noted his suspicions of Störk's diagnoses. In at least one case, Störck gave none of the "pathognomonic Signs of a Scirrhus" – at least not the appearances to convince his English critic (p. 33).
91 Andrée, *Observations*, viii.

but also avoid "a large History of Cases." He could do so, Freke implied, because of his "twenty years at St. Bartholomew's" as surgeon. With his extensive experience he could best choose cases to illustrate "such Diseases, and their Cure, as I think I can shew a mechanical Cause for, from the several Redundances of Nature and Accidents."[92] Such claims and cases, in short, enhanced hospital men's images as skilled – and observant – practitioners, yet ultimately had meaning only when displayed in particular case accounts, be they charitable or fee-based, "public" or private.

The men elected to hospital posts at St. Thomas's, St. Bartholomew's, Guy's, the Westminster, St. George's, the London, and the Middlesex between 1700 and 1760 comprised a diffuse group among the metropolis's elite physicians and surgeons. From poets and classical pedants to mechanical philosophers and dissecting surgeons, these practitioners blended with their social peers and aspired to the circles of their social betters. Success hinged on cultural acceptance, which, in the competitive marketplace of eighteenth-century practice, had as much – or more – to do with style as with medical skill. In this context, publishing to "advance" medical knowledge and therapeutics was merely one tactic London men could try, and nearly half the staff physicians and just over a quarter of the hospital surgeons did so. Some, like the surgeons Claudius Amyand and William Cheselden and the physicians Richard Mead, James Jurin, and John Andrée, were fairly prolific. Others, such as Dr. James Hawley, with whom this chapter opened; Dr. Nicholas Munckley; and John Dobyns (surgeon, St. Bartholomew's, 1719–30), were content with one or two articles or pamphlets. The minority of staff men who reached out to a public through print have nevertheless allowed me to sketch their intellectual interests and approaches to knowledge, however disingenuous it may be to let their work represent the beliefs and practices of all the general charities' physicians and surgeons.

The Royal Society's activities, particularly seen through the *Philosophical Transactions,* suggest how much the medical men accepted into the Society's rooms shaped their investigative methods to the Fellows' beliefs about valid and useful knowledge. The Royal Society itself was still an innovative forum in early-eighteenth-century London, the place for the public confirmation of matters of fact, right reasoning, and polite consensus. Its journal extended the "public" to letter writers and unknown readers, creating new genres for writing short pieces about the natural world. Neither the Royal Society nor its *Philosophical Transactions* were the only arenas for intellectual dispute and agreement, of course, given the British universities,

---

92 John Freke, *An Essay on the Art of Healing,* vii–viii; See also, Donald Monro (physician, St. George's, 1758–86), *An Essay on the Dropsy and its Different Species,* 3rd ed. (London: A. Millar, 1765), ix–x; John Brisbane, *Select Cases,* v.

the London corporations and college, coffeeshops, and the expanding world of print in the metropolis. Yet in its rooms and journal, members of the Royal Society constantly articulated and reconfirmed (more by example than by philosophical analysis) contemporary standards for (new) knowledge. There hospital men, in company with those recognized as "gentlemen" both as social beings and as disinterested observers, pursued popular theoretical themes and introduced case commentaries as studies in natural knowledge.

For London hospital men in the first half of the eighteenth century (and later, as I argue in the following chapters), the confirmation of "the case" as knowledge had a significant place in their struggle for intellectual and occupational authority. Caught up in their rivalries, their ambivalent use of the ancients as timeless experts, and their allegiance both to theoretical systems for "rational" practice and to the Royal Society's celebration of Baconian "matters of fact," both medical and lay people constructed the short case history as a valuable contribution to knowledge separable from learned texts and on-the-spot experience. It was a place to display expertise and appropriate character, careful observations and rational deductions, detachment and kindness. During this period, a hospital post offered London physicians and surgeons some occupational status (as depicted on their title pages), public notice, and, if evoked, grounds to claim experience. Yet they did not need to walk a charity's wards to discover clinical facts or to try out new treatments: all patients, public or private, offered insights – and even "experiments" – for the astute gentleman scholar. And, composed with care, with restrained interpretations, and a certain erudition, case commentaries were safe.

7

London hospital men and a medical community, 1760–1815

In the preface to their first volume of *Medical Observations and Inquiries* (1757), a "Society of Physicians in London" praised the publications of the Royal Society and the Parisian Academy of Sciences, yet noted that their scope "does not allow them to insert several things . . . calculated only for the improvement of physick." Furthermore, the anonymous editor(s) continued, some

> important cases . . . cannot decently be read in mixed company, and there are others, of the merits of which, physicians only can be adequate judges, and which would appear neither entertaining nor instructive to philosophers or mathematicians.[1]

"Mixed company," a phrase that evokes audiences of men and women, suggests that these physicians had extraordinary delicacy about presenting medical details to nonmedical men, unless prim ladies indeed visited the Royal Society meetings. Note how the physicians claimed to be the only "adequate judges" of their experiences. They could share the "entertaining" or "instructive" case with educated folk, but they were the appropriate interpreters of such matters of fact. Asserting their unique expertise had, of course, always marked medical practitioners, however much they negotiated their authority with patients and peers. So the editor(s) went on to explain the particular grounds for *their* valuable work:

> The persons who formed this Society, were either such as had the care of hospitals, or were otherwise in some degree of repute in their profession; and consequently had frequent opportunities of making observations themselves, and of verifying, in the course of their practice, the discoveries of others. When difficult cases occurred to any of them, the rest were consulted; and that method of cure, which appeared most likely to be attended with success, was tryed, and the event communicated.[2]

The Society of Physicians, the second medical society in London and the first in the metropolis to publish a collection of cases and essays, nicely

1 *Medical Observations and Inquiries* I (1757): viii–ix.
2 *Medical Observations and Inquiries* I (1757): iv.

remarked upon two of the three main points of this chapter. First, the overt appeal to fellow practitioners as "adequate judges" of medical experience marked a claim central to the proliferation of medical societies and journals for the rest of the century. Locating part of the ongoing process of abstracting knowledge from cases and other reports in face-to-face encounters among medical men reaffirmed them as both contributors and evaluators of medical facts. Defining *who counted* as "adequate judges" in various societies and publications could both open and restrict this category to specific kinds of practitioners. For the midcentury Society of Physicians their self-conscious description had pointed inclusions and omissions. They really did not mean that all "physicians" had their skills, much less all practitioners. Quite the contrary. They were men of "repute," serving in hospitals or in extensive practice. They made many observations and sought to verify claims. They, moreover, *consulted* with each other, evoking a network that operated outside their collective discussions in the society meetings. And they omitted any nods to the Royal College of Physicians, either in the preface or in authors' identifications in the table of contents and heads of articles. This subtle snub spoke volumes about their notion of "adequate judges," the import of which I discuss later.

Second, the "Society of Physicians" established themselves as men of practice because they sought "new truth" in clinical experience. They published only those cases, the editor(s) asserted, "such as shall appear of use and importance." They eschewed "hypothetical disquisitions" or those with "rather a tendency to shew the parts and erudition of the writer."[3] This rhetorical move aligned these men with those who saw improvement in medicine coming from the bedside, not from learned texts and commentaries. With the brief case history established as a worthy genre in the *Philosophical Transactions,* a publication still serving to entertain and instruct "philosophers and mathematicians," these medical practitioners could use it to further their own place as producers of new, *useful* knowledge. For the rest of the century, medical men, from London pupils to colonial correspondents, thrived on this newly privileged stance. Through the publication of societies' collections and, later on, nonaffiliated journals, moreover, such contributions from experience became public. Accessible to medical and lay readers, but overtly aimed at practitioners, such journals regularly displayed current practice, discoveries, and information, all ostensibly "good" work. As I stressed in the previous chapter, case histories provided a wealth of detail not only on how to treat patients, but also on how medical men behaved – at least how they chose to recount their actions and observations. In the following pages, I discuss the range and types of medical periodicals, and lay out when and where practitioners

3 *Medical Observations and Inquiries* I (1757): xi, xii.

could both assert themselves as benefiting medicine and read about others who seemed to do so successfully.

The Society of Physicians in 1757 did not address the third issue at stake in this chapter, for it arose as a consequence of the trends just sketched. London medical societies and periodicals opened the possibility to "advance" knowledge to an extensive, diverse population of practitioners. Men "of some degree of repute in their profession" managed to contain this potential nightmare of leveling by deciding just who was allowed to participate in medical society meetings and publications. Yet they still had a problem of how to demarcate themselves from those without much "repute" whose accounts of experience they ostensibly welcomed. One strategy, which the Society of Physicians used, was to qualify who *they* were, such as those who "had the care of hospitals." The FRS, too, served as a distinct badge of status for elite medical men throughout the century, for the Fellowship remained socially restricted. Thus authors who had the FRS nearly always displayed these initials on their cases and essays for the medical press. Yet fostering a connection with "science," especially the gentlemanly science of the Royal Society, had even further import by the last decades of the eighteenth century. For hospital men, the Royal Society and its *Philosophical Transactions* remained the place to present and to publish on the medical sciences. They occasionally included their work on human anatomy, comparative anatomy, animal chemistry, and physiology in medical journals, but for the most part not until the early nineteenth century. The Royal Society, with its perpetual social exclusivity, enhanced the role of certain practitioners as a core intellectual elite, as "men of science."[4] And the "adequate judges" of their work, work that was carefully distanced – but not totally detached – from the bedside, were obviously their peers at the Royal Society. Natural historians and natural philosophers gave these practitioners' investigations a cultural authority no medical group could rival.

These three issues – the identity of "adequate judges," case histories as a focus for new knowledge, and the role of the Royal Society in making medical "men of science" – all figure in this chapter's basic argument. Put succinctly, between 1760 and 1820 a new sort of medical community appeared in London. It had multiple expressions, and certainly many constituent parts, yet enough of a distinct historical presence for me to apply this term as an embracing metaphor. In a narrow sense, the London medical community literally existed in the medical societies and journals I set out later. Their members and authors, together with the gamut of ward-walking pupils, lecture attenders, teachers, consultants, and hangers-on,

---

4 Benjamin Brodie gave this phrase to Sir Joseph Banks for his typology of Fellows of the Royal Society. See n. 67.

constituted interlocking networks of practitioners that constantly decentered the corporate communities of physicians, surgeons, and apothecaries. The public venues for medical knowledge – lectures, societies, and journals – were the new elements in eighteenth-century metropolitan life that layered collective experience onto the usual routines of practicing, reading, and discussing that had always been available to literate medical men. It was this quasi-official organizing that created a medical community. In a very important second sense, however, this community also was (and is) a rhetorical one. Conjured up in the prefaces to medical journals, displayed in printed lists of medical societies' members, evoked by case histories published in journals by correspondents, this community included not only the practitioners who did contribute, but also those who *could have* participated in the making and disseminating of medical knowledge. These were the pupils who stayed silent in meetings, the provincial practitioner who never got around to sending in his interesting case, the hospital surgeon who showed up to medical gatherings and took students on ward rounds but did not publish. Casting this wide community in such subjective places puts it where it belongs: in the shadowy realm of unnamed listeners, actors, and readers. It was as real, nonetheless, as the more concrete networks, for this sense of the community included the universalized surgeon–apothecary, the Edinburgh graduate in provincial practice, the dispensary man, and the hospital snob, all of whom early-nineteenth-century reformers marshaled into medical politics.

Elaborating on where, and how, matters of medical authority were played out in these decades reveals the gradual formation of an alternative medical hierarchy, one potentially distinct from that embodied in London's medical corporations. As I indicated in Chapter 3, the Royal College of Physicians, Surgeons' Company, and Society of Apothecaries maintained their traditional places as formal centers of power among physicians, surgeons, and apothecaries. Within these groups the ruling councils chose certain men to join their self-perpetuating elites. In a narrow sense these practitioners were the leaders of their professions by corporate definition. I argue in this chapter that authority over "good" knowledge within the broader medical community did *not* necessarily depend upon a practitioner's rank within a corporate institution, but rather upon participation in medical societies, lecturing, and publishing of useful knowledge. Such insider meritocracy conferred respect upon active teachers and investigators and promised a degree of professional status for ordinary practitioners that was partly independent of mere popularity among private patients.

The differences between the values and standards associated with corporate rank and those with community respect underlay reformers' criticism of these institutions during the late eighteenth and early nineteenth centuries. Yet the reform movements faltered, thwarted by the continuing influence that the councils of the Royal College of Physicians and the Royal College of Surgeons had over their members and among London's lay elite. At the end of this chapter, I explain why this was so. From the 1780s on into the nineteenth century, the ruling members of both the Royal College of Physicians and the Royal College of Surgeons invited hospital men to join them, drawing physicians and surgeons who had quite visible roles in hospitals, medical teaching, societies, and publications into their folds.[5] Authority in the medical community thus became deeply intertwined with corporate interests and professional power.

PUBLIC PLATFORMS: PUBLISHING AND STATUS

Casting hospital men as a particularly visible and influential group within London's medical community rests in part upon their collective image during this period. In the sixty years between 1760 and 1819, hospital physicians and surgeons began to look more like the top of a modern academic and professional hierarchy than they had during the first six decades of the century.

Four working generalizations emerge from the data collected on these men. First, the proportion of staff men who published on medical topics, lectured, or obtained the FRS grew from half for the period from 1700 to 1760 (Table 6.1) to three-fourths by the 1790s to 1820s (Table 7.1). A clear majority of hospital men thus displayed themselves as "improvers" of knowledge (whether they actually put much energy into it is a different question). Second, among all the physicians in the Royal College of Physicians, hospital Licentiates particularly stand out as a publishing group in the later decades (Table 7.2). They constituted a subset of hospital physicians increasingly compelled to compete with their FRCP colleagues for status, as more Fellows had begun to seek – and to get – hospital positions, as explained in Chapter 2.[6] Third, hospital surgeons made a major shift in their collective presence. By the later decades, staff surgeons looked

---

5 For the power of hospital men in the nineteenth century, see Ivan Waddington, "General Practitioners and Consultants in Early Nineteenth Century England: The Sociology of an Intra-Professional Conflict," in *Health Care and Popular Medicine in Nineteenth Century England,* ed. John Woodward and David Richards (New York: Holmes & Meier, 1977), 164–88; M. Jeanne Peterson, *The Medical Profession in Mid-Victorian London* (Berkeley: University of California Press, 1978).

6 On average, 1.7 Fellows and 6.7 Licentiates entered the RCP annually between 1780 and 1799; for the period from 1800 to 1815, the average number of new members rose to 2.3 and 10 per year, respectively. Twenty-two of the seventy-eight new Licentiates (28 percent) between 1805 and 1809 had received the MD degree prior to 1800, in a period of heightened discussion about reform and licensing. The sheer number of graduated MDs in Britain – especially from Edinburgh – also increased during these decades, another story of competition and status. See Lisa Rosner, *Medical Education in the Age of Improvement* (Edinburgh: Edinburgh University Press, 1991).

Table 7.1. *Physicians and surgeons elected to St. Bartholomew's, St.
Thomas's, the Westminster, Guy's, St. George's, the London,
and the Middlesex hospitals, 1760-1819*

Position	Elected	Published	FRS	Lectured	Did only one	Did all three
Physicians						
1760-1789	53	51% (27)	51% (27)	34% (18)	74% (39)	15% (8)
1790-1819	48	63% (30)	38% (18)	49% (22)	77% (37)	17% (8)
Surgeons						
1760-1789	35	40% (14)	43% (15)	29% (10)	54% (19)	23% (8)
1790-1819	25	60% (15)	40% (10)	36% (9)	68% (17)	28% (7)
Totals						
1760-1789	88	47% (41)	48% (42)	32% (28)	66% (58)	18% (16)
1790-1819	73	62% (45)	38% (28)	42% (31)	74% (54)	21% (15)
1760-1819	161	53% (86)	43% (70)	37% (59)	70% (112)	19% (31)

remarkably like staff physicians in the overall percentages of those publishing and becoming Fellows of the Royal Society (Table 7.1). The rise of the surgeon to academic parity with hospital physicians had a major part in the dynamics of the medical community as it emerged in London. Lastly, hospital men's individual careers varied considerably over these years, and the other side of the proportions need to speak for a moment: in broad terms, 30 percent of hospital men – one-fourth of the physicians and two-fifths of the surgeons – did *not* publish, lecture, or get the FRS between 1760 and 1820. Whatever hospital service may have done to connect practitioners with public platforms, it hardly compelled them to stand on them. Indeed, the patterns depicted here resulted from quite complex interactions among medical men and their peers, patients, patrons, and pupils. These patterns influenced new expectations of appropriate professional routes to fame and fortune, but they by no means monopolized the paths to success in the early nineteenth century.

Looking at the London medical population defined by Samuel Foart Simmons's *Medical Register* of 1783 further clarifies how numerical profiles can offer a partial view of the professions and publishing. Simmons's compilation of the *Medical Register* was a private venture to make regular

Table 7.2.   *Physicians and publishing, 1760-1819*
            By year of entry into the Royal College of Physicians

| | 1760-1779 | | 1790-1819 | | |
	Hospital	Other	Hospital	Other	Total
Fellows	24	16	36	39	115
Published	10 (42%)	11 (68%)	24 (67%)	19 (49%)	64 (57%)
Licentiates	36	97	17	195	345
Published	24 (67%)	49 (51%)	16 (94%)	64 (33%)	152 (44%)
Extralicentiates	0	35	0	42	77
Published		11 (31%)		11 (26%)	22 (28%)
Non-RCP	4		1		5
Published	2 (50%)		0		2 (40%)
Total	64	148	54	276	
Published	36 (56%)	71 (48%)	39 (74%)	94 (34%)	
	V		V		
All physicians	212		330		542
Published	107 (50%)		134 (41%)		241 (44%)

Note: The data include all physicians who entered the Royal College of Physicians between 1760 and 1819, as Fellows, Licentiates, or Extralicentiates. The five hospital physicians who did not become FRCP or LRCP obtained their posts during this period; the one elected in 1793 would likely have obtained the FRCP, as he had a Cambridge MB, but he died in 1794. The hospital category covers physicians to St. Bartholomew's, St. Thomas's, the Westminster, Guy's, St. George's, the London, and the Middlesex hospitals, excluding physician-accoucheurs to the Middlesex.

practitioners known to the public. Historians have noted that this text has definite weaknesses, arising from Simmons's quite personal method of collecting practitioners' names, especially for provincial practice.[7] This incomplete list nevertheless still serves as a way into the otherwise impene-

7 On the weaknesses of Simmons's register, particularly for provincial practitioners (who are not included here), see Joan Lane, "The Medical Practitioners of Provincial England in 1783," *Medical History* 28 (1984): 353–71; Mary Fissell, *Patients, Power and the Poor in Eighteenth Century Bristol* (Cambridge: Cambridge University Press, 1991), 201–2.

Table 7.3. *Medical Register of 1783: London physicians*

	Hospital: in post or retired[a]	Dispensary affiliation (listed)	Other	Total
Fellows	12	1	8	21
Published	3 (25%)	0	6 (75%)	9 (43%)
Licentiates	16	16	20	52
Published	6 (38%)	8 (50%)	5 (25%)	19 (37%)
Extralicentiates	0	0	2	2
Published	0	0	2 (100%)	2 (100%)
Non-RCP	2	18	39	59
Published	0	9 (50%)	10 (27%)	19 (32%)
Total	30	35	9	134
Published	9 (30%)	17 (49%)	23 (33%)	49 (37%)

Note: Identifications of membership category in the Royal College of Physicians are based on the information provided by Munk's *Roll*, not the affiliations given in Simmons's *Medical Register*, which are unreliable.

[a]Includes current and retired staff men to St. Bartholomew's, St. Thomas's, the Westminster, Guy's, St. George's, the London, and the Middlesex hospitals. Publication numbers do not include articles in collections or periodicals.

trable mass of medical men in the metropolis. Simmons's list of London physicians is particularly valuable because he included physicians who had not bothered to obtain the Licentiate or Fellowship of the Royal College of Physicians; his extensive list of surgeons, in contrast, covered only members of the Surgeons' Corporation. Tables 7.3 and 7.4 depict the publishing portraits of these occupations as they were in 1783, though the data are limited to authors who managed to produce monographs or pamphlets, not journal articles.

From the perspective of the *Medical Register,* hospital men have an intriguing image. Simmons listed 134 physicians (Table 7.3), of whom half had no institutional affiliation. The rest were, or had been, on the staff of one of the general hospitals or were identified as physicians to dispensaries and specialized charities. As of 1783, the general hospital men had published the least compared with the other groups. Since 44 percent of the London physicians on Simmons's list were not then licensed by the College (although some later trotted in to sit the examinations), and a third of *them* published, compared with 40 percent of the RCPs, membership in the College clearly did not necessarily appeal to those who published on medi-

Table 7.4. *Medical Register of 1783: Members of the Surgeons'*
Corporation

Distribution					
London	Provinces	Military/ colonial	Abroad	Not given	Total
271 (36%)	251 (41%)	95 (14%)	48 (7%)	98 (13%)	763 (100%)

Publication[a]			
	Surgeons	Published	Percentage of the total number who published
London			
General hospitals	35[b]	43% (15)	41%
Dispensaries, asylums, other hospitals	17	12% (2)	5%
Other	219	5% (10)	27%
Provincial/other			
Provincial/Military hospitals	15	13% (2)	5%
Other	379	2% (8)	22%
Totals			
London	271	10% (27)	73%
Provincial/Other	394	3% (10)	27%
Total with known locations	665	6% (37)	100%

[a]Publication as of 1783, for those with locations given: Total = 665
[b]Includes current and retired staff men to St. Bartholomew's, St. Thomas's, the Westminster, Guy's, St. George's, the London, and the Middlesex hospitals. Publication numbers do not include articles in collections or periodicals.

cal topics.[8] For the surgeons, Simmons's list carries different implications. Since he restricted it to members of the Surgeons' Corporation (Table 7.4), it likely omitted many men who considered themselves regular prac-

8 Seventeen of the fifty-nine non-RCP physicians (29 percent) later obtained the Licentiate, eleven of them by 1786. Among the non-RCP authors in this sample were: John Millar,

titioners and included some surgery in their rounds. Counting only those listed with London addresses, hospital surgeons in 1783 had published in far greater proportion to their number in the sample than either surgeons to dispensaries or other hospitals, or those without such charity affiliations. London's hospital surgeons comprised 13 percent of the London men, yet represented 56 percent of metropolitan surgeons who produced books or pamphlets. While the nonpublishing "others" cannot be simply labeled as the surgical rank and file, the overt prominence of the hospital men in the list certainly shows that they stood out from most surgeons in ways that hospital physicians in the early 1780s did not.

The *Medical Register* itself testifies to an attempted organization of regular practitioners into a medical profession with multiple hierarchies. Simmons's very arrangement of his text reveals a mapping of the medical community in which the new elements of eighteenth-century medical life were laid out in conjunction with the old. Simmons began with London, first giving accounts of the corporate bodies, their ruling courts, and their memberships in expected order: physicians, surgeons, apothecaries. (In the section for physicians, moreover, the entire medical entourage of the Royal Family, from physicians to dentists, came first.) Throughout the rest of the text, Simmons used symbols with the names he gave to denote physicians' and surgeons' suitable corporate identity (or lack thereof). This method ironically managed both to highlight those with corporate affiliations and to show that not all regular men bothered with them. Simmons then briefly described, with the names of staff, every medical charity in the metropolis; he followed this with information on London medical societies, listing their members; finally, he printed the names and courses of London's medical lecturers. Provincial practitioners, arranged by county, came next – in no doubt of their peripheral relationship to London. Simmons's inclusion of medical charities, societies, and lecturers placed them with the traditional corporate bodies as major parts of medical life in the metropolis, with their nuances of status and public prominence.

One of Simmons's most suggestive items followed his preface, facing the first page on London and the Royal College of Physicians: an advertisement for his *London Medical Journal*, extolling the virtues of the medical press.

GATHERINGS OF LIKE-MINDED MEN

Medical societies, like literary and philosophical ones, originated in gatherings of like-minded individuals determined to discuss particular topics on a

MD, physician to the Westminster General Dispensary, who wrote *A Discourse on the Duty of Physicians* in 1776 and never joined the RCP, and William Black, who wrote *Observations Medical and Political on the Small-Pox* (London: J. Johnson, 1781) and *An Historical Sketch of Medicine and Surgery* (London: J. Johnson, 1782). Black did not get the LRCP until 1787.

regular basis.[9] In the coffeehouse culture of eighteenth-century London, all sorts of informal groups coalesced and dispersed, a few becoming clubs or societies. Their members thrived on talk within the fluid sociability of urban life. The Pow-Wow Club, for example, which began in the 1780s, was a circle of John Hunter's various medical friends. They met once a month in the Thatched House Tavern, and the group continued after Hunter's death. While "ostensibly for the purpose of scientific conversation on natural history," Dr. John Yelloly (London, 1807–18) recalled, they really met for pleasure and did not bother with minutes, papers, or publications.[10] The "Gentlemen educated at the London Hospital" similarly met at the London Tavern to have dinner once a year, a lovely example of esprit de corps among the amorphous crowd of hospital pupils.[11] Distinguishing "societies" from other associations, in the end, depends upon the group's self-identification and, inevitably, on the existence of records.

Every London medical society thus has its own story, a version of founding, success, or decline, frequently embellished with the association's own rhetoric on how it promoted professional aims (see Table 7.5).[12] Like the Royal Society before them, medical societies did indeed encourage an exchange of information, ideas, and cautious criticisms. "The object," proclaimed the Medical Society of London, "is to give practitioners in medicine frequent opportunities of meeting together, and conferring with each other, concerning any difficult or uncommon cases which may have

9 James E. McClellan III, *Science Reorganized: Scientific Societies in the Eighteenth Century* (New York: Columbia University Press, 1985), 41–54; Nicholas Hans, *New Trends in Education in the Eighteenth Century* (London: Routledge and Kegan Paul, 1951), 163–80. For the context of scientific societies in Britain from the 1780s to the 1850s, see Jack Morrell and Arnold Thackray, *Gentlemen of Science: Early Years of the British Association for the Advancement of Science* (New York: Oxford University Press, 1981), 2–46.

10 Bransby B. Cooper, *The Life of Sir Astley Cooper*, 2 vols. (London: J. W. Parker, 1843), 2: 243; quotation from a letter written by John Yelloly.

11 See, for example, *Times*, 25 Sept. 1794.

12 Susan C. Lawrence, " 'Desirous of Improvements in Medicine': Pupils and Practitioners in the Medical Societies at Guy's and St. Bartholomew's Hospitals, 1795–1815," *Bulletin of the History of Medicine* 59 (1985): 89–104; George Peachey, *A Memoir of William and John Hunter* (Plymouth, UK: William Brendon & Son, 1924), 79–90. Cuthbert E. Dukes, "London Medical Societies in the Eighteenth Century," *Proceedings of the Royal Society of Medicine* 53 (1960): 699–706; A. Batty-Shaw, "The Oldest Medical Societies in Great Britain," *Medical History* 12 (1968): 233–44; Sir Humphrey Rolleston, "Medical Friendships, Clubs and Societies," *Annals of Medical History*, n.s. 2 (1930): 257–64; G. Newton Pitt, "Reflections on John Hunter as a Physician and his Relation to the Medical Societies of the Last Century," *Lancet* (9 May 1896): 1270–2; James J. Abraham, *Lettsom: His Life, Times, Friends and Descendents* (London: W. Heinemann, 1933), 124–38, 152–7, 182–3, 216–26; J. R. Wall, "The Guy's Hospital Physical Society (1771–1852)," *Guy's Hospital Reports* 123 (1974):159–70; Lloyd G. Stevenson, "The Siege of Warwick Lane, Together with a Brief History of the Society of Collegiate Physicians (1767–1798)," *Journal of the History of Medicine* 1 (1952): 105–21; Sir George Clark, *A History of the Royal College of Physicians of London*, 3 vols. (Oxford: Clarendon Press, 1966), 2: 552–73; *Laws and Regulations of the Medical Society founded [at Great Queen Street] in 1779* (London, 1783).

Table 7.5. *London medical societies, 1746-1819*

Name	Dates	Publication
Society of Naval Surgeons	1746-62?	
"A Society of Physicians"	1752-84	*Medical Observations and Inquiries*
Society of Collegiate Physicians	1767-98	
Society Instituted for the Improvement of Physical Knowledge [?]	1767	*Select Papers on the Different Branches of Medicine* (1 vol.)
Guy's Hospital Physical Society	1771-1852	
Physico-Medical Society	1771-?	
The Medical Society (of London)	1773-	*Memoirs of the Medical Society of London*
Middlesex Hospital Medical Society	1774-	
Great Queen Street Medical Society	1779-88?	
"A Society of Physicians" [?]	1781-3?	*London Medical Journal*[a]
Society for the Improvement of Medical Knowledge	1782-90?	*Medical Communications*
Society for the Improvement of Medical and Chirurgical Knowledge	1783-1818	*Transactions of the Society for the Improvement of Medical and Chirurgical Knowledge*
Lyceum Medicum Londinense	1785-1805/9?	
The Medical and Physical Society of St. Bartholomew's Hospital	1795-1827	
"A Private Medical Association"	1798	*Medical Records and Researches* (1 vol.)
Society of Physicians of London Instituted for the Improvement of Medical Knowledge	1798-1801	
Medical and Chirurgical Society	1805-	*Transactions of the Medical and Chirurgical Society*
Westminster Medical Society	1805-1850	[occasionally called the "Western" Society]
"A Society of Practical Physicians"	1811	*Selection of Interesting Cases* (1 vol.)
Hunterian Society	1819	

[a]Only volumes 1 and 2 claim an origin with "A Society of Physicians."

occurred; or communicating any new discoveries in medicine which have been made, either at home or abroad."[13] They offered predictable places to meet other practitioners, to consult on cases, and to build occupational networks and friendships. Some, like the Medical Society of London and Guy's Hospital Physical Society, encouraged the advancement of medical knowledge by offering prizes for the best essay on set topics: "Is nutrition performed by the arteries or the Nerves?" "In what points of view [ought]

13 *Statutes of the Medical Society of London Instituted 1773* (London, 1790), preface, n.p.

the human body be considered so as to speak of it intelligibly yet consistent only with truth & reality?"[14] The manuscript records that survive for a few groups also show how such societies gave practitioners sites to worry, in professional privacy, over treatments, ignorance, and failures.[15]

All of the medical societies over these decades had a part in the constant creating and reshaping of the medical community as they offered their "insiders" and "outsiders" ways to define themselves within the ranks of the capital's healers. All, through their activities and self-perpetuating memberships, made regular medical men. To join, a man had to be nominated and acknowledged in some way, whether informally by a member's introduction, more officially through an election, or by consensual acclaim as a "distinguished" person.[16] In doing so, the men who created and maintained medical societies interpreted "the" medical profession and subtly negotiated status within it. In the process of holding meetings centered on current medical issues, and discussing ongoing cases and new discoveries, moreover, these societies also shaped and channeled the oral culture of medical knowledge.[17] In those rooms, pupils and practitioners literally learned how to speak about their work: to choose "interesting" cases and to narrate them, to formulate short essays on particular topics, to present them, and to discuss them. The very sameness of the meetings, as glimpsed through the brief accounts given in minute books, attests to the ongoing construction of a medical culture by practitioners drawn together from bedsides, lecture podiums, libraries, ward chats, consultations, and dissecting rooms. When offering case histories and papers, in short, participants simultaneously imitated previously printed knowledge; defined themselves as the appropriate observers, critics, and authors of such knowledge; and then reinscribed some of this knowledge in published journals and texts.

Of particular concern for my argument are the various ways that these metropolitan societies built their constituencies, defined their purposes, and

---

14 Minutes of the Guy's Hospital Physical Society, 7 Dec. 1776, 11 vols., 1775–1825, 1835–52, Guy's Hospital Medical School, Wills Library; *Statutes of the Medical Society of London . . . 1773*, preface; Abraham, *Lettsom*, 218; Dukes, "London Medical Societies," 705; see *New London Medical Journal* 1 (1792): 229, for a printed announcement of the Guy's society's prize questions for the year.

15 See especially Minutes of the Guy's Hospital Physical Society; Minutes of the St. Bartholomew's Medical and Physical Society, 1799–1815, St. Bartholomew's Hospital Medical School Library; S. Lawrence, " 'Desirous of Improvements'," discusses these at length.

16 See, for example: Minute books of the Lyceum Medicum Londinense, 1792–1805, 4 vols., WIHM MS MSL MS 140a-d, 140a: 19 Oct. 1792; Medical Society of London, *Statutes*, 4–7; *Laws and Regulations of the Medical Society founded [in Great Queen Street]*, 17; Proceedings of the Society for the Improvement of Medical and Chirurgical Knowledge from its foundation in 1793 to its Dissolution in July [1817], WIHM MS 5282, 5 June, 2 July 1793.

17 Rosner, *Medical Education in the Age of Improvement*, 119–134, has an excellent discussion of the Royal Medical Society of Edinburgh in this context; see also, Kathryn Hunter, *Doctors' Stories: The Narrative Structure of Medical Knowledge* (Princeton, NJ: Princeton University Press, 1991).

transferred medical experience from the individual to the community. Roughly arranged, London's medical organizations fall into four categories. First, some groups were started for activist ends. The Society of Collegiate Physicians (1767) was a unique early example, followed by various reforming associations decades later. These later ones are not counted as medical societies in that their aims were, and remained, institutional and legislative change, but such groups articulated the regular practitioners' professional awareness that medical societies per se helped to create (see Chapter 3). Second, hospital practitioners, pupils, and their local colleagues established societies at London's hospitals and anatomical theaters, emphasizing the place that such associations had in teaching. Third, London practitioners created the ostensibly broader-based Medical Society of London and, later on, the Medical and Chirurgical Society. Finally, clusters of medical men organized much smaller and more select societies, notably the Society for the Improvement of Medical Knowledge and its contemporary, the Society for the Improvement of Medical and Chirurgical Knowledge.

A core group of the Society of Physicians who introduced this chapter organized the Society for Collegiate Physicians in 1767, in an attempt to reform the Royal College of Physicians. Despite their self-promotion as men of repute, at midcentury members of the Society of Physicians were still on the fringes of London's medical elite, which was primarily composed of RCP Fellows. All but one of the known early participants in the Society of Physicians were Licentiates of the RCP (and the Fellow, Richard Brocklesby, had started off as a Licentiate before managing to incorporate his MD at Cambridge).[18] After publishing two volumes of papers, these Licentiates quite likely felt the gap between their professional work and occupational status more intensely than before.[19] In 1765 the Royal College

18 The early members of this society at least included those who were listed in the first volume of the *Medical Observations and Inquiries* with their addresses so that others could communicate with them. Thus, using the first two volumes (1757, 1762), I counted as members all who had items communicated *to* them or published without a reference that they "communicated" their work: John Silvester (London, 1749–64, FRS 1747), George Maccaulay, Gowin Knight (Westminster, 1748–52, FRS 1745), Samuel Pye, John Clephane (St. George's, 1752–8, FRS 1746), John Fothergill (FRS 1763), William Hunter (FRS 1767), Michael Morris (Westminster, 1761–91, FRS 1764), John Pringle (FRS 1745), Richard Brocklesby (FRS 1746), Alexander Mackenzie, Thomas Dickson (London, 1759–84, FRS 1770). Richard Brocklesby obtained his first MD from Leiden and he became LRCP in 1751. He then incorporated at Cambridge the Dublin degree awarded him, and made FRCP in 1756. William Munk, *The Roll of the Royal College of Physicians of London*, 2nd ed., 4 vols. (London: Royal College of Physicians, 1878), 2: 201–3.

19 Clark, *Royal College of Physicians*, 2: 555–9. Clark claims that the first "Society of Physicians" began in order to challenge the RCP's "professional organization," as Dr. Schomberg's controversy over becoming a LRCP was well under way and Dr. John Clephane's refusal to pay his LRCP fees had just begun. This may be so, for certainly early members participated in these episodes. Yet the *Medical Observations and Inquiries* in 1757 and 1762 ignores all such overt political wrangling, which I believe is significant for how these physicians *wished to be seen* by the literate public.

of Physicians revised its statutes, aiming, in its historian's words, "to take particular care to preserve the dignity of the society" and keep control of the College in the Fellows' hands. Shortly thereafter, a controversy erupted over a Licentiate's examination, and the failed candidate, Dr. Letch, took the College to court. This was the overt reason for several men of "repute" in the Society of Physicians – notably John Fothergill, William Hunter, Thomas Dickson (London, 1759–84), John Silvester (London, 1749–64), Michael Morris (Westminster, 1761–91), Alexander Russell (St. Thomas's, 1759–68), and William Watson – to form the separate "Society for Collegiate Physicians." This group took up Letch's case, but much more broadly championed the Licentiates' claim to be members, with voting rights, of the Royal College of Physicians.[20] The rebellion between 1767 and 1771 occurred not because Licentiates only then realized that the Fellows controlled the RCP (as they had known from the beginning) or objected to the ways the RCP treated particular physicians and scorned non-Oxbridge MDs (as they did), but, I suggest, because they had a grounding in collective experience centered on the "advancement" of medical knowledge separate from their stodgy corporate body. Ultimately unsuccessful with this attempt to be recognized and to have the Fellowship open to non-Oxbridge MDs, by the mid-1770s this feisty set settled down into a medical discussion group, with papers, cases, and dinners.[21]

Medical reforming societies remained but glitter in a few eyes until the rank and file similarly discovered such collective experience in the later eighteenth century. This process probably occurred in the metropolitan societies that embraced a wide range of practitioners, particularly the ones I have labeled the "teaching" societies. Historians have long attributed the foundation of the first London teaching society, created at Guy's in 1771, to William Saunders (Guy's, 1770–1802), who imported his experience with the Edinburgh Medical Society to London. Guy's and St. Thomas's pupils, hospital staff, and local practitioners frequented the Guy's Hospital Physical Society's Saturday evening meetings. In 1774, a similar society appeared at the Middlesex, a more convenient place for West End students, and that at St. Bartholomew's emerged in 1795. John Sheldon, surgeon to

---

20 Stevenson, "The Siege of Warwick Lane"; Ivan Waddington, "The Struggle to Reform the Royal College of Physicians, 1761–1771: A Sociological Analysis," *Medical History* 17 (1975): 107–26; Alexander Russell and William Watson appear as contributing (not "communicating") authors in the third volume (1767) of the *Medical Observations and Inquiries*.

21 The Fellows also helped diffuse the Licentiates' claims by raising four LRCPs to the Fellowship – although none was a man of "repute" of the Society of Physicians. See Clark, *Royal College of Physicians*, 2: 564. Dr. Isaac Schomberg, a source of considerable controversy in the 1750s, was one of those made a Fellow (2: 548–51). The others were Richard Jebb, physician to the Westminster, 1754–62, and to St. George's, 1762–69, FRS 1765; Donald Monro, physician to St. George's, 1758–86, FRS 1766; and James Greive, physician to St. Thomas's, 1762–73, FRS 1769.

the Westminster and extramural lecturer, started a society at his Anatomical Theatre on Great Queen Street in 1779; John Hunter, surgeon to St.
George's and a lecturer, began his Lyceum Medicum Londinense at his
house and theater on Castle Street in 1785; the Western Medical Society
met at an unspecified "Anatomical Theatre" in 1807–8. John Hunter's
group struggled on after he gave it up in 1792 (and died in 1793), perhaps
meeting at St. George's or the Great Windmill Street Theatre until about
1805. The hospital groups managed to survive well into the nineteenth
century, with staff interest maintaining their continuity for fluctuating
groups of pupils.[22]

These societies allowed all sorts of medical men (and a few nonpractitioners) to join, give papers, and discuss cases. Designed, as Mr. Fernan-
dez, secretary to the Western [Westminster] Medical Society, put it, "for
promoting the objects of medical students (& Medical Inquiry)," the societies had multiple purposes in sharing and discussing medical experiences
and theories, as manuscript minutes attest.[23] What distinguished these societies from others, however, was their emphasis on pupils as active members among local and hospital practitioners. Indeed, at Guy's Hospital
Physical Society "ordinary" members included both pupils and undistinguished local men, an important reminder that students were not necessarily cast as uninteresting beginners. "Honorary" members, nevertheless,
included hospital men and other distinguished practitioners, such as lecturers, as a matter of course. As ordinary members could achieve honorary
status by giving case commentaries and papers, these societies' organizers
explicitly linked moving up in rank to contributing to knowledge. The
rules of the Lyceum Medicum Londinense elaborated further, distinguishing four levels of members: honorary, practitioners, students who "had
attended a hospital and one course of anatomy and the practice of Physic,"
and raw beginners.[24] Roughly speaking, then, the loose hierarchy present
at gatherings of teaching societies placed hospital and other reputable
men – defined, in part, by other reputable men's consensus – at the head
of the meetings and as the honored members. Others, the ordinary folk,
performed with, for, and among them, becoming regular medical men as
those with occupational authority accepted them and their contributions.

The teaching societies thus collected and reaffirmed the medical commu-

22 Minutes, Lyceum Medicum Londinense, 24 Feb. 1792.
23 Proceedings of the Western Medical Society, 4 Dec. 1807. NLM MS B 100. Since at least
   James Wilson, Benjamin Brodie, and William Brande (all of whom were active in the
   meetings) were associated with the Great Windmill Street Theatre, the society may have
   met there. Several of the Society's members, such as Henry Jeffreys, Thomas Stockwell,
   and Thomas Cobham, were perpetual pupils at St. George's and, for the former two,
   House Surgeons to St. George's in 1804 and 1809 respectively; see S. Lawrence, " 'Desirous of Improvements.' "
24 Newton-Pitt, "Reflections on John Hunter," 1273, from the Society's Laws of 1792.

nity that centered on the hospitals and anatomical theaters in the last three decades of the eighteenth century. Their institutional homes lent authority to their internal rankings, placing hospital practitioners and teachers over those who came to learn from them and extending that influence from the wards and lecture rooms to these new professional sites.[25] As some of these medical societies, notably Guy's Hospital Physical Society and Sheldon's Great Queen Street Society, adopted the category of "corresponding members," moreover, student (and other) visitors to London maintained their associations with these metropolitan centers. In 1783, for example, Sheldon's society claimed at least 64 corresponding members after its first four years, along with 66 ordinary members in London, 18 honorary members, and 12 "foreign honorary" men (including Linneaus). In 1804, the Guy's society named 659 members on its published list, of whom 365 (55 percent) were labeled as ordinary corresponding members, living in the provinces, colonies, or America.[26] Whether or not corresponding members actually corresponded with London matters less than the publication of membership rosters that included their names and locations. These men, such lists proclaimed, had connections with *these* groups, and *these* groups, connected to hospitals or theaters, conveyed knowledge. Perhaps the "corresponding" folk had some, too.

In contrast to the teaching societies, the two general medical societies admitted only men in practice, not pupils or nonpractitioners. Dr. John Coakely Lettsom founded the Medical Society in 1773. Lettsom, an ardent Quaker physician who had recently married into a fortune, had begun his philanthropic career a few years earlier by establishing the General Dispensary on Aldersgate Street. Ensconced in a house in Crane Court, off Fleet Street, and then (1788) in nearby Bolt Court, the Medical Society soon started a library; created a Council composed of three physicians, three surgeons, and three apothecaries; and made laws. Often hailed as an egalitarian society because it included physicians, surgeons, and apothecaries, in contrast to most earlier associations, Lettsom's group probably started out – and certainly became – more restrictive in its membership than the teaching societies. Despite its overtly representative administration and

25 For students' references to attending medical societies, see Hampton Weekes, letters to his father 15 Nov. 1801, 11 Jan. 1802, in John M. T. Ford, ed., *A Medical Student at St. Thomas's Hospital, 1801–1802: The Weekes Family Letters, Medical History*, Supplement No. 7, 1987, 76, 107; John Green Crosse, Diary, 1811–1814, 7 Nov. 1811, 17 Oct. 1812, and passim, Norfolk Record Office (NRO) MS 468; Frederick G. Parsons, *The History of St. Thomas's*, 3 vols. (London: Methuen & Co., 1932–6), 2: 251.
26 S. Lawrence, " 'Desirous of Improvements'," 91–2; *Laws and Regulations of the Medical Society founded [at Great Queen Street]*, v–ix; *Laws of the Physical Society held at Guy's Hospital . . . to which are annexed a list of the officers and members* (London, 1803), 1–29; the list itself is dated 1804.

membership, the Medical Society was dominated by physicians well into the nineteenth century.[27]

Divided both publicly and privately by internal disagreements, the Medical Society ironically figured as a group officially committed to "improv[-ing] the medical art" and to welcoming those versed in "sciences connected to medicine," yet unable to maintain stability among its members. In a notable fracas, for example, Dr. John Whitehead, a Quaker physician and president of the Medical Society, lobbied its members for support for his election as physician to the London Hospital in 1784. He resigned as president in a huff when some supported his rival (also a member) and, shortly afterward, the society expelled him for continuing to criticize other members.[28] Another major confrontation in 1805 between the president, Dr. James Sims (who had by then served as president for twenty years), and some prominent members led to the secession of a splinter group that included several hospital men, such as Astley Cooper and Dr. William Babington of Guy's. These men, among others, then formed the Medical and Chirurgical Society. The superficially benign story of its origin, published in 1809, digs pointedly at the parent body:

The want of a Society, founded upon liberal and independent principles, and conducted with the propriety and dignity which are worthy of the medical profession, had long been acknowledged: and a few physicians and surgeons in the year 1805, held a meeting for the purpose .... They invited many gentlemen of eminence to join them, and thus a Society was formed, which they soon had the satisfaction to see, comprised a very respectable portion of the professional rank and talent of the metropolis.[29]

The "respectable portion" of medical men who would conduct a society with "propriety and dignity" had a rather different profile from that of the Medical Society of London. The Society's first council had fourteen current or retired hospital men (ten physicians, four surgeons), two nonhospital lecturers, and twelve FRSs among its twenty members; prominent physicians, retired from hospital posts, served as presidents between 1805 and 1815: William Saunders (Guy's), Matthew Baillie (St. George's), Sir Henry Halford (Middlesex), and Sir Gilbert Blane (St. Thomas's). In its first five years, moreover, the new association listed only one apothecary as a member – Mr. Everard A. Brande, apothecary to the King and Queen.

27 All physicians had to belong to the RCP or have a university degree; all surgeons had to be members of the Corporation of Surgeons. The Society explicitly excluded "proprietors of empirical nostrums." *Memoirs of the Medical Society of London* I (1787): x–xii. The presidents from 1773 to 1808 were Drs. Nathaniel Hulme, John Millar, John Lettsom, John Whitehead, John Relph, and James Sims, at various times. All except Relph were dispensary physicians and most were Quakers.
28 Abraham, *Lettsom*, 222–5.
29 *Transactions of the Medical and Chirurgical Society* I (1809), i–ii.

Nearly 60 percent of the members who lived in London were hospital men, dispensary staff, lecturers, and medical attendants to the royal household, compared with 24 percent of the London-based members of the Medical Society in 1789–91.[30]

The two general societies thus embodied divergent perspectives on "the" medical profession, although both defined regular medical practitioners and claimed all metropolitan men as their potential constituencies.[31] Lettsom and his friends created the Medical Society when only two other groups existed, both with delimiting names (Collegiate Physicians, Guy's Hospital). It openly embraced the three traditional categories and kept nonhospital, Licentiate physicians as presidents. Its vague hierarchy downplayed not only any presumed social or intellectual monopoly of the London corporate bodies, but also that of hospital men and lecturers. It implicitly represented, in short, the middling sorts of the growing urban rank and file. Decades later, the Medical and Chirurgical Society claimed a professional elitism, one explicitly based on its members' decisions about eminence. Its physicians and surgeons (and a few apothecaries) had institutions, connections, and abbreviations: MD, FRS, Esq. Its hierarchy summed up a newly configured medical profession, with these men at the top. On them rested, as they knew, "the claims which [the Society] possesses to professional patronage."[32]

In the years between 1773 (the Medical Society) and 1805 (the Medical and Chirurgical Society), hospital men and their close colleagues developed the networks of authority that gave them confidence enough to claim their collective eminence in the early nineteenth century. They did so, as discussed, through the teaching societies. In an equally important step, they consolidated their self-defined control over new knowledge created within their circles by meeting in small groups of peers. These select groups not only intertwined social functions with medical ones, meeting in some sense as friends, but also fostered close connections by *excluding*

30 In the published membership lists for 1805–9, the Medical and Chirurgical Society had 98 members. Eighty of these lived in, or close to London, with 24 hospital men (30 percent), and 23 dispensary staff, lecturers, or royal attendants (29 percent). The Medical Society of London, from its 1789–91 lists, had 284 members, of whom 130 had London addresses. Of these, 8 were hospital men, 18 served dispensaries, and an additional 5 lectured – and all of these were physicians or surgeons. Counting only physicians and surgeons, moreover, to compare with the Medical and Chirurgical Society, reduces the London total to 99, giving the following proportions: 8 percent hospital, 18 percent dispensary, and 5 percent other lecturers, for a total of 31 percent of the "teaching" establishment among the London physicians and surgeons in the society, or 11 percent of the entire (284) membership. *Transactions of the Medical and Chirurgical Society* 1 (1809): ix–xiii; "List of Members," *Memoirs of the Medical Society of London* 1 (1787); 3 (1791).

31 Most probably some of their members chose particular societies for political and religious reasons, as suggested by the Quaker presence in the Medical Society; uncovering such allegiances requires a great deal more prosopographical investigation.

32 *Transactions of the Medical and Chirurgical Society* 1 (1809): i, ix–xiii.

others. Leaving out pupils, rank-and-file practitioners, even hospital colleagues, established and reinforced their self-defined image as men *really*
concerned to promote good work. The two select societies begun in 1782–
83 exemplify these nuances of professional merit and exclusion. Samuel
Foart Simmons started the Society for the Improvement of Medical
Knowledge in 1782 as a break-away group from the Medical Society of
London. Simmons, a dispensary physician, was a consummate entrepreneur on the London medical scene, founding journals and creating (as I
have described) the 1783 *Medical Register*.[33] John Hunter (St. George's) and
Dr. George Fordyce (St. Thomas's) initiated their association, the Society
for the Improvement of Medical and Chirurgical Knowledge, in 1783,
when each had solid reputations in publishing, lecturing, and hospital
teaching. Both groups deliberately stayed small (about seventeen for the
former, a mandated twelve for the latter); both admitted only physicians
and surgeons living in London, most of whom had institutional connections; both overtly aimed to improve knowledge through discussions and
publication; both even met at Slaughter's Coffee-House in St. Martin's
Lane, not far from several West End lecture theaters.[34]

Whether or not Simmons's group was self-consciously defined to include
only certain types of practitioners, according to published lists from 1782–
3 his society had hospital men only from the Westminster (two), the
Middlesex (three), and St. Thomas's (four), in addition to several dispensary men, physicians to lying-in charities, and midwifery lecturers.[35] In
contrast, the manuscript minutes from the Society for the Improvement of
Medical and Chirurgical Knowledge leave no doubt about their views:
"No person is eligible who has not been in regular practice as a Physician
or Surgeon upwards of five years, or who is not Physician or Surgeon to
St. Thomas's, St. Bartholomew's, St. George's or Guy's Hospitals." (The
omission of those from the Westminster, the Middlesex, or the London
raises the specter of a subtle hierarchy among the hospitals that remains
tantalizing at best.) Existing members proposed and balloted for new ones,
and their rules demanded a unanimous vote and secrecy: "No person shall
be acquainted with his being proposed as a member of this Society until he

33 Simmons, an Edinburgh MD and 1778 LRCP, served as physician to the Westminster
   General Dispensary from 1780 and to St. Luke's Hospital (for the insane) from 1781.
34 Newton-Pitt, "Reflections on John Hunter," 1272; Dukes, "London Medical Societies,"
   704. Neither of these accounts is very accurate. *London Medical Journal* 3 (1782): 216–17;
   Samuel Foart Simmons, ed. *The Medical Register* (London, 1783), 39, 221; Proceedings of
   the Society for the Improvement of Medical and Chirurgical Knowledge, passim.
35 *London Medical Journal* 3 (1782): 216–17; *Medical Register*, 39, 221. The hospital men were
   Westminster: Dr. George Hicks (1775–92), Henry Watson (surgeon, 1762–93; previously
   surgeon to the Middlesex, 1751–62); Middlesex: Samuel Howard (surgeon, 1759–1810),
   Dr. James Carmichael Smyth (1775–89), John Wyatt (surgeon, 1765–97); St. Thomas's:
   Dr. Adair Crawford (1783–95), Dr. William Keir (1780 to his death in 1783), George
   Chandler (surgeon, 1783–1822), and Henry Cline (surgeon, 1784–1812).

be elected."[36] Notably, moreover, none of the St. Thomas's men in Simmons's society were ever proposed for membership in Hunter's and Fordyce's clique; indeed, the hospital men invited in over the course of its existence were its founders' allies. Three staff surgeons and one physician embodied the Hunterian succession: John Hunter, Everard Home, Dr. Matthew Baillie, and Benjamin Brodie from St. George's. The four St. Thomas's physicians show the Fordycean network: George Fordyce, Gilbert Blane, William Lister, and William Charles Wells. The only odd hospital man here was David Pitcairn, a physician who retired from St. Bartholomew's in 1793; no members came from Guy's. The nine other members elected over the course of the Society's existence had lecturing and personal connections to these first men, such as James Wilson, Baillie's lecturing partner at Great Windmill Street.[37] After 1812, moreover, with the stability and apparent success of the broader Medical and Chirurgical Society (which this select group had helped to start), Hunter's and Fordyce's successors relaxed into a dining club that finally dispersed in 1817.

Under both these societies' imposing titles, in short, lay concrete connections among individuals across the metropolis in the 1780s and 1790s. Their professional intimacies delineated subtle boundaries, suggestive hints about who mattered. More significantly, these alliances, far from simply displaying these men's preexisting medical authority, show them learning to express it and practice it through collective experience. Of all the practitioners in London during these decades, *these* men – factions of hospital staff, dispensary men, and lecturers – simultaneously had the self-importance to present themselves as arbitrators of knowledge and the insecurity to turn to one another to confirm it. This dynamic process, played out across London in all the medical societies' rules, meetings, controversies, and agreements, was the core of the London-centered medical community emerging between 1760 and 1815. At these sites, practitioners turned inward. Acceptance from one another repeatedly trans-

36 Proceedings of the Society for the Improvement of Medical and Chirurgical Knowledge, 3; all of the members signed these "laws": see p. 7.
37 The absence of Guy's and St. Bartholomew's men is intriguing. This pattern, among men otherwise thought to be close colleagues and friends, strikes again at simple assumptions about how to draw connections between practitioners based on sketchy evidence. I think it is quite probable, nevertheless, that the one-volume publication of *Medical Records and Researches* by "A Private Medical Association" in 1798 emerged from three of the very active, but junior, Guy's men left out of other associations. This proclaimed "private" group consisted of Astley Cooper (lecturing on anatomy at St. Thomas's, but soon to be a Guy's surgeon), William Babington (apothecary turned assistant physician at Guy's), and John Haighton (who lectured on physiology at Guy's, taught midwifery, and was physician to the Eastern Dispensary). *Medical Records and Researches* 1 (1798), see title page and table of contents. All the papers are either by these three men, or communicated to them from provincial practitioners. As at least three (of eight) of these had been pupils at Guy's or St. Thomas's (Richard Brown Cheston, John Richard Farre, and James Barlow), I suspect this volume resulted from very direct "communications" among practitioners well-known to Cooper, Babington, or Haighton.

formed them into regular medical men and made what they did and how they theorized into regular medicine. With a few important exceptions (such as Matthew Baillie), moreover, medical society physicians were Licentiates of the Royal College of Physicians, seeking recognition apart from the Royal College and its Fellows. From the 1780s on, Licentiates joined elite surgeons (and some apothecaries), finding collegiality across traditional occupational divisions.

The regular medicine created and confirmed in medical societies arose from that defined by texts and lectures, shaped within the medical marketplace, and constantly negotiated with patients. Yet the inward turns provided among peers in societies momentarily detached practitioners from lay approbation and shifted them toward medical approval. The shifting hierarchies within and among London's medical societies associated rank with occupational experience and knowledge, both its production (e.g., preparing papers) and its display (e.g., giving cases). The collections of papers and cases published in societies' transactions and journals turned this collective experience outward, replaying acceptable, polished contributions for reading practitioners and the curious laity.

DIFFUSING USEFUL KNOWLEDGE

Broadsides, pamphlets, chapbooks, almanacs, newspapers, and periodical publications all mark the emergence of a scattered and sometimes ephemeral print culture in early modern England. By the mid-eighteenth century, regular newspapers, magazines, and journals, as much as crowded streets and markets, informed urban life. Printing and bookselling had become considerable businesses as well as trades, creating the "Grub Street" writer subsisting on wits and market-centered patronage.[38] As I noted in Chapter 6 of the earlier decades of the century, medical publication was – and continued to be – deeply embedded in the broader stories of production, distribution, and marketing that accompany the expansion of commercial society. Medical periodicals, like so many other ventures in the eighteenth century, depended upon the exigencies of buying and selling. How much, and in what specific ways, their market lives affected the relative success or failure of various journals remain to be investigated. Yet, because so little is known about the production, financing, and readerships of most of these

---

38 Alvin Kernan, *Samuel Johnson & the Impact of Print* (Princeton, NJ: Princeton University Press, 1987), has an excellent survey discussion of the creation of a "print culture" in eighteenth-century London. See also David A. Kronick, *A History of Scientific and Technical Periodicals*, 2nd ed. (Metuchen, NJ: Scarecrow Press, 1976), 33–76, for a discussion of the emergence and forms of specialized periodicals in the seventeenth and eighteenth centuries. I regret that at the time I completed this manuscript I had not read Roy Porter's "The Rise of Medical Journalism in Britain to 1800," in *Medical Journals and Medical Knowledge: Historical Essays*, ed. W. F. Bynum, Stephen Lock and Roy Porter (London: Routledge, 1992), 6–28. Porter has argued along similar lines.

volumes, it is worth a strong reminder that their lifespans hinged not only upon the significance of their contents, but also upon a host of mundane chores consuming individuals' hours and pocketbooks.

Specialized periodicals offer a way to see what London medical men presented to other practitioners, and the public, as "useful" knowledge. Just as the *Philosophical Transactions* gave a public face to the Royal Society, so too did medical journals provide character sketches of eighteenth-century medical occupations. Like issues of the *Philosophical Transactions*, as well, these volumes sometimes display a bewildering hodgepodge of material. This diversity had the same overt purpose and vitality as the Royal Society's productions. Here was new knowledge of all sorts, channeled into London, evaluated as reliable in some fashion, and pronounced worthy of public exhibition.

Roughly categorizing medical periodicals according to how their organizers gathered and evaluated appropriate material offers one way to connect them to the metropolitan medical community that produced and sustained them. First, as already mentioned, medical societies collected papers and cases from their members' contributions at meetings, from corresponding members, and, in some groups, from nonmembers acquainted with those who belonged. I include the Royal College of Physicians' *Medical Transactions,* whose first volume appeared in 1767, among the society-based publications, although the role of meetings and membership at the College is unclear.[39] Second, from the 1780s, a few enterprising men, notably Samuel Foart Simmons, began "general" journals that relied on information provided by practitioners who simply chose to submit it. As many journals did not identify particular editors on their title pages, such volumes present an illusory sense that they arose from a disembodied profession. All of these *look* like medical journals, even when the editor was anonymous, because they primarily contained original articles by named authors. In addition to these publications, however, medical men, printers, and booksellers produced numbers of periodical texts for the medical market that ranged from derivative collections to a quasi-pamphlet literature about health. At the end of the century, medical editors started a few review periodicals devoted to summarizing and commenting upon the growing output of the medical press.[40] Not nearly enough historical work

39 Clark, *Royal College of Physicians,* 2: 579–80; The published papers were noted as "read at the College" on particular dates in the *Medical Transactions'* volumes, but the organization – and membership – of such meetings requires further investigation. Certainly information communicated to named Fellows of the Royal College appeared in their collections; whether such pieces were read to those who met is not clear. See *Medical Transactions of the Royal College of Physicians* 1 (1767), table of contents.

40 See, for an example of the former, *The British Physician, treating of our diet and common nourishment,* which managed five numbers in 1716; for the latter, see *The Medical and Chirurgical Review,* begun in 1794, and *The London Medical and Surgical Spectator; or Monthly*

has gone into either popular or review texts to place them neatly within sets distinguished by their creators or intended audiences; I bypass them here in favor of those most evidently constructed by and for regular practitioners around the original work of their peers.

When the Society of Physicians published its first volume of *Medical Observations and Inquiries,* it replicated for London medical men collections already familiar to readers of the *Philosophical Transactions,* the Edinburgh *Medical Essays and Observations,* or various foreign periodicals. Its rhetoric and format exemplify those of most societies' volumes that appeared throughout the eighteenth and early nineteenth centuries. Promoted as a collective endeavor on the title page, it contained papers selected, the Society claimed, from those given in their meetings, clearly implying their joint judgment on their value.[41] The Society, moreover, deliberately eschewed "hypothetical disquisitions" and essays with "rather a tendency to shew the parts and erudition of the writer" rather than useful knowledge.[42] The papers followed with the authors' names, degrees, and location specified. By imitating other periodicals (like the *Philosophical Transactions*), those devoted to medical topics in London quickly established a fairly stable genre, albeit one that anonymous editors felt called upon to justify repeatedly in prefaces over the next sixty years. In 1805, for example, the "president and council" of the Medical and Chirurgical Society, the voices used to introduce its first volume of *Transactions,* hoped that the "medical public" agreed that their publication "support[ed] the claim of respectability and usefulness, which they [were] desirous that it should possess" (p. ii).

In 1763–4, "Gentlemen of the Faculty" produced three volumes of *The Medical Museum, or a Repository of Cases, Experiments, Researches and Discoveries, Collected at Home and Abroad*; a "Society Instituted for the Improve-

Register of Medicine in its various branches: Containing Original Communications; Cases and Reviews in Medicine, Surgery, Midwifery, and Pharmacy; with a variety of Miscellaneous Matter, and other Professional Intelligence 1 (1808), "address." W. R. Lefanu provides a complete list of those considered medical periodicals in his *British Periodicals of Medicine, 1640–1899,* rev. ed. (Oxford: Wellcome Unit for the History of Medicine, 1984). For an extended discussion on how to categorize medical periodicals, in the context of scientific ones, see Kronick, *Scientific and Technical Periodicals,* 18–30. I have chosen to rely on the fairly simple division among society-based, general, and "collected" periodicals for the London literature in the eighteenth century.

41 How much selection went into any society's choice of papers for publication is rarely known. At least the Society for the Improvement of Medical and Chirurgical Knowledge did not publish *all* of the papers submitted to the group, some deemed not ready, others withdrawn from such consideration. See Proceedings of the Society for the Improvement of Medical and Chirurgical Knowledge, 4 June, 6 Aug. 1799. On this latter date, "The form of Dr. [John] Hunter's Paper & the Subject of it were thought not adapted to the plan of the Transactions published by the Society." Dr. Hunter's paper concerned "the means of preserving Troops from infectious Fever" (2 July 1799).

42 *Medical Observations and Inquiries* 1 (1757): xii.

ment of Physical Knowledge" followed with its *Select Papers on the Different Branches of Medicine* in 1767. Locating the authority for these works in "gentlemen of the faculty" and a "society" suggests how important such models were. Yet neither volume identifies its organizers with any additional detail. Whereas the physicians behind the *Medical Observations and Inquiries* listed their addresses next to their names in the table of contents, the editors of *The Medical Museum* and *Select Papers* stayed hidden. Both journals, in fact, primarily contain more or less acknowledged extracts from other texts.[43] In 1781, the *London Medical Journal* similarly began with the title page acknowledgment to "A Society of Physicians" and included essays "read" and "communicated to" the group. In the third volume this attribution disappeared, and, with the fourth volume in 1783, all the papers were "communicated" to Samuel Foart Simmons himself, a major presence in the journal all along. At some point, in short, the invisible society behind the publication became the single editor, who nevertheless submerged his identity within the format of a collective project.

Simmons's journal was the first medical periodical that lasted more than one or two years. The initial issues appeared monthly, then, with the third volume, quarterly. From the start, it included sections for unattributed book reviews and medical news, such as announcements for other medical societies and publications, not just communicated papers or (as with the earlier ventures) copied extracts.[44] The *London Medical Journal* thus emulated productions like *Gentleman's Magazine,* a periodical full of current events, book notices, correspondence, and essays, but set its medical news around a central core of original papers specifically aimed at medical men. That the *London Medical Journal* survived, and continued with its mixed format, suggests that practitioners welcomed its abstracts. Including brief accounts of the *Philosophical Transactions* and the *Memoirs of the Royal Medical Society of Paris,* for example, made keeping up to date convenient. At some point in the next decades, as review journals proliferated, their very convenience made being current no longer a social luxury, but a growing

43 See, for example, the first two volumes of *The Medical Museum* from 1763. A few pieces that look original were actually reprints, particularly from work in the *Philosophical Transactions* by prominent men. See, for example, Richard Grindall's "Case of the Efficacy of Bark in a Mortification," *Philosophical Transactions* 50 (1757): 379–83, which appeared as "A Remarkable Case of the Efficacy of Bark in Mortification," *The Medical Museum,* 2 (1763): 171–5. The third volume seems to have some original essays, such as W. Perfect (surgeon), "An Attempt to Improve Medical Prognostication," 3 (1764): 287–312. In the *Select Papers on the Different Branches of Medicine* (1767), the articles are highly derivative. See, for example, pp. 44–58, drawn from Alexander Reid's translation of Henri-Francis Le Dran's text, *Consultations on the Disorders that Require the Assistance of Surgery* (London: Robert Horsefield, 1766).

44 *The London Medical Journal* 1 (1781): iii–iv; 2 (1781): iii–iv; 3 (1782), title page. Simmons's journal may well have been informally connected with the Medical Society of London, or a subset of physicians from it. I have found no independent reference to this group of practitioners.

necessity for medical practitioners in touch with the metropolis.[45] During the 1790s, other general journals appeared, beginning labyrinthine trails as these changed their names, merged, and divided. Other medical societies, notably the Medical Society of London and the two associations for "improving" medical knowledge, also started printing sporadic collections in the 1780s and 1790s. In 1793, practitioners within the orbit of London printers could have purchased three distinct medical journals or society transactions; in 1815, they could buy five, not to mention specialized review periodicals and those from other cities and nations.

All of these publications depict networks of communication, occupational relationships, and *what counted* as medical knowledge.[46] The distribution of authors among them displayed a profession weighted toward London hospital men in the "select" transactions and toward provincial practitioners in the general journals and the *Memoirs of the Medical Society of London*.[47] Even a cursory look at tables of contents, or a glance through these volumes, shows that London's general society and ostensibly nonaffiliated journals provided a generous place for the rank-and-file medical man to share his experience as a contribution to knowledge. Thus Mr. Cook, a surgeon at Barking, sent in "An Account of a remarkable Fracture of the Scull [*sic*], by a pistol-ball," and John Covey, apothecary in Basing-

---

45 "Historical Sketch of the Progress of Medicine, Surgery and Chemistry in the Year 1808," *Annual Medical Review and Register* 1 (1809): 302–20; that for 1809 appeared in 2 (1810): 415–20; Aesculapius [Laurence H. Potts], *Oracular Communications, Addressed to Students of the Medical Profession* (London: Cox, 1816), 95.

46 In his extremely influential article, "Medical Knowledge and the Patronage System in 18th Century England," *Sociology* 8 (1974): 382, N. D. Jewson perpetuated the idea that medical periodicals did not appear until the 1820s and 1830s. He emphasized that the "network of relationships" necessary for the improvement of medical knowledge was simply not possible before the late eighteenth century and hardly realized until much later.

47 Using the identifications usually provided in the journals' tables of contents allows for a rough numerical profile of the distribution of authors. This table summarizes the data for sampled periodicals between 1780 and 1800, according to number of authors, not number of contributions. Counting articles shifts the profile even further toward London hospital men in the select societies' publications.

Medical press: authors' locations, 1780–1800

	London hospital	London other	Provincial colonial	Other & unknown	Total
Select[a]	31% (18)	32% (19)	27% (16)	10% (6)	59
General society[b]	2% (1)	14% (9)	52% (33)	20% (13)	64
General[c]	6% (4)	17% (11)	53% (35)	23% (15)	65

[a] *Medical Communications* (Society for the Improvement of Medical Knowledge), 1784, 1790; *Medical Transactions of the Royal College of Physicians*, 1785; *Transactions of the Society for the Improvement of Medical and Chirurgical Knowledge*, 1793, 1800.
[b] *Memoirs of the Medical Society of London*, 1789, 1795.
[c] *London Medical Journal*, 1782, 1784, 1788; *Medical Facts and Observations*, 1793, 1795.

stoke, Hampshire, offered "Observations and Facts relative to the Practice of Inoculations of the Small-Pox" to Simmons's *London Medical Journal,* apparently on their own initiative.[48] What the *Philosophical Transactions* had done in exhibiting a community of gentlemen linked by a metropolitan center, the eighteenth-century medical journals did for a nascent medical community. Whatever hidden decisions editors made to include or exclude material, the published results provided the appearance of networks at once open to any correspondent, yet in fact restricted to those regular practitioners who could "improve" knowledge.

OBSERVING PRACTITIONERS AND MEN OF SCIENCE

Medical societies and periodicals diffused the useful knowledge that individuals provided them. And, at least in terms of the number of articles, that knowledge resided in case histories.[49] Investing specific experience with the aura of advancing or improving the scope of medical knowledge had been, as I noted in Chapter 6, a common rhetorical claim for decades. From the mid-eighteenth century, medical men acted upon this Baconian tenet, as it smoothly moved from the *Philosophical Transactions* to medical journals. By the 1780s, case histories had all but disappeared from the concerns of the Royal Society for their new home in medical publications. The proliferation of societies and journals thus supported a quasi-democratization of medical investigation, in which any attentive and literate practitioner could participate: "The observing practitioner has various opportunities of improving the profession by attention to the facts which come daily within his view, and by the management of the materials which are already in his possession."[50] Even at midcentury, the Society of Physicians could congratulate itself that "many able practitioners [have been] incited to observe and enquire" through its meetings and collections.[51] As a genre, the case history provided a way to encapsulate a diverse range of experiences and insights, celebrating the primacy of this direct clinical observation. Such accounts, as the *Medical Observations and Inquiries* noted in 1757, truly allowed practitioners "to revive the Hippocratic method of composing narratives of particular cases, in which the nature of the disease, the manner of treating it, and the consequences, are to be specified."[52]

48. *London Medical Journal* 4 (1783): 72–3; 7 (1786): 180–6.
49 At least 45 percent of all articles in a series of sampled journals (from 1757 to 1814) were centered on case reports. A further 18 to 30 percent focused on specific therapies and relied on references to experience, although they may or may not have included accounts of particular patients. The remainder, in rough categories, covered discussions of military medicine, anatomy and morbid anatomy, chemistry, physiology, and broad discursive essays.
50 *Transactions of the Medical and Chirurgical Society* 1 (1809): ii–iii.
51 *Medical Observations and Inquiries* 4 (1771): v.
52 *Medical Observations and Inquiries* 1 (1757): ix.

Opening the advancement of medical knowledge to provincial apothecaries and ordinary surgeons helped to create a new medical community concerned with peer acceptance. Yet this process also challenged medical elites, whose authority had partially rested upon claims to mastery of medical theory and practice and hence to the means to improve it. The Fellows of the Royal College of Physicians recognized this threat in the 1760s, as Licentiates both produced the *Medical Observations and Inquiries* and attacked the Fellows for unwarranted exclusivity. Concerned Fellows then inaugurated their *Medical Transactions of the Royal College of Physicians,* ostensibly "ready to receive any Medical Papers that shall be presented to them, in order to publish the most useful." In practice a small number of Fellows filled its volumes with their essays.[53] Critical of "abstract reasonings," the early editors nonetheless reminded its readers that "whatever important additions or exceptions to the general practice may be contained in those cases [of routine experience], would be much better drawn out by the author himself, and presented without giving along with them a tiresome account of common appearances, with which everyone is supposed to be well acquainted."[54] Members of the College presumably would indeed be "well acquainted" with "common appearances," not to mention horrified at being considered "tiresome." The judgment necessary for such nice discriminations between the common and the important details, in short, undercut the full Hippocratic method and returned *real* contributions to learned physicians. The Royal College, of course, could not control medical publishing, but it could add the voices of its Fellows to the growing din.

During the last decades of the century, the very success of medical societies and journals encouraged elite practitioners to turn their investigative attention to the medical sciences. While the community at large read about new work in chemistry, morbid anatomy, and physiology, only men with sufficient time and resources could pursue research problems in these fields. Doing science thus served, once again, to distinguish an intellectual elite from the rank and file. Hospital men certainly did not abandon case histories, for these sustained their clinical prestige, participation in medical societies, teaching, and consultations. A solid minority, however, especially surgeons and Licentiate physicians, produced papers noticeably different from the familiar case histories dominating medical journals. In prefaces to medical periodicals throughout the second half of the eighteenth century, editors had primarily called for communications on "useful cases"

53 *Medical Transactions of the Royal College of Physicians* 1 (1767): vi; The first four volumes of the *Medical Transactions* contained ninety-nine articles by forty-nine named authors; six (12 percent) of these wrote forty-five (45 percent) of the pieces: Mark Akenside, Matthew Baillie, Sir George Baker, William Heberden, Sr., William Heberden, Jr., and John Latham, all Fellows. All but Baker and Heberden, Sr. were hospital physicians.
54 *Medical Transactions of the Royal College of Physicians* 1 (1767) and 2 (1772), "advertisement."

and added, rather as an aside, an invitation for those on "such other matters as may tend to the improvement of medical science."[55] General journals routinely promised "accounts of every important discovery and improvement that shall be made in medical science" as part of the medical news provided to, not implored from, their readers.[56] In contrast, the editors of the *Transactions of the Medical and Chirurgical Society* in 1809 called for "researches in anatomy, physiology and that part of chemistry which is immediately connected with some of the branches of medicine," and received responses from a few men already actively investigating problems only tangentially connected to clinical work.[57] James Wilson, anatomy lecturer, contributed "A Description of two Muscles surrounding the membraneous part of the Urethra"; Alexander Marcet, physician to Guy's, offered "A Chemical Account of Various Dropsical Fluids"; John Yelloly, physician to the London, presented the collaborative study he did with Astley Cooper, surgeon to Guy's, on "the Propagation of the Nervous Influence."[58] Compared with the rare surfacing of original science essays in medical periodicals of the 1780s and 1790s, such work became a small but regular part of medical journals in the early nineteenth century.[59]

Much of London men's original work on anatomy, physiology, and chemistry between 1760 and 1815, however, was not to be found in medical periodicals. Observing, recording, practicing rationally, appealing to the sciences – all these informed the rhetoric of the medical press. Yet, at least in London medical circles, the production and display of *new* work abstracted from the details and direct concerns of clinical experience re-

55 *London Medical Journal* 1 (1781): v.
56 *Medical Facts and Observations* 1 (1791): vii; *New London Medical Journal* 1 (1792): v; Simmons, in both the *London Medical Journal* and its successor, *Medical Facts and Observations*, provided articles extracted from the *Philosophical Transactions, Journal de Chirurgie, Memoirs of the American Academy of Arts and Sciences, Transactions of the Royal Society of Edinburgh*, and other publications. These appear in the tables of contents as though direct submissions by the author (not under "medical news"), with the source given after the article's title.
57 *Transactions of the Medical and Chirurgical Society* 1 (1809): iv; see also the "Advertisement" in the *Edinburgh Medical and Surgical Journal* 1 (1805): 3–4.
58 *Transactions of the Medical and Chirurgical Society* 1 (1809): 175–81, 181–221; 2 (1811): 340–82. The Liverpool physician John Bostock contributed significantly in chemistry and physiology to the *Transactions of the Medical and Chirurgical Society*. Bostock was the son of a Liverpool physician of the same name. Born in 1773, he took an Edinburgh MD in 1798. He moved to London in 1817 and gave up medicine to devote himself full time to chemistry and physiology (*Dictionary of National Biography*). See, for example, his "Experiments and Observations on the Serum of the Blood," *Transactions of the Medical and Chirurgical Society* 2 (1811): 161–79, and "On the Nature and Analysis of Animal Fluids," 4 (1813): 53–72; June Goodfield, *The Growth of Scientific Physiology* (London: Hutchinson, 1960), 81–4, discusses Bostock.
59 In the 1820s, practitioners began specialized volumes for the medical "sciences," such as *Transactions of the Medico-Botanical Society* (1821–37) and the *Journal of Morbid Anatomy* (1828). These did not survive long, yet hint at the patterns of clinical and scientific specialization that would explode with new journals in the 1860s to 1880s. LeFanu, *British Periodicals*.

mained within the Royal Society and its *Philosophical Transactions*. As medical groups took up the exploration of improvements using case histories, elite medical men sought and maintained a presence within the Royal Society by continuing their connections to gentlemanly interests.[60] For some, notably the youthful Thomas Young in his work on optics, but also physicians like George Fordyce, who pursued a few topics in mechanics and nonmedical chemistry, gentlemanly concerns were hardly limited to medical subjects.[61] By the 1780s, those probing medical problems had turned from the pragmatic details of clinical experience to investigations connected with comparative anatomy, human anatomy, chemistry, and physiology.[62] Everard Home (surgeon, St. George's, 1787–1827), for instance, reminded the *Philosophical Transactions'* readers that case references served "general science" when they "brought to light facts of importance in the animal oeconomy." George Pearson (physician, St. George's, 1787–1828) made a pointed aside that he had omitted "conclusions . . . relate[d] to the agency of medicines . . . [that] of course do not properly fall within the views of the Royal Society" in his chemical study of urinary concretions.[63]

The emergence of "men of science" in the Royal Society in this period is

60 London medical men who pursued experimental work in physiology, chemistry, and comparative anatomy tended to publish their results in medical journals only when beginning their careers, transferring their papers to the Royal Society when better established. For example, John Haighton published his early physiological investigations, "An attempt to ascertain the powers concerned in vomiting," in the *Memoirs of the Medical Society of London* 2 (1789): 250–61, 512–6. By the early 1790s, after being well established as a practitioner and lecturer on physiology at Guy's, he submitted his experimental work to the *Philosophical Transactions,* while continuing to use the medical periodicals for discussion of specific cases. See his "An Experimental Inquiry Concerning the Reproduction of Nerves," *Philosophical Transactions* 85 (1795): 190–201 and "An Experimental Inquiry Concerning Animal Impregnation," *Philosophical Transactions* 87 (1797): 159–96, both communicated by Maxwell Garthshore. Haighton, despite his active research, was never elected to the Royal Society.

61 George Fordyce, "Account of a New Pendulum," *Philosophical Transactions* 84 (1794): 2–20; George Pearson, "Experiments and Observations, Made with a View of Ascertaining the Nature of the Gaz [*sic*] Produced by Passing Electric Discharges Through Water," *Philosophical Transactions* 87 (1797): 142–58.

62 Not only did case histories decline in the *Philosophical Transactions,* but they also seem to have vanished from the Royal Society's meetings by the 1790s. A close examination of the Society's Journal Books (vol. xxxiv, 1789–1792) from January to June 1792, for example, did not turn up any case histories either presented to the meetings or submitted by letters. The Society did, however, regularly receive London's medical journals for their library; see the entry of 8 Nov. 1792 for an example.

63 Everard Home, "Observations on the Changes which Blood undergoes, when extravasated into the urinary Bladder," *Philosophical Transactions* 86 (1796): 486; George Pearson, "Experiments and Observations, tending to show the Composition and Properties of Urinary Concretions," *Philosophical Transactions* 88 (1798): 28; the manuscript version of Pearson's paper contains the identical comment: Letters and Papers, Decade XI, no. 38, Royal Society of London; Caleb H. Parry, MD, "On a Case of nervous Affection cured by Pressure of the Carotids; with some physiological Remarks," *Philosophical Transactions* 101 (1810): 89–95.

as yet underexplored territory. In the late 1820s to 1840s, those seeking to reform the Royal Society, to make it more "scientific" and "professional," created a powerful image of the earlier institution as moribund, amateur, and frivolous compared with an ideal of serious science seen operating in Continental academies and institutes. Complaints about the constraints of practice on medical men's time, and moans about the lack of opportunities for professional scientists to survive and do research in Britain's economy of amateurs, must not obscure the issues at stake for medical men between the mideighteenth and the early nineteenth centuries.[64] To challenge the hegemony of learned physicians over theoretical medical knowledge, which still emanated from university professors and a Continental elite favored by state patronage, London men needed to demonstrate that they, *as practitioners*, could *do* science. Indeed, the very skills obtained through their education and training, honed by their experiences, recognized through their work as lecturers and consultants, and freed from incessant toil by the support of students and well-off patients gave certain London men multiple grounds for their work in the medical sciences.

Under Sir Joseph Banks, president of the Royal Society from 1778 to 1820, members of the Society still dabbled in all branches of natural history and natural philosophy. Banks frowned on independent, specialized scientific societies, hoping to maintain the Royal Society's hegemony in the face of splintering competition. Yet he encouraged certain groups, such as the Linnaean Society (1788), the Royal Institution (1799) and medical societies, as they attracted constituencies that supported the Royal Society's place and prestige.[65] The latter associations, in particular, centered on practical problems in agriculture and medicine, topics that indeed balanced the Royal Society's ostensibly detached and intellectual aims.[66] From the perspective of London medical men in these decades, the Royal Society's continued embrace of gentlemen distanced from mere pragmatic concerns allowed the FRS to mark an elite among them. This elite, even more than earlier in the eighteenth century, enjoyed and fostered the intertwining of the social status and intellectual merit that getting the Fellowship evoked. According to retrospective accounts, in the 1780s Banks tried to make election more select – that is, more completely under his suzerainty. Benja-

64 D. S. L. Cardwell, *The Organization of Science in England* (London: Heinemann, 1972), 37–8, 60–5; Morrell and Thackray, *Gentlemen of Science*, 33, 41–52.

65 Roy M. MacLeod, "Whigs and Savants: Reflections on the Reform Movement in the Royal Society, 1830–48," in *Metropolis and Province*, ed. Ian Inkster and Jack Morrell (Philadelphia: University of Pennsylvania Press, 1983), 55–63. Morris Berman, *Social Change and Scientific Organization* (Ithaca, NY: Cornell University Press, 1978), xx–xxi, emphasizes that the Royal Society was a locus classicus for the gentleman–amateur tradition throughout the early nineteenth century; David Miller, "The Royal Society of London, 1800–1835: A Study in the Cultural Politics of Scientific Organization," Ph.D. dissertation, University of Pennsylvania, 1981, esp. chs. 1–3.

66 See Miller, "The Royal Society of London", 9–60, for the larger commercial interests apparent in Banks's support of botanical research and exploration.

min Brodie (surgeon, St. George's, 1808–40) recalled that Banks envisioned "two classes: – the working men of science, and those who, from their position in society or fortune, it might be desirable to retain as patrons of science."[67] Brodie noted, to support his claim, that Everard Home (surgeon, St. George's, 1787–1827) once suggested Dr. Henry Vaughan, FRCP and hospital physician (Middlesex, 1793–1800), to Banks. The President rejected Vaughan's possible nomination, as "he would not allow a gentleman to be qualified for admission merely because he was a fashionable physician." Brodie continued, "After some years Dr. Vaughan inherited a fortune, and became Sir Henry Halford. Sir Joseph then said he might now be admitted as belonging to the other class."[68] Described in his nomination certificate as a "zealous promoter of the Objects of Science," Sir Henry had the Earl of Winchilsea among his signatories, and obtained his FRS in 1810.[69]

Unlike vague gentleman–promoters, practitioners to royalty, or those simply "well versed in various branches of knowledge," most of the surgeons and Licentiate physicians proposed, such as Benjamin Brodie, William Charles Wells (physician, St. Thomas's, 1795–1817), and Alexander Marcet (physician, Guy's, 1802–19), had explicit references to their previous research activity in their nomination certificates.[70] They were gentlemen – but also Banks's "working men of science." Precisely because

67 Quoted from a letter of Sir Benjamin Brodie to Charles Weld, 7 Apr. 1848, in C. R. Weld, *A History of the The Royal Society*, 2 vols. (London: J. W. Parker, 1948), 2: 153; see pp. 151–69 for a membership controversy and Banks's power in 1783–4; MacLeod, "Whigs and Savants," 60–1.

68 Brodie to Weld, quoted in Weld, *The Royal Society*, 2: 153–4. This passage is also quoted in N. G. Coley, "The Animal Chemistry Club: Assistant Society to the Royal Society," *Notes and Records of the Royal Society of London* 22 (1967): 185, n. 54. See also, Henry Lyons, *The Royal Society, 1660–1944* (Cambridge: The University Press, 1944), 198–9, 204–5.

69 Nomination certificates, Royal Society of London, VI.156; for Halford's life, see Munk, *Roll*, 2: 427–35.

70 Nomination certificates, Royal Society of London, V.146 (quotation from Dr. James Robertson's certificate, 1790); VI.158 (Brodie, 1810); V.215 (Wells, 1793); VI.136 (Marcet, 1808). Thomas Keate (surgeon, St. George's, 1787–1813) and Dr. Christopher Pemberton (physician, St. George's, 1800–8), represent the Royal Society's gentlemanly approbation of royal service or social lineage. Thomas Keate's nomination notice of 1793 introduced him as "Surgeon to the Queen, and Prince of Wales, Inspector General of regimental Infirmaries, Surgeon to Chelsea and St. George's Hospitals, a Gentleman well versed in Natural Knowledge"; Christopher Pemberton was simply "desirous of becoming a member" in 1796. Since he was, according to Munk, "a grandson of the lord chief justice Pemberton" and had an impeccable education, his nomination apparently needed no elaborations. Nomination certificates, Royal Society of London, V.226, V.285; Munk, *Roll*, 2: 450. Thomas Young, in contrast, exemplifies the rare "man of science" as young genius in the Royal Society. Young ("the marvel of his age") acquired a considerable reputation for his work in vision and optics and was elected FRS when twenty-one (1794), before his Göttingen MD (1796), his later Cambridge MD (1806), or his service as physician to St. George's (1811–29). Munk, *Roll*, 3: 80–8; George Peacock, *Life of Thomas Young MD FRS* (London: J. Murray, 1855); nomination certificate, Royal Society of London, V.232.

Banks's "classes" were defined by insiders' awareness of social networks, not by distinct titles like "ordinary" and "honorary," the categories of working men and patrons could blur for mutual reinforcement. Even when, as the physician Augustus Granville reported, Londoners joked that the FRS meant "Fees Raised Since," from the mid-eighteenth to the early nineteenth centuries medical men clearly risked such envious ridicule for a share in the Society's aura of respectability and responsibility to advance knowledge.[71] Hospital surgeons, in particular, found a scholarly home in the Royal Society and its *Philosophical Transactions,* one in which they, too, could offer theoretical insights from observations, experiments, and learned texts. John Hunter, FRS 1767 (St. George's, 1768–73); William Blizard (London, 1780–1833); John Abernethy (St. Bartholomew's, 1787–1827); Astley Cooper (Guy's, 1800–25); and Benjamin Brodie were among the hospital surgeons who contributed work on comparative anatomy, human anatomy, and physiology that distanced them from mere surgical practice, yet depended upon their dissecting expertise (see Chapter 8). Being gradually acknowledged as gentlemen *and* "working men of science" *and* surgeons during the last half of the eighteenth century made these men the primary evidence for the "rise of the surgeon" that historians have identified in this period.[72] Later knighthoods or baronetcies (Blizard, Cooper, Brodie) further associated professional and social (and political) success with the FRS and "contributions" to knowledge.[73]

Within the purview of the Royal Society, various activities exemplify how certain London hospital men – and surgeons in particular – could

---

71 Augustus B. Granville, *Autobiography . . . being Eighty-Eight Years in the Life of a Physician,* ed. Paulina B. Granville, 2 vols. (London: Henry S. King, 1874), 1: 66; also quoted in MacLeod, "Whigs and Savants," 60.

72 See, for example, Oswei Temkin's classic article, "The Role of Surgery in the Rise of Modern Medical Thought," *Bulletin of the History of Medicine* 25 (1951): 248–59. In 1830, Augustus Granville, in his polemical *Science without a Head; or, The Royal Society Dissected* (London: Farnborough, Gregg, 1969: facsimile reprint of the first edition), used an analysis of the current membership to claim that many physicians were still elected for social reasons, while surgeons were underrepresented and were generally elected only after demonstrating considerable scientific interests (39–46). See also, John Harley Warner, "The Idea of Science in English Medicine: The 'Decline of Science' and the Rhetoric of Reform, 1815–45," in *British Medicine in an Age of Reform,* ed. Roger French and Andrew Wear (Cambridge: Cambridge University Press, 1991), 136–64.

73 All of the following hospital surgeons honored by the Crown, according to the *DNB,* had the FRS and published at least one article in the *Philosophical Transactions:* William Blizard, FRS 1787, was knighted in 1803; Benjamin Collins Brodie, FRS 1810, and serjeant–surgeon to William IV, was awarded a baronetcy in 1834; Anthony Carlisle, who served the Westminster from 1793 to 1840, was made FRS in 1804, acted as surgeon extraordinary to the Prince Regent, and was knighted in 1821; Astley Cooper, FRS 1802, was knighted in 1820 and made surgeon to George IV in 1828; Everard Home, FRS in 1787, was made serjeant–surgeon to George III in 1808 and created a baronet in 1813; William Lawrence, assistant surgeon to St. Bartholomew's from 1813 and full surgeon from 1824, obtained the FRS in 1813, was made serjeant–surgeon to Queen Victoria in 1857, and was belatedly created a baronet in 1867.

present themselves not just as "men of science" meeting in congenial company, but specifically as men of the *medical* sciences. The Croonian lectures on muscular motion, for instance, reveal this shift. As I noted in Chapter 6, this endowed lectureship began during the enthusiasm for mechanical explanations of how muscles worked; it was intended to combine experimental observations with learned interpretations. During the mid-eighteenth century, the lecture was given sporadically, and was rarely published or even kept in a manuscript version.[74] It became a more or less standard event again after 1775, when the Council annually appointed John Hunter to give the lectures until 1782; regular publication of the lectures in the *Philosophical Transactions,* however, did not start until 1795. Of the six men who gave the eighteen known lectures in the first half of the century, all were physicians, the first three Fellows and the last three Licentiates of the Royal College of Physicians.[75] In contrast, between 1775 and 1815, the Royal Society heard thirty-four lectures by fourteen men: seven physicians gave eight of them (in 1784–8, 1809–10), while the seven surgeons presented twenty-six. Needless to say, the list of surgeons contains names by now familiar. John Hunter (eight lectures), William Blizard (one), Everard Home (nine), John Abernethy (one), Anthony Carlisle (three) and Benjamin Brodie (two) all had posts to the general hospitals and taught in London when they became the Croonian lecturer. John Pearson (two) served as surgeon to the Lock Hospital and lectured on surgery in London; neither of his presentations was published in the *Philosophical Transactions,* however.[76]

Later lecturers more or less followed John Hunter's ideas and methods, affirming repeatedly that, for example, "the power of muscles to act is a simple property superadded to them by life," and then discussing the possible materiality of this property as revealed empirically through experi-

---

74 The Royal Society's minute books and journals have no mention of the Croonian lecturer for 1752, 1753, 1759, 1760, 1762–74. Those given from 1751–58 (1751 by Dr. James Parsons; 1754–8 by Dr. Charles Morton) were not published and no manuscript versions exist in the Royal Society's archives. Royal Society of London, *Adjudication of the Copley, Rumford and Royal Medals and Appointment of the Bakerian, Croonian and Fairchild Lectures* (London: Royal Society of London, 1831), 50.

75 *The Record of the Royal Society,* 3rd ed. (London: For the Royal Society, 1912), 217–18; Dr. James Douglas's 1742 lecture was actually given by his son, William Douglas.

76 The physician–lecturers were Samuel Foart Simmons, LRCP; Edward Whittaker Grey (sometimes spelled Gray), a nonpracticing MD who served as librarian to the British Museum; George Fordyce, made an FRCP by special election in 1787, physician to St. Thomas's; Gilbert Blane, LRCP and physician to St. Thomas's; Matthew Baillie, FRCP and physician to St. George's; Thomas Young, in 1808 a candidate for the FRCP; and William Hyde Wollaston, FRCP, who failed to get elected physician to St. George's in 1800 and was one of the rare physicians who left medical practice for successful full-time work in chemistry. Munk reported that "one of his great discoveries, the malleability of platinum, produced him, it is said, as much as thirty thousand pounds." At the time of his Croonian lecture (an idiosyncratic essay on seasickness), Wollaston was a secretary to the Royal Society. Munk, *Roll,* 2: 439.

ments.[77] Not all of the lecturers actually performed their own experiments, and few used specimens to demonstrate particular points. The physicians still tended to give more textually based and abstract lectures, as Edward Grey (1785) did when he discussed Albrecht von Haller's ideas about irritability and sensibility, and Thomas Young (1809) did when he configured the arteriovenous system as a hydraulic model complicated by the elastic and muscular powers of the arterial coats.[78] It was the surgeons, in contrast, who most overtly displayed their training in anatomy and their surgical expertise using experimental physiology and Hunter's insistence on comparative anatomy as a means to investigate "life." In his first lecture, for instance, Hunter's protégé Everard Home reported on hydatids, seeing them as primitive moving forms with "no visible muscular structure," to establish that action "does not depend upon any particular structure." In a similar fashion, Anthony Carlisle discussed his experiments on fish to illuminate "the Arrangement and Mechanical Action of the Muscles."[79] Connecting surgical interests to the broader phenomena of muscular motion through the objects of natural history allowed these practitioners to proclaim their detachment and concern for science outside mere clinical encounters, yet to focus on problems with theoretical import for their disciplines.

The formation in 1808 of the Animal Chemistry Club as a semiformal "assistant" society to the Royal Society further exhibited surgeons' roles as "working men of science." This group, which began as a casual one among a few Fellows, brought together a handful of chemists and surgeons to explore animal chemistry.[80] Physician–chemists, such as Humphrey Davy,

77 Report on Matthew Baillie's Croonian lecture, Journal Books, Royal Society of London, vol. xxxiv, 17 Nov. 1791; report on Everard Home's Croonian lecture, 11 Nov. 1790; report on John Abernethy's Croonian lecture, vol. xxxvi (1795–9), 23 Nov. 1797, and the full manuscript version in Letters and Papers, Decade XI, no. 37, Royal Society of London.
78 Edward Grey read his Croonian lecture, "An examination into Haller's Theory of Muscular Motion," in 1785; it was not published. A precis appears in the Journal Books, Royal Society of London, vol. xxxii, 18 Dec. 1785; Thomas Young, "The Croonian Lecture on the Functions of the Heart and Arteries," Philosophical Transactions 99 (1809): 1–31; see also George Fordyce, "The Croonian Lecture on Muscular Motion," Philosophical Transactions 78 (1788): 23–36.
79 Everard Home, "The Croonian Lecture on Muscular Motion," Philosophical Transactions 85 (1795): 202–20; the lecture was given in November 1790. Anthony Carlisle, "The Croonian Lecture on the Arrangement and Mechanical Action of the Muscles of Fishes," Philosophical Transactions 96 (1806): 1–12; see also Anthony Carlisle, "The Croonian Lecture on Muscular Motion," Philosophical Transactions 95 (1805): 23–6.
80 Coley, "The Animal Chemistry Club," 173–85; Granville, Science without a Head, 25. Granville quoted from an account of the Anniversary Meeting, 30 Nov. 1809. Banks, he reported, applauded the collaboration of anatomists and chemists, with their own special fields, to "promote the advancement of animal chemistry." See also Gwen Averley, "The Social Chemists: English Chemical Societies in the Eighteenth and Early Nineteenth Century," Ambix 33 (1986): 99–128.

and apothecary–chemists, such as William Brande, collaborated with Everard Home and Benjamin Brodie. These two hospital surgeons were especially noticeable, moreover, as they were the ones, along with Brande, whose papers – labeled as submitted from the Society for the Improvement of Animal Chemistry – were published in the *Philosophical Transactions.* Together Home (four), Brodie (four), and Brande (four) presented the dozen articles that appeared between 1809 and 1816. Brodie's work on animal chemistry, particularly his research on poisons, moreover, shaped the topic he chose for his Croonian lecture of 1810. In it he addressed the "Influence of the Brain on the Action of the Heart, and on the Generation of Animal Heat," a problem connected to his ongoing investigation into what happened when he applied poisons to various vessels and nerves, using rather complex vivisectional techniques.[81]

Brodie's projects aptly capture the ways a young hospital surgeon aimed his public work at different audiences, one focused on the "observing practitioner" and the other on "men of science." Elected assistant surgeon to St. George's in 1808, when he was twenty-five, Brodie soon participated in both the Society for the Improvement of Medical and Chirurgical Knowledge and the Medico-Chirurgical Society. In their publications, Brodie presented case commentaries, discussing the import of specific, unusual patient histories and, more broadly, referring to hospital cases for his work on diseases and injuries of joints.[82] In this part of his life, he displayed an image of the rational surgeon concerned with clinical practice. At the same time, however, with Everard Home's patronage, his first paper was read before the Royal Society, and he soon obtained the FRS with considerable medical support on his nomination certificate.[83] Brodie

---

81 Benjamin Brodie, "The Croonian Lecture, on Some Physiological Researches Respecting the Influence of the Brain on the Action of the Heart, and on the Generation of Animal Heat," *Philosophical Transactions* 101 (1811): 36–48, esp. p. 47; Benjamin Brodie, "Experiments and Observations on the Different Modes in which Death is Produced by Certain Vegetable Poisons," *Philosophical Transactions* 101 (1811): 178–208; "Further Experiments and Observations on the actions of Poisons in the Animal System," *Philosophical Transactions* 102 (1812): 205–27; "Further Experiments and Observations on the influence of the Brain in the generation of Animal Heat," *Philosophical Transactions* 102 (1812): 378–93. The sequence of Brodie's research work appears in his manuscript notebook, Physiological Experiments and Observations, 1810, 1811, MS 40, St. George's Hospital Medical School Library. He began recording his experiments on 2 May 1810 and gave the Croonian lecture in December of that year; see in particular the experiments performed on 13–28 Sept. 1810.

82 The members of the Society for the Improvement of Medical and Chirurgical Knowledge elected Brodie to their select group a few months after his election as assistant surgeon to St. George's. Proceedings, 5 July 1808. Brodie's major articles were "Case of Abscess in the Brain, which discharged matter by the Ear," *Transactions of the Society for the Improvement of Medical and Chirurgical Knowledge* 3 (1812): 106–14, a case read to the Society on 4 July 1809, and "Pathological Researches respecting the Diseases of the Joints," *Transactions of the Medical and Chirurgical Society* 4 (1813): 208–77.

83 Nomination certificates, Royal Society of London, VI.158.

continued to use the Royal Society and the *Philosophical Transactions*, not the medical press, for reports on his experimental physiology.

Whatever the personal and social motives for Brodie's choices, in the end they revealed and reinforced how certain members of the London medical elite operated. They interwove their prominent positions within the medical community as "observing practitioners" making useful contributions with their respectable niches in the Royal Society as "men of science." Despite the different emphasis on the sources and utility of medical experience to advance knowledge, these venues complemented each other for the emerging London elite of hospital men and their colleagues. In both arenas, hospital men exhibited expertise – by practicing, studying learned texts, performing experiments, circulating with nonmedical gentlemen, and writing for publication – that enhanced their visibility among practitioners and lay audiences alike.

In this chapter I have explored the emergence of a medical community around medical societies and the publication of medical transactions, collections, and general journals. This community has resonances, of course, with past occupational associations: the textual communities of practitioner–readers, especially those among learned physicians; the social connections inherent in urban or country neighborhoods where practitioners might turn to each other as allies, not rivals; or the professional organizations of guilds, fellowships, and colleges of the early modern period. The scene I have sketched for eighteenth-century London, however, marked a shift of dynamics and scale. While the medical community was linked to non-London men through correspondence, reports on other publications, and an elusive audience of readers, at its core it depended upon the possibility of face-to-face discussions and debates. It had no formal limits and was continuously re-created through the interaction of various groups, social and occupational networks, rivals, competitors, pupils, patrons, and friends.

As was the case for members of the early Royal Society, gatherings of self-proclaimed peers into societies allowed them to make decisions about *who* and *what* counted by their very existence as public places for professional judgment. Medical societies and periodical publications thus offered ways to construct the regular practitioner and to gather physicians, surgeons, apothecaries, men-midwives (and all the hyphenated versions) in shared rituals of producing, presenting, and publishing medical knowledge. The vague boundaries for participating, especially compared with university study or corporate membership, permitted common neighborhood practitioners to become the rank and file within a broadly based profession while hospital men and their circles of close teaching and researching colleagues became the new elite. What might have been a recipe for medical revolution – the formation of a large, articulate community with its own respected and increasingly powerful leaders – was, of course, nothing of the sort. The older professional and social elites of the Royal College of Physicians and the Corporation/Royal College of Surgeons judiciously welcomed hospital men into their ranks. The very men who could have seriously contested the corporations' legitimacy as effective licensing bodies, speaking for their pupils and for ordinary members of medical societies, instead enjoyed the trappings of traditional corporate power.

In a masterly move, for instance, the Council (all Fellows) of the Royal College of Physicians, voted itself the power – through the President – to propose two Licentiates annually for admission to the Fellowship, although later bylaws considerably restricted this practice. The names of the few Licentiates created Fellows *speciali gratia* from 1784 to 1790 included a roll call of well-connected hospital physicians active in the medical community: Richard Huck Saunders, FRCP 1784 (Middlesex, 1766–8; St. Thomas's, 1768–77); Robert Knox, FRCP 1786 (Middlesex, 1769–82); George Fordyce, FRCP 1787 (St. Thomas's, 1770–1802); James Carmichael Smyth, FRCP 1789 (Middlesex, 1775–89); and William Saunders, FRCP 1790 (Guy's, 1770–1802).[84] Among the Oxbridge Fellows, too, were a small number of hospital men who lectured, presented case histories, and investigated topics in the medical sciences like energetic Licentiates: Matthew Baillie (St. George's, 1787–1800); John Latham (Middlesex, 1789–93; St. Bartholomew's, 1793–1802), and Clement Hue (lecturer at St. Bartholomew's from 1810, elected physician in 1823). Latham, indeed, not only served in the College's administration along with Baillie during the reform movements of the early nineteenth century but was President of the RCP from 1813 to 1820 and oversaw the College's response to the Apothecaries' Act.[85] Latham joined the Medical Society of London in 1789, lectured, and taught on hospital wards, and wrote case commentaries for the College's *Transactions*. His career moved him through the medical community into prominence in one of the most conservative and traditional medical corporations in all of Britain.

Hospital men and lecturers predominated even more among the corporate leadership of the Company, then College (1800), of Surgeons. Nearly all of the Surgeons' twenty-three Masters between 1780 and 1820 had served one of the general hospitals; most had published at least one article in the medical press; several lectured; four received knighthoods.[86] Hospital men had held a majority in the Court of Assistants and the Court of

84 Clark, *Royal College of Physicians*, 2: 571–2. The other two were Drs. William Watson and John Hunter; Hugh Smith, physician to the Middlesex, 1756–64, was proposed, but not accepted by the council.
85 Munk, *Roll*, 2: 394, 404; Clark, *Royal College of Physicians*, 2: 647.
86 Cecil Wall, *A History of the Surgeons' Company, 1745–1800* (London: Hutchison's Scientific and Medical Publications, 1937), 226–7; Sir Zachary Cope, *The Royal College of Surgeons of England, A History* (London: A. Blond, 1959), 340. See Appendix I.E.

Examiners for most of this period, and by the early 1800s many of these men had also published. The Naming several of those elevated to the Court of Assistants between 1800 and 1815 sets up familiar echoes: William Blizard (1800), Henry Cline (1800), Everard Home (1801), John Abernethy (1810), Astley Cooper (1815), Anthony Carlisle (1815).[87]

Such interconnections suggest the ways that hospital men who belonged to both old and new elites managed professional stability. They also balanced the slightly different roles required to be "observing practitioners" and "men of science." These ultimately became more specialized tracks, with the former leading to quantitative clinical research and the latter to the biomedical laboratory. Yet in the late eighteenth and early nineteenth centuries, these paths commingled for medical men looking toward the top. And they had to. Neither could serve alone for acceptance into the multiple circles that gave key actors – from John Hunter and George Fordyce to Alexander Marcet and Benjamin Brodie – the range of social, intellectual, and professional authority that allowed them to act as elite practitioners. The "observing practitioner," sanctioned much earlier by the Royal Society, located his medical knowledge in the case experience given to peers in societies and the medical press. The "man of science," equally present in the earlier Royal Society as the physician–philosopher and learned–surgeon, continued within this prestigious group, yet increasingly laid claim to the medical sciences – particularly anatomy, physiology, and animal chemistry – that foregrounded both occupational expertise and erudition. Whether or not hospital men consciously contributed to this disjunction is beside the point; their choices created and re-created their status as producers of both "good" clinical practice and "good" medical science. Any regular medical man could aspire to the first; only a few medical gentlemen could manage the second.

---

87 Cope, *Royal College of Surgeons,* 341; Cline and Blizard were both elected to the Corporation of Surgeons' Court of Assistants in 1796 and reappointed on the transition to the College of Surgeons under its new charter.

8

Hospital men make medical knowledge, 1760–1815

"[L]ast night a nasty little dog was in the dissecting room shut up there for some experiment or other & made free with the Os Cuboides & the falanges of the little Toe, for wh. I have substituted part of an other foot," wrote Hampton Weekes, a resident apothecary's pupil at St. Thomas's, to his father on 10 November 1801.[1] Busy making anatomical preparations to send home, Hampton evinced complete disinterest in what that "experiment or other" might have been about, much less concern for the fate of the dog. Hampton later warned his family: "These things I suppose you will not circulate for what I tell you on this head I conceive goes no farther."[2] Hampton, happily participating in the clinical and anatomical rituals at St. Thomas's and Guy's, was quite blasé about the notion of animal experiments, yet clearly aware others might not have such enlightened views. Hampton, in short, even as a pupil on the fringes of hospital men's investigations, identified with the culture of "men of science." He acquired those tidbits of theory that extended his repertoire not only into talk of constitutions and ultimate causes for disease, but also into experiments and science.[3] He savored those delicious moments of *knowing* more about nature than others did: "I tell Dick ye source of animal heat is acertained ask him if he knows it," he wrote to his sister, Mary Ann, "This is a chemical operation— ."[4] Students like Weekes not only accepted hospital men's authority, but also valued their instructors' appeals to rational practice and scientific knowledge.

During the late eighteenth century, cultural currents – political radicalism, religious dissent and reform, bourgeois sensibility, moral earnestness, utilitarianism, and romanticism – shaped the meaning and practice of

1 Hampton to his father, 10 Nov. 1801, in John M. T. Ford, ed., *A Medical Student at St Thomas's Hospital, 1801–1802: The Weekes Family Letters*, Medical History, Supplement No. 7, 1987, 72.
2 Hampton to his father, 10 and 15 Nov. 1801, in Ford, ed., *A Medical Student*, 72, 75.
3 See Chapter 5 for one of Hampton's comments on his chemistry lectures.
4 Hampton to Mary Ann Weekes, 28 Mar. 1802, in Ford, ed., *A Medical Student*, 145; See also, Hampton to his father, 5 Aug. 1802 (p. 207); 29 Nov. 1802 (p. 238).

science. Recent studies of politics, theology, science, and medicine, especially those by Adrian Desmond, Simon Schaffer, Jan Golinski, John Gascoigne, and Roy Porter, make such connections clear. From the broader perspective of lay society, these scholars have shown that talking about chemistry, comparative anatomy, and physiology always – however indirectly, even innocently – had epistemological, spiritual, and political implications. Each of these fields ultimately required its investigators to hold metaphysical beliefs about the attributes of matter and the existence of vital powers. And such beliefs always – however obliquely – involved culturally contentious assumptions about God's action in the material world and the possibilities of human understanding of divine, natural, and social order.[5]

Hampton Weekes, however, worried not at all about epistemological uncertainties, threats to his religiosity, or coarsening of his moral sensibilities when he studied anatomy or chemistry. And why should he have felt these concerns? He spent most of his time living within London's medical community dissecting body parts, observing ward patients, following hospital men's instructions, hearing lectures, going to meetings of medical societies, and drinking porter with other pupils. He was comfortably surrounded by those who encouraged his curiosity and enjoyed his comradery. In his accounts of business as usual among hospital men, students, and patients, Hampton reveals the intense matter-of-factness of most London medical work. To avoid controversy, these men practiced and taught him safe science – "facts" apparently stripped of their dangerous moral or philosophical implications. And Hampton learned, as his story about the "nasty little dog" reveals, to protect this community from outsiders who just might not understand how *normal* it all was.

Hampton's offhand comments aptly capture both the tone of hospital men's work during these decades and the major point of this chapter. In order to convey the ways that hospital physicians and surgeons made new knowledge, I return to the image of "safe" work: work that appeared to be prudent, uncontroversial, and culturally appropriate for members of a social and professional elite. In this chapter I argue that hospital men had both to demonstrate *and* to preserve their positions as elite physicians and

5 Roy Porter, *Doctor of Society: Thomas Beddoes and the Sick Trade in Late-Enlightenment England* (London and New York: Routledge, 1992); Simon Schaffer, "States of Mind: Enlightenment and Natural Philosophy," in *The Language of Psyche,* ed. George S. Rousseau (Berkeley: University of California Press, 1990), 233–90; John Gascoigne, *Cambridge in the Age of Enlightenment: Science, Religion and Politics from the Restoration to the French Revolution* (Cambridge: Cambridge University Press, 1989); Adrian Desmond, *The Politics of Evolution: Morphology, Medicine and Reform in Radical London* (Chicago: University of Chicago Press, 1989); Jan Golinski, *Science as Public Culture: Chemistry and Enlightenment in Britain, 1760–1820* (New York: Cambridge University Press, 1992); Susan Faye Cannon, *Science in Culture: The Early Victorian Period* (New York: Dawson and Science History Publications, 1978); Robert E. Schofield, *Mechanism and Materialism: British Natural Philosophy in an Age of Reason* (Princeton, NJ: Princeton University Press, 1970).

surgeons throughout all of their public activities, which certainly included what they wrote for publication in medical journals and in the *Philosophical Transactions*. In their clinical work, this requirement had two significant implications. First, hospital men did not rely entirely upon charity patients under ward supervision for the observations they offered on interesting cases, despite the advantages of access to a supervised population of sick people. Quite the contrary: they needed to display practice among the well-to-do as well as among the poor to demonstrate their own social and clinical status. Second, hospital physicians and surgeons had to consult with one another whenever cases crossed the complex boundary between "internal" and "external" disorders. As hospital staff and as attendants to high-ranking patients, both physicians and surgeons had to stick to "pure" practice. And "pure" practitioners worked within the complex interactions of consultations and collaborations.

The display of appropriate roles for "pure" practitioners, furthermore, had important implications for just what counted as "good" knowledge for these men, how to make it, and how to talk about it. Physicians were experts on "internal" disorders and concentrated on the diagnostic skills needed to understand and treat these constitutional diseases. Those who pursued experimental projects, in turn, chose chemistry as the discipline suitable for physicians. Chemistry not only had associations with learned physic, but also focused attention on the analysis of bodily substances of considerable import for "internal" conditions: blood, urine, and mucus. Surgeons were experts on "external" disorders and those below the surface that were both perceptible to the touch and accessible with the knife. They collected observations of surgical diseases and of morbid structures. Surgeons eager to be men of science, in turn, chose experimental projects that demonstrated their specific knowledge and skills, working particularly on experimental surgery and experimental physiology. When aspects of their observational and experimental work overlapped, moreover, physicians and surgeons consulted each other in science as they did in medical practice.

Nowhere was this division of labor more apparent than in the fact that hospital physicians called upon hospital surgeons to perform the autopsies and vivisectional experiments that interested them. Unlike the peculiar circumstances in Paris, where lowly staff physicians like Bichat worked tirelessly among hospital corpses to probe the subtle manifestations of disease in organic parts and hence more vociferously championed a clinico-anatomical method in the early 1800s, in London corpses belonged to surgeons. In London, at least, it was in elite *surgeons'* interests to discourage physicians from encroaching upon their intellectual and professional territory, as much as – or more than – it may have been in elite physicians' interests to protect a cultural self-image as men with clean hands. Collegiality and consultations thus maintained the conceptual distinctions both between "internal" and "external" conditions, and between chemistry and anatomy, that were so much a part of physicians' and surgeons' professional identities.

So far, I have portrayed the hospital physicians and surgeons who inhabit this chapter as "safe" primarily because they minded their social and professional manners, deferring to each other's areas of expertise as a matter of mutual convenience and public legitimation of their elite status. But I believe that the notion of "safe" knowledge characterizes not only staying within one's own clinical and scientific territories, but also the way that most hospital men wrote about their work. Given the radical currents and political import that certain sorts of science had in these decades – especially anything that hinted at crude materialism – hospital men adopted a descriptive style that emphasized their commitment to matters of fact, not to speculation. Most of them simply do not include nods to God or social order; when hints do appear, they are – with a few important exceptions – politically bland and theologically benign.[6]

Silence, in this context, was safe. And, I believe, silence about anything other than basic descriptions of phenomena was a significant element of the ongoing rhetorical construction of "objectivity." I briefly explore in a later section of this chapter the way that hospital men participated in the long process by which "good" science became "objective" not necessarily by the way it was done, but by the way it was appropriately reported to others. London's hospital men in these decades by no means began this process, nor did they finish it. Rather, as active clinicians, teachers, lecturers, and researchers, they gave the detached, unemotional, third-person narrative authority through their own positions in the medical community. And this authority was central to the entrenchment of "objectivity" in science's flight from philosophy and politics.

My argument rests on the notion that doing safe science helped elite practitioners to "advance" knowledge without jeopardizing their social positions by possibly offending hospital governors and wealthy patients. In his 1843 biography of his uncle, Sir Astley Cooper, Bransby Cooper recounted a revealing tale of Astley's dance with dangerous opinions, complete with a particularly apposite moral. In the late 1780s and early 1790s, when he lectured on surgery at St. Thomas's, Astley Cooper favored democratic reform and even supported the early years of the French Revolution. Benjamin Harrison, the powerful treasurer of Guy's, took

6 For the theological implications of late-eighteenth- and early-nineteenth-century science, see: Neal Gillespie, "Divine Design and the Industrial Revolution: William Paley's Abortive Reform of Natural Theology," *Isis* 81 (1990): 214–29; P. M. Heimann, "Voluntarism and Immanence: Conceptions of Nature in Eighteenth Century Thought," *Journal of the History of Ideas* 39 (1978): 271–83; John Gascoigne, "From Bentley to the Victorians: The Rise and Fall of British Newtonian Natural Theology," *Science in Context* 2 (1988): 219–56.

Astley aside one day and warned him that he would not get elected surgeon to Guy's if he persisted in holding such political views. Bransby proudly reported that his uncle then not only embraced but also taught the wisdom of reticence. "As the duties of a surgeon extend alike to men of all parties and views," Astley Cooper cautioned his pupils, "it must be most unwise for him to attach himself to any one particular set, and thus render adverse to him all maintaining contrary opinions."[7] Cooper was, of course, elected to Guy's.

Cooper's advice applied, I believe, to any sort of views that might render a practitioner "adverse" to those he needed for his livelihood. I close this chapter with my version of a well-known public dispute between two hospital surgeons, John Abernethy and William Lawrence, to illustrate the real dangers Lawrence faced when Abernethy attacked him for promoting the sort of science that led directly to immorality and corruption. Yet this episode was only a dramatic instance of the larger theme running throughout this chapter: hospital physicians and surgeons made knowledge – be it clinical or experimental – in ways that reinscribed and displayed their status as elite practitioners both within the medical community and among lay men and women. And, even as secure as most of them undoubtedly were within their circles of patients, pupils, and friends, they needed to protect this status – and so they tried to be safe.

TO OBSERVE – AND "MAKE THE TRYAL"

The cultural value accorded to careful observation supported the proliferation of case histories and accounts of therapies that engaged medical societies and dominated the medical press from the 1770s on.[8] The attuned practitioner was a natural historian, one who recounted "with fidelity the rise, Progress, & the events of such diseases" granted to him by simple experience.[9] Such passive observation was suitable for nearly any occasion

7 Bransby B. Cooper, *The Life of Sir Astley Cooper, Bart.*, 2 vols. (London: John W. Parker, 1843), 1: 298. The irony of such "impartial" wisdom from one securely enfolded in an elite social and professional position probably spoke more loudly to the rank and file in the 1840s, when Bransby published the biography, than it had in the early 1800s, when Astley lectured. Already having medical success and power made it easy for the Coopers to advise detachment from "politics" – meaning beliefs that challenged the status quo – compared with those who had little enough of either.
8 Heading quotation from William Bromfield, *Chirurgical Observations and Cases*, 2 vols. (London: T. Caddell, 1773), 1: 9.
9 William Saunders, Oration on the Improvement of Medicine, 1790, Royal College of Physicians (RCP) MS 529, n.p.; "Advertisement," *Edinburgh Medical and Surgical Journal* 1 (1805): 6; S. J. Peitzman, "Bright's Disease and Bright's Generation – Toward Exact Medicine at Guy's Hospital," *Bulletin of the History of Medicine* 55 (1981): 309; Russell Maulitz, *Morbid Appearances: The Anatomy of Pathology in the Early Nineteenth Century* (New York: Cambridge University Press, 1987), 114–16; Robert Kilpatrick, " 'Nature's Schools': The Hunterian Revolution in London Hospital Medicine, 1780–1825," Ph.D. dissertation,

where interesting events might occur, whether in private or public practice.[10] Articles on single cases, on multiple cases of people beset with the
same condition or given similar treatment for related illnesses and traumas,[11] and on hundreds of institutional cases reduced to tabular form,[12] all

University of Cambridge, 1989, explores the concept of natural history in medical knowledge. I have not seen this dissertation, however.
   I use "natural history" in the eighteenth-century sense of collecting detailed descriptions
as well as in the sense of seeking a *taxonomy* for such descriptions. These are intimately
connected, as Foucault stressed in both *The Birth of the Clinic* and his *Archeology of
Knowledge*. Yet those looking at specific objects did not necessarily aim to make taxonom-
ies; the potential to use "internal" as well as "external" characters, and the attention to
seeing change in an organism over its lifespan, were integral to much of what natural
historians did in the eighteenth century. So the metaphor incorporates more epistemological possibilities than just making grand organizations for "nature."
10 James Carmichael Smyth, "Three Instances of Sudden Death, with Appearances on Dissection," *Medical Communications* 2 (1790): 466. Several elite medical men, most notably
   William Heberden, Sr. (FRCP 1746), a physician unattached to any hospital or dispensary,
   found plenty to note among his private cases. Heberden is well known, for example, for
   describing the clinical course of angina pectoris for the first time. Ernest Heberden,
   William Heberden: Physician in the Age of Reason (London: Royal Society of Medicine
   Services, 1989), 122–6; Heberden's first paper on this topic was "Some Account of a
   Disorder of the Breast," *Medical Transactions of the Royal College of Physicians* 2 (1772): 59–
   67. See also: "Is There Any Certainty in Medical Science?" *Edinburgh Medical and Surgical
   Journal* 1 (1805): 427, 429.
11 Alexander Russell, "An Account of Some Experiments made with the Decoction of the
   root of the Mezereon, in Cases of Venereal Nodes," *Medical Observations and Inquiries* 3
   (1767): 189–228; Everard Home, *Observations on Cancers connected with Histories of the
   Disease* (London: G. & W. Nicol, 1805); Brodie, "Pathological Researches," 207–77;
   among nonhospital men, see, for example, the ebb and flow of cases in which practitioners
   tried digitalis: [S. F. Simmons], "An Account of the Effects of the Digitalis Purpurea in
   Dropsy," *London Medical Journal* 6 (1785): 55–60. John C. Lettsom, "Of the Digitalis
   Purpurea in Hydroptic Diseases," *Memoirs of the Medical Society of London* 2 (1789): 145–
   76; William Currie, "Observations on the Digitalis Purpurea, or Fox Glove," *Memoirs of
   the Medical Society of London* 4 (1795): 10–16; William Hamilton, *Observations on the Preparation, Utility and Administration of the Digitalis Purpurea, or Foxglove* (London: Longman,
   Hurst, Rees and Orme, 1807), and its favorable review in the *Edinburgh Medical and Surgical
   Journal* 4 (1808): 215–9.
12 Ulrich Tröhler has detailed the ways that some eighteenth-century British medical men –
   particularly dispensary and military practitioners – sought inductive certainty through
   numerical studies. Ulrich Tröhler, " 'To Improve the Evidence of Medicine': Arithmetical
   Observation in Clinical Medicine in the Eighteenth and Early Nineteenth Centuries,"
   History and Philosophy of the Life Sciences 10, supplement (1988), 31–40; idem, "Britische
   Spitäler und Polikliniken als Heil- und Forschungsstätten 1720–1820," *Gesnerus* 1 (1982):
   115–31; further details can be found in idem, "Quantification in British Medicine and
   Surgery, 1750–1830, with Special Reference to Its Introduction into Therapeutics", Ph.D.
   dissertation, University College London, London University, 1978, 48–72, and summarized 447–73. Only one hospital physician, Gilbert Blane of St. Thomas's, published a
   study including large-scale numerical data from hospital practice: "Observations on the
   Comparative Prevalence, Mortality & Treatment of Different Diseases," *Transactions of
   the Medical and Chirurgical Society* 4 (1813): 89–143. Thomas Beddoes, "Introduction," in
   his *Contributions to Physical and Medical Knowledge, Principally from the West of England*
   (Bristol: Biggs & Cottle, 1799), 7–13. The only other London hospital practitioner I have
   found who did a broad quantitative study between 1760 and 1815 was William Heberden,
   Jr. (physician, St. George's, 1793–1803), who relied entirely on the London Bills of

served the same laudable goal: to contribute individual men's experiences to the common pool of medical knowledge.[13]

To be of interest, however, case histories had to contribute observations beyond the usual routines of unproblematic practice. Which experiences were common and which unusual were judgments themselves constructed during medical training, discussions in medical societies, and articles in medical journals. In this sense, the medical community created the dynamic interchanges that sustained practitioners' ongoing participation in making "good" clinical knowledge.[14] The aura of long or extensive experience lent weight to practitioners' clinical observations and conclusions among their peers. Having seen many patients, senior medical men were presumably well prepared to recognize unusual or particularly illustrative cases and to proclaim the wisdom of their impressionistic inductions. Here hospital physicians and surgeons had a decided advantage for reasons indicated in Chapter 6: hospitals offered large numbers of patients presumably under closely supervised treatment. Indeed, the belief that the inpatient hospital allowed medical men more control over their patients, and hence more certainty about their observations of symptoms and the effects of medicines, had become a fairly commonplace point in medical circles by the 1770s.[15] Throughout the later eighteenth century, hospital practitioners continued to evoke a hospital's presence as a vital source for clinical authority, a place where they accumulated quantities of observations to a degree

Mortality to discuss the relationship between cold winters and health: "Of the Influence of the Cold Upon the Health of the Inhabitants of London," *Philosophical Transactions* 86 (1796): 279–84. For a surgeon's quantitative work, see Charles Bell, *Surgical Observations. Being a Quarterly Report of Cases in Surgery, treated in the Middlesex Hospital, in the cancer Establishment and in Private Practice* (London: Longman, Hurst, Rees, Orme and Brown, 1816).

13 As I explained in Chapter 4, contemporary texts and clinical lecturers presented plenty of examples for aspiring authors to follow.

14 Gilbert Blane, *Elements of Medical Logick* (London: T. and G. Underwood, 1819), 91; William Hillary, *An Enquiry into the Means of Improving Medical Knowledge* (London: C. Hitch and L. Hawes, 1761), x–xvi, 254–9; James Sims, *A Discourse into the Best Method of Prosecuting Medical Inquiries, delivered before the Medical Society of London* (London: J. Johnson, 1774), 72–80, 89–101; Joseph Hooper, *A Discourse on the Best means of improving the Science of Medicine delivered at the Anniversary of the Medical Society of London* (London: J. Phillips, 1788), 26–31; George Fordyce, "An Attempt to Improve the Evidence of Medicine," *Transactions of the Society for the Improvement of Medical and Chirurgical Knowledge* 1 (1793): 243–94; [anon.], "Is there any certainty in Medical Science?" 427–9; Benjamin Brodie, "An Essay on the Principles of Science," read to the Academical Society, 1802, MS 17, St. George's Hospital Medical School Library.

15 I have covered the early-eighteenth-century discussion of hospitals as places for clinical observations in Chapter 6; see also: Francis Home, *Clinical Experiments, Histories and Dissections* (Edinburgh: W. Creech; London: J. Murray, 1780), vi; Joseph Warner, *Cases in Surgery, with Remarks*, 2nd ed. (London: J. & R. Tonson & S. Draper, 1754), 142–5; George Fordyce, "Observations on the Small Pox, and the Causes of Fevers," *Transactions of the Society for the Improvement of Medical and Chirurgical Knowledge* 1 (1793): 1–17 (Fordyce read this paper on 5 Dec. 1783).

simply unavailable to most medical men. They did not need to specify just how many cases of a particular condition they had seen or how many times they might have successfully used a debatable remedy for the assertion of hospital experience to have considerable rhetorical force.[16]

Of course hospital physicians and surgeons *did* see lots of patients on the wards.[17] With the expansion of ward-walking after the 1760s and the introduction of publicized clinical lectures in the 1770s, more and more members of the medical community knew how many patients a hospital man could attend on his rounds and the ways that he could arrange his observations into proper case histories. Surgeons especially took advantage of the concentration of interesting and difficult external conditions, as patients with severe injuries, growths, and ulcers sought refuge and care in hospital wards. A few hospital surgeons, including Percival Pott (St. Bartholomew's, 1745–87), Joseph Else (St. Thomas's, 1768–80), and John Abernethy (St. Bartholomew's, 1787–1827), wrote on specific disorders in part to use the diverse manifestations revealed in hospital cases to detail the natural histories of common afflictions, including head injuries, testicular hydroceles, and tumors.[18] Even in hospital men's work on quite narrowly defined conditions, their references to choosing exemplary cases to illustrate a point suggested that hospitals provided more experiences than one man could possibly recount, yet which nonetheless added to the author's certainty about his generalizations. In this sense, hospitals endowed a man with clinical authority merely by their presence in his prose.

Hospital men's ward observations had certainty, moreover, because they could claim – when it suited them – that cases in institutions were "public" ones. "The following cases [were] selected from many others," wrote Alexander Russell in 1767, "as the least complicated and, being hospital

---

16 Donald Monro, *An Essay on Dropsy and its Different Species*, 3rd ed. (London: A. Miller, 1765), ix–x; John Latham, *On Rheumatism and Gout; A letter addressed to Sir George Baker, Bart.* (London: T. N. Longman, 1796), 4–5; see also Joseph Else, *An Essay on the Cure of the Hydrocele of the Tunica Vaginalis Testis*, 3rd ed. (London: John Wilkie, 1776), 66, 73; William Saunders, *A Treatise on the Structure, Economy and Diseases of the Liver*, 3rd ed. (London: W. Phillips, 1803), Part II; George Fordyce, "Some Observations upon the Combination of Medicines," *Transactions of the Society for the Improvement of Medical and Chirurgical Knowledge* 2 (1800): 315.

17 Trying to estimate how many cases hospital men paid attention to largely depends upon the existence of extensive clinical notes for adequate evidence. To date I have found very few sets of hospital men's records. Benjamin Brodie, however, kept several case books for his hospital and private practice in the nineteenth century, and these beg for close analysis. See, among others, Cases, MS 30–7, St. George's Hospital Medical School Library; Timothy Holmes, *Sir Benjamin Collins Brodie* (New York: Longmans, Green & Co., 1898), 37–8.

18 Percival Pott, *Injuries of the Head [1760]*, in *Chirurgical Works*, ed. James Earle, 3 vols. (London: J. Johnson, 1790), 1: 255–70; Else, *An Essay on the Hydrocele*; John Abernethy, *Surgical Observations on Tumours and Lumbar Abscesses* (London: Longman, Hurst, Rees, Orme, and Brown, 1811).

patients [at St. Thomas's], most under public inspection."[19] Thomas Gataker, surgeon to St. George's, was rather more blunt in 1764:

> The opportunities for experiments in private practice are not always sufficient, and are confined to the limits of one man's understanding and knowledge, as well as liable to the bias of partiality or interest.[20]

As the century wore on, any reader of medical journals could well wonder about practitioners' biases, given the conflicting results of treatments found in clinical reports.[21] The puffing case histories used to advertise medical wares in the daily press, moreover, demonstrated how easily the language of sincerity and veracity could be put to fallacious use; anyone could claim experience. The notion of abuse – possible or actual – of "one man's . . . knowledge" gave the anonymous comments in the 1809 "Hints to Young Practitioners and Observations for the Benefit of Those Whom They May Concern" a particularly biting edge. In his directions for quick success the satirist advised: "Write monthly reports of diseases in newspapers or magazines, swell out the list according to your own fancy. . . . Intersperse your observations with some extraordinary cases which occurred in your private practice, no matter whether you forge them or not."[22] The familiar assurances of truth – such as giving the names of those who consulted or witnessed the case – still had some rhetorical power for observers of singular conditions and therapeutic successes. The appeal to hospitals, and to other sites for communal charity practice, thus promised a strong antidote to fraud, if not to error, with medical students and other practitioners subjecting patients to "public inspection."

A practitioner's possible abuse of his truthfulness when reporting cases paled in comparison to his possible abuse of his patients, however. Gataker's casual reference to "experiments" in the preceding quotation raised uncomfortable connotations of overly speculative and dangerous practice, whether for charity cases or for those in private homes, as I noted in Chapter 6. For the rest of the century, doing "experiments" or "trials" continued to evoke the manipulative interests of the elite and the cruel coldness of the natural philosopher. Both practitioners and patients confronted the still inescapable tensions between risk and security in any clinical investigation beyond the benign description of customary practice, freak accidents, or unusual diseases watched by the powerless observer.

The outspoken dissenter, John Aikin, when a surgeon in Chester in

---

19 Russell, "An Account of some Experiments," 196.
20 Thomas Gataker, *Essays on Medical Subjects* (London: R. & J. Dodsley, 1764), xlv.
21 Lettsom, "Of the Digitalis Purpurea," 145–76. Comparing his poor results with those of other authors, Lettsom remarked, "I am at loss to explain the different results of our experiments" (p. 169).
22 "Hints to Young Practitioners and Observations for the Benefit of Those Whom They May Concern," *Edinburgh Medical and Surgical Journal* 5 (1809): 336.

1771, boldly proclaimed that the "improvement of medical knowledge is greatly indebted to hospitals for the opportunities they afford of *experimental practice*." The word "experiment," he noted, "occasions great outcries and prejudices among the vulgar; and . . . it is apt to startle some well disposed persons of a superior class." Nevertheless, Aikin continued, all improvement "has its original foundation in *experiment*."[23] Dr. Francis Home, a professor at the University of Edinburgh and a clinical lecturer at the Royal Infirmary, deliberately tempered the polemical effect of "experiment" in comments he made in 1780. The hospital practitioner certainly "can try different and new methods of cure, provided he has a probability of success, and proceeds with proper caution." For Francis Home, hospitals allowed practitioners to make the observations of disorders and the effects of various medicines that practitioners needed in order to improve medicine. In this sense, he articulated, once again, the eighteenth-century sense of the case as a story in natural history. Yet, Home commented, such observations "are real experiments in this branch of natural knowledge, and tend to make medicine as certain as most other sciences."[24]

In their own ways, both Aikin and Home tried to defuse the radical connotations of "experiment." If "experiment" could mean the very cautious introduction of new methods by men capable of recognizing and acting with "proper caution," then it could indeed convey the aura of benign science moving to and from the bedsides of sick people. It is Francis Home's sense of "experiment" as both improving and prudent that captures London men's rhetorical use of the term, however cavalier they may actually have been with trials on their patients in the wards or in operating theaters. Hospital physicians and surgeons certainly tried different medications and new operations on their charity cases and reported these openly in the medical press.[25] But the cynical conclusion that they exploited these vulnerable patients more than others must be tempered because of the way that these practitioners tried the very same innovations on their private patients, sometimes *before* using them in the hospitals. Dr.

23 John Aikin, *Thoughts on Hospitals; with a letter to the author by Thomas Percival* (London: Joseph Jackson, 1771), 29, 75–6; Guenter Risse, *Hospital Life in Enlightenment Scotland* (Cambridge: Cambridge University Press, 1986), 21–2.

24 Home, *Clinical Experiments*, vi–viii; Guenter Risse discussed the same authors within the Edinburgh context; see his *Hospital Life*, 191; Mary E. Fissell, *Patients, Power, and the Poor in Eighteenth Century Bristol* (Cambridge: Cambridge University Press, 1991).

25 See, for a range of examples, Thomas Dickson, "Of the Use of Blisters, applied to the region of the os sacrum, in the cure of Incontinence of Urine, and Palsies of the lower extremities," *Medical Observations and Inquiries* 2 (1767): 311–20; idem, "Observations on the Cure of an Haemoptoë, and upon riding on Horseback for the Cure of Phthisis," *Medical Observations and Inquiries* 4 (1771): 206–14; William Blizard, "Experiments and Observations on the External Use of Emetic Tartar," *London Medical Journal* 8 (1787): 57–60; William Charles Wells, "On the Presence of the red Matter and Serum of Blood in the Urine of Dropsy which has not originated from Scarlet Fever," *Transactions of the Society for the Improvement of Medical and Chirurgical Knowledge* 3 (1812): 231–9.

Michael Morris, for instance, wrote that he first tried using Peruvian bark on his own children when they had whooping cough and, hopeful about its beneficial effects, then tried it on a case at the Westminster Hospital and on a private patient.[26]

As much as some hospital men used their charity posts to claim authority based on extensive experience, the close supervision and "public inspection" of patients, and judicious experimentation, they nevertheless continued to report extensively on cases from private practice. For staff physicians and surgeons who wanted not only to produce "good" clinical observations, but also to preserve their elite status as they described their practice and their patients in the medical press hospital work had significant liabilities. One of the drawbacks of inpatient practice concerned the quality and completeness of observations made only in hospitals. As critics of hospitals pointed out, such institutions were "unnatural" environments for the proper observation and treatment of diseases that were heavily influenced by local conditions and personal life-styles.[27] This argument, which was especially favored by champions of dispensaries and domiciliary care, rarely bothered hospital men explicitly, although it likely prompted some to include examples of relatively poor patients seen in their homes for salutary contrasts and similarities. Hospital men commented far more often on the problems of learning about patients' previous histories and their conditions after they left the charities. When trying to grasp the natural history of a condition or efficacy of a treatment, however much distorted by either charity or civilization, observing the poor in hospitals had a decided disadvantage.

"Experiments made in public, as in hospitals," noted Thomas Gataker, "though in general most useful, must for a time at least, leave the event in suspence [sic]."[28] Daniel Lysens, who had been a physicians' pupil at St. Thomas's in 1754–5, tried the decoction of elm bark on cutaneous diseases in his provincial practice.

26 Michael Morris, "An Account of the Effects of Castor, and the Peruvian Bark, in the Hooping Cough," *Medical Observations and Inquiries* 3 (1767): 281–6; Nicholas Munckley, "The History and Cure of a dangerous Affection of the Oesophagus," *Medical Transactions of the Royal College of Physicians* 1 (1767): 165–74; Dickson, "Observations on the Cure of the Haemoptoë," 208–9; Dale Ingram [a lecturer], *A Strict and Impartial Enquiry into the Cause and Death of the late William Scawen, Esq. of Woodcote-lodge, in Surrey* (London: T. Caddell, 1777), 5–7; John Hunter, "A Case of Paralysis of the Muscles of Deglution, cured by an artificial Mode of conveying Food and Medicines into the Stomach," *Transactions of the Society for the Improvement of Medical and Chirurgical Knowledge* 1 (1793): 182–8; Everard Home, "Cases and Observations, which shew that Inflammation is sometimes communicated from the Dura Mater to the Pericranium," *Transactions of the Society for the Improvement of Medical and Chirurgical Knowledge* 3 (1812): 122–57.
27 For some of the pragmatic objections to hospitals see Donna T. Andrew, *Philanthropy and Police: London Charity in the Eighteenth Century* (Princeton, NJ: Princeton University Press, 1989), 104–9; see also Chapter 2, this volume.
28 Gataker, *Essays on Medical Subjects*, xlv, 11.

Observing these great effects of the medicine in the hospital, seldom, if ever heard of after their discharge [*sic*], I determined to make use of the first opportunities that offered, to find out, whether such cures were permanent.[29]

Having seen patients for ten years, he could report on two cases in which the cure eventually worked. Later in the century, Astley Cooper made a regular habit of following his interesting surgical cases home from Guy's, continuing to care for them without charge so that he could report on their later recovery or death.[30]

Working only with the poor was the second drawback to an exclusive emphasis on hospital patients. After all, interesting and useful cases occurred in the homes of the middling sort, the gentry, and the aristocracy, where hospital men spent a great deal of their time earning money.[31] While practitioners gave neither the names of their private patients nor identifying personal details in case reports, they nevertheless clearly considered them suitable objects for clinical inquiry. But there were significant social as well as intellectual reasons to recount the histories of private patients. Stories of elite patients confirmed and strengthened a hospital man's professional status, respectable practice, marketplace success, and gentlemanly expertise. Everard Home, for example, dotted the pages of his 1805 book on cancer with clinical details on unnamed "ladies" and "gentlemen," along with "Margaret Dalton" and "William Barker" seen at St. George's. He left no doubt about the distinguished calls on his time.[32] (That the late John Hunter and other distinguished practitioners had attended some of the cases he described presumably ensured Home's probity as well as his surgical pedigree.) Contemporaries knew that such displays in clinical accounts deliberately served to flaunt an author's well-to-do clientele. Dr. John Latham, physician to St. Bartholomew's, observed that

it necessarily falls to my lot, in the discharge of my public duty (*for I would not be thought vain and ostentatious by arguing from what I may observe in private practice*) to see annually a great number of patients afflicted with this disease [rheumatism].[33]

Latham's appeal to his "public duty" – and to his modesty – had its own disingenuous resonances, of course. His study concerned gout, the

29 Daniel Lysens, "Letter to Dr. Adee on Elm Bark," *Medical Transactions of the Royal College of Physicians* 2 (1772): 206–7.
30 See, for example, Astley Cooper, "A Case of Aneurism of the Carotid Artery," *Transactions of the Medical and Chirurgical Society* 1 (1809): 1–10. For Cooper's explicit use of private patients for long-term observations, see "Some Observations on Spina Bifida," *Transactions of the Medical and Chirurgical Society* 2 (1811): 323; Wells, "On the Presence of the red Matter," 213–39.
31 See, for example, Richard Warren, "Of the Bronchial Polypus," *Medical Transactions of the Royal College of Physicians* 1 (1767): 407–26; Home, *Observations on Cancers*; Brodie, "Pathological Researches."
32 Home, *Observations on Cancers*, 215–16, 237–42, and passim.
33 Latham, *On Gout and Rheumatism*, 25; my emphasis.

paradigmatic disease of the rich, as much as rheumatism, all too familiar to the poor.[34]

Throughout the process of making clinical knowledge, London hospital men moved within the opportunities and constraints of their charity posts and private practices. Producing good knowledge from patients meant making careful observation of ailments and injuries, while gaining that extensive experience so useful for repute and respect. At the same time, improving clinical medicine meant waiting for patients who could contribute to a problem already at hand: another possible trial of a medicine, another body with rheumatism, or dropsy, or angina pectoris, or hydrocele. In portraying medicine as akin to other fields in natural history, eighteenth-century authors conveyed not only the sense that diseases interacted with an environment and passed through various stages, but also the image of the practitioner as a relatively passive observer. He made "trials," moreover, much as the horticulturist did – as reasonable interactions with the "natural" course of growth or decline, to help nature along, not to provoke disease, disorder, or death.

From this perspective, reporting on patients' case histories was a culturally safe way to contribute to the improvement of medical knowledge. If done with prudence and good judgment – appropriately displayed in the author's account, of course – even doing "experiments" marked the conscientious practitioner who took advantage of suitable opportunities to help present and future sufferers.

CLINICAL TERRITORY: WHOSE CASE? WHOSE KNOWLEDGE?

For elite practitioners in London, the narration and analysis of clinical experience demanded due respect for the boundaries between the physicians' and surgeons' areas of expertise. Ordinary surgeon–apothecaries practiced both physic and surgery – not to mention midwifery and the preparation of medicines. But – by definition – "pure" physicians and surgeons called each other in for consultations and patient care rather than adopt their colleagues' techniques or instruments.[35] Consultations, in turn,

34 Roy Porter, "Disease Framed: Disease Fantasized? The Case of Gout," Fielding H. Garrison Lecture, American Association for the History of Medicine annual meeting, 1 May 1992.

35 John Gregory, *Observations on the Duties and Offices of a Physician; and on the Method of Prosecuting Enquiries in Philosophy* (London: W. Strahan and T. Caddell, 1770), 11–40; Thomas Kirkland, "Essay on the Inseparability of the Different branches of Medicine," in his *An Inquiry into the Present State of Medical Surgery*, 2 vols. (London: J. Dodsley, 1783, 1786), 1: 1–145; Mary E. Fissell, "Innocent and Honorable Bribes: Medical Manners in Eighteenth Century England," in *The Codification of Morality: Historical and Philosophical Studies of the Formalization of Western Medical Morality in the Eighteenth and Nineteenth Centuries* (Dordrecht: Kluwer Press, 1993), 19–25; George Clark, *A History of the Royal College of Physicians of London*, 3 vols. (Oxford: Clarendon Press for the Royal College of

shaped how clinician–narrators constructed what they observed and the methods they used to establish them. Decisions to consult were thus simultaneously and inextricably social and conceptual ones.[36]

In hospitals, the taking-in diagnosis labeled the patient as medical or surgical, with moves between categories later decided by the physicians and surgeons. Social power, in most cases, merged with professional authority: the patient ended up in an appropriately labeled bed, given certain kinds of treatment.[37] In private practice, at least among those who could afford a choice, the patient (or his or her family) determined the initial problem, what sort of medical people to call in, and whether or not to follow their medical advice. In this dynamic, the ill person's notion of his or her disorder as "internal" or "external" intertwined with the practitioner's, leading to accord or conflict, depending upon each one's perceptions and categories.

From hospital men's accounts of both ward and private patients, in practice the distinctions between internal and external rested on traditional associations between "general" diseases, especially those that affected most of the body (such as fevers), and physicians' prescriptions, and between injuries or cutaneous conditions and surgeons' treatments with instruments and surface unguents.[38] In practice, elite physicians did not operate, splint, or bandage; surgeons did. The converse, that "pure" surgeons did not write prescriptions for medicines taken internally, was more contentious, since many surgeons believed that such remedies were necessary for surgical care; but no one doubted that such behavior was the sine qua non of physicians' work.[39]

Physicians, 1966), 2: 610–11; Dorothy Porter and Roy Porter, *Patient's Progress: Doctors and Doctoring in Eighteenth Century England* (Stanford, CA: Stanford University Press, 1989), 79–82; Thomas Percival, *Medical Ethics* (Manchester: Russell, 1803).

36 For examples of consultations, see: John Silvester, "An Account of a Woman who was cured of a Spasmodick Contraction of the lower jaw, commonly called a Lockt-jaw, occasioned by the laceration of the tendon of one of her fingers," *Medical Observations and Inquiries* 1 (1757): 1–7; Alexander Russell, "A Case of an almost universal Emphysema," *Medical Observations and Inquiries* 3 (1767): 397–9; William Cooper, "A Case of the Caesarean Section," *Medical Observations and Inquiries* 4 (1771): 261–71; Fordyce, "An Attempt to Improve the Evidence of Medicine," 255; Alexander Marcet, "A Case of Hydrophobia," *Transactions of the Medical and Chirurgical Society* 1 (1809): 132–56; Benjamin Brodie, "Case of Abscess in the Brain, which discharged Matter by the Ear," *Transactions of the Society for the Improvement of Medical and Chirurgical Knowledge* 3 (1812): 106–14; John Yelloly, "History of a Case of Anesthesia," *Transactions of the Society for the Improvement of Medical and Chirurgical Knowledge* 3 (1812): 96; William Lawrence, "On Some Affections of the Larynx, which require the Operation of Bronchotomy," *Transactions of the Medical and Chirurgical Society* 6 (1815): 221–56; William Saunders, Lectures on the Theory and Practice of Physic, c. 1788, 57, St. Thomas's Medical School Library; John Abernethy, The Principles and Practice of Surgery, 1808, 33–5, WIHM MS 814.

37 See Chapter 2.

38 For an apt example, see Henry Thomson, "A Remarkable Case of the Softness of the Bones," *Medical Observations and Inquiries* 5 (1776): 259–60.

39 John Abernethy, The Principles and Practice of Surgery, 1808, 43; Resolutions of the Court of Examiners of the Royal College of Surgeons, vol. 1 (1763–1824), 17 May 1822.

The distinctions between internal and external disorders played out in elite physicians' and surgeons' conduct literally shaped how they could perceive a patient's body and disease. A clearly external condition, London lecturers stated regularly, was one that had obvious, accessible signs that simply *were* the disorder. Wounds, broken bones, most ulcers, tumors, skin diseases, and the like could hardly be mistaken. Whatever the underlying cause, even the patient knew what was amiss and, if well socialized, saw a surgeon. And surgeons touched the patient; they had, of course, since antiquity. Close inspection, probing fingers, hand pressure, manipulation of limbs and flesh – all of these were entirely obvious and accepted elements of surgical diagnosis and treatment among practitioners *and* the ill or injured, quite aside from the application of knives or saws.[40]

A great many of hospital surgeons' investigative projects, in fact, centered on conditions already *known* to be anatomically localized and accessible to surgical inspection and intervention. John Hunter, one of the more speculative of eighteenth-century surgeons, forayed into the general physiology and pathology of inflammation and healing. But his contemporaries and surgical offspring tended to turn Hunter's explanatory musings back onto questions with practical agendas. Even when they theorized about underlying physiological processes, these surgeons tried to guide their students and readers through the complexities of diagnosis and prognosis primarily to help them decide whether to operate or to employ less radical treatment. Joseph Else, Percival Pott, James Earle, and, rather later, Astley Cooper, for example, *all* wrote on diseases of the testis, replete with details of morbid anatomy, to help the practitioner – and patient – deal with the delicate problem of removing this organ and adjacent parts.[41] Similarly,

---

40 Susan C. Lawrence, "Educating the Senses: Students, Teachers and Medical Rhetoric in Eighteenth-Century London," in *Medicine and the Five Senses,* ed. William Bynum and Roy Porter (Cambridge: Cambridge University Press, 1993), 154–78, esp. pp. 171–5. Of course visual inspection and touching had to be acceptable to the patient; see, for example, the discussion in William Collyns's correspondence with Lucas Pepys. Collyns, a provincial surgeon, complained in a letter to Sir Lucas Pepys (physician, Middlesex, 1769–75) in 1799, that he had a difficult time with Lord Courtenay over his lordship's "hemorrhoids," first diagnosed by "conversation." Collyns "strongly pressed his Lordship to permit me to examine the part, this from delicacy was objected to." His discomfort continuing, Courtenay finally allowed the surgeon to look, and, from Collyns's account, Pepys obviously suspected venereal disease. The eminent physician advised Collyns that "there is *no Use* in giving *the Disease* any Name," but to insist upon a course of mercury for the reluctant noble. William Collyns to Lucas Pepys, 1799; Pepys to Lucas, 1799, in William Collyns, Letterbook 1787–1838, RCP MS 226. These are copies of Collyns's letters, and do not have precise dates.

41 Percival Pott, *Treatise on the Hydrocele, or Watery Rupture, and other Diseases of the Testicles, its coats and Vessels,* in *The Chirurgical Works of Percival Pott,* 3 vols. (London: J. Johnson, 1790), 2: 171–388; Else, *An Essay on the Hydrocele*; James Earle, *A Treatise on the Hydrocele containing an examination of all the usual methods of obtaining relief in that disease* (London: J. Johnson, 1791); Thomas Ramsden, *Practical Observations on the Sclerocele and other Morbid Enlargements of the Testicle* (London: Wilkie and Robinson, 1811); Astley Cooper, *Observations on the Structure and Diseases of the Testis* (London: Longman, Rees, Orme, Brown, & Green, 1830).

Everard Home and John Abernethy paid close attention to tumors and cancers, another set of external conditions long familiar to surgeons, to lay out current methods of diagnosis that might assist with difficult decisions about where, when, and whether to operate.[42] With studies like these, hospital surgeons upheld and reinscribed their expertise with external disorders, albeit with due concern for constitutional symptoms and treatment by regimen and drugs.

At midcentury, Dr. Donald Monro inelegantly summarized the opposite of external conditions: "internal diseases are the same kind to external only they can't come under the notice of the senses."[43] At least, that is, to the physician's sense of touch. Physicians used their vision, and the look of the patient formed an important part of a clinician's skill. Beyond that (and a bit of smell, sound, and taste), physicians relied on the feel of the patient's pulse, and his or her verbal account of sensations and dysfunctions. These premodern physicians, as historians have frequently claimed and criticized, did *not* touch their patients to gain any other sort of information.[44] Because probing and touching contact smacked of manual labor, earlier physicians kept their distance from their patients in order to enhance their status as educated gentlemen who directed others' work. By the later eighteenth century, I believe, this distance continued to demonstrate that a practitioner knew the appropriate bedside manners for an elite physician among genteel patients.

In general, moreover, eighteenth-century concepts of disease stressed the importance of internal imbalances, whether of the body's fluids, nervous powers, nutritive actions, or basic discordance with the environment, that provided a theoretical basis for the physician's customary detachment; his polite detachment, in turn, reinforced the idea that internal diseases arose from imbalances. When the "cause" of disease had no particular site, even when the ill body responded with localized anatomical changes, such manifestations were secondary to the physician's primary aim to cure the real problem.[45] From this perspective, looking for internal abnormalities by

42 Home, *Observations on Cancers;* John Abernethy, *Surgical Observations, Containing a Classification of Tumors, with Cases* (London: Longman and Rees, 1804); see also: Brodie, "Pathological Researches"; Benjamin Brodie, *Pathological and Surgical Observations on the Diseases of the Joints* (London: Longman and Co., 1818).

43 Donald Monro, Practice of Physic, 1758, 2 vols., 1: 87, NLM MS B 47; see also George Fordyce, Lectures on the Theory and Practice of Physic, 1787, 3, WIHM MS 2401; S. Lawrence, "Educating the Senses," 172–5.

44 Charles Newman, "Diagnostic Investigation before Laennec," *Medical History* 4 (1960): 322–9; Michel Foucault, *The Birth of the Clinic,* trans. H. M. Sheridan Smith (New York: Vintage Books, 1973), 6–9; Kenneth Keele, *The Evolution of Clinical Methods in Medicine* (London: Pitman Medical, 1963); Stanley Reiser, *Medicine and the Reign of Technology* (Cambridge: Cambridge University Press, 1978), ch. 1.

45 See, for example, David Macbride, *Methodological Introduction to the Theory and Practice of Physic* (London: W. Strahan, 1772); A. H. T. Robb-Smith, "Morgagni and English Medicine," *Proceedings of the XXIII International Congress of the History of Medicine (1972)* (Lon-

physical manipulation was not just socially undesirable; it was medically irrelevant. Dr. Thomas Young (St. George's, 1811–29) of natural-philosophy fame, presented an innocently telling example of this in his work on consumption in 1815. In his learned text, full of discussion of his wide reading, including French authors' accounts of morbid anatomy, Young described Auenbrugger's method of percussion. This technique, he noted, was perhaps best at "ascertaining the parts of the lungs most immediately affected." But, he continued, watching the patient take a deep breath gave just as much useful clinical insight about impaired respiration, and was certainly easier.[46]

Much historical reflection on the links between generalized internal dis-orders and physicians' distance from the patient, on the one hand, and those between localizable external conditions and surgeons' touching, on the other, has tended to cast these tactics as quite separate – even oppos-ing – conceptual approaches. Among London's elite physicians and sur-geons, however, "internal" and "external" views of the body and its dis-orders supported each other across the traditional occupational lines. The ways that they addressed overlapping problems of causes and perceptions reveals that physicians and surgeons often *agreed* that external conditions were the obvious ones for which physical examination was pertinent, while internal ones had more "constitutional" causes and symptoms, only discoverable through the pulse, general appearance and interrogation.[47] From midcentury on, several hospital surgeons, including Samuel Sharp, Percival Pott, Joseph Warner, John Hunter, and John Abernethy, began to insist ever more vehemently that a good surgeon avoided operating if possible, and cured, instead, by regimen and medicines. To do this sur-geons not only benefited from understanding disease through medical

don, 1974), 18–31; Malcolm Nicolson, "The Metastatic Theory of Pathogenesis and the Professional Interests of the Eighteenth-Century Physician," *Medical History* 32 (1988): 277–300; idem, "Giovani Morgagni and Eighteenth-Century Physical Diagnosis," in *Medical Theory and Surgical Practice*, ed. Christopher Lawrence (London: Routledge, 1992), 101–34.

46 Thomas Young, *A Practical and Historical Treatise on Consumptive Diseases, deduced from Original Observations, and collected from authors of all Ages* (London: Thomas Underwood, 1815), 22–3; see also, Charles Badham, "Practical Observations on the Pneumonic Dis-eases of the Poor," *Edinburgh Medical and Surgical Journal* 1 (1805): 170.

47 S. Lawrence, "Educating the Senses," 172–5; the ways that physic and surgery supported each other conceptually and pragmatically need much further research. The *rhetoric* of observation and diagnosis throughout eighteenth-century texts seems to support my gen-eral assertion. See, for example, Robert James, *The Modern Practice of Physic, As Improved by the Celebrated Professors, H. Boerhaave and F. Hoffman*, 2 vols. (London: J. Hodges, 1746), particularly vol. 2, which covers local inflammations; John Rutherford, Clinical Lectures of John Rutherford [at Edinburgh, 1750], MS 1, 1–17, St. George's Medical School Library; Midwifery was an extremely important field for the overlap of "internal" and "external" conditions and examinations but cannot be addressed in sufficient detail in this book.

theory, but also from learning to pay attention to the patient's constitution.[48]

Hospital physicians, in turn, touched their patients on the rare occasions when they inquired about external disorders. In Dr. Alexander Russell's hospital trials of "the Root of the Mezereon" for venereal nodes, for instance, he described a consultation with a St. Thomas's surgeon about a patient, Robert Page.

> I then examined the limb more narrowly with Mr. Cowell, the surgeon, and found that, although nothing appeared to the eye, yet in pressing the fingers along the *tibia,* a roughness was felt on that part where the tumor had formerly been, and the patient complained of pain upon our touching that part.[49]

Donald Monro, John Latham, and William Charles Wells (St. Thomas's, 1795–1817), among others, mentioned touching and palpating hospital and private patients in particular circumstances, impelled by diagnostic curiosity. With or without the presence of surgeon-colleagues, London hospital physicians sought enlightenment from physical examination, nevertheless, only when an internal condition clearly had external signs and they had reason to want more than the patient's account of what she or he noticed about such symptoms.[50]

During the second half of the eighteenth century, the scope of what information an "external" sign might offer expanded. Those who lectured on anatomy and ran dissecting rooms had extensive experience with the internal ravages of disease even when simply teaching normal structures and functions. Postmortem examinations became much more common by the end of the century, as well. More significantly, however, trained practitioners increasingly used more precise, technical anatomical language

48 John Freke, *An Essay on the Art of Healing* (London: W. Innys, 1748), 53–5; James Earle, "A Short Account of the Life of the Author," *The Chirurgical Works of Percival Pott,* ed. James Earle, 3 vols. (London: J. Johnson, 1790), 1: xxiii; Samuel Sharp, *A Critical Inquiry into the Present State of Surgery* (London: J. & R. Tonson and S. Draper, 1750); Joseph Warner, *An Account of the Testicles, their Common Coverings and Coates; and the Diseases to which they are liable; with the method of treating them* (London: L. Davis, 1774), 26–35; John Hunter, *A Treatise on the Blood, Inflammation and Gunshot Wounds,* 2 vols. (London: George Nicol, 1793); John Abernethy, *Surgical Observations on Tumours and Lumbar Abscesses* (London: Longman, Hurst, Rees, Orme, and Brown, 1811).

49 Russell, "An Account of Some Experiments," 223–4.

50 Mark Akenside, "Observations on Cancers," *Medical Transactions of the Royal College of Physicians* 1 (1767): 64–92; Donald Monro, "An Account of Some Uncommon Cases," *Medical Transactions of the Royal College of Physicians* 2 (1772): 353–5; John Latham, "Remarks on Tumors which have been mistaken for diseases of the Liver," *Medical Transactions of the Royal College of Physicians* 4 (1813): 47–54; William Charles Wells, "On Rheumatism of the Heart," *Transactions of the Society for the Improvement of Medical and Chirurgical Knowledge* 3 (1812): 384–7; for an elite nonhospital physician's work, see Robert Bree [FRCP], "On Painful Affections of the Side from Tumid Spleen," *Transactions of the Medical and Chirurgical Society* 2 (1811): 84–101; and see also George Fordyce, *A New Treatise on the Practice of Physic taken from Dr. Fordyce's Lectures* (c. 1775?), 2 vols., 2: 523, 535–7, WIHM MS 2396–7.

for describing both clinical and postmortem appearances.[51] In their attention to these details, many medical men commented on the way that internal conditions had perceptible "external" signs quite useful for diagnosis, if not for treatment. While the "feel" of dropsies, encysted swellings, enlargements of abdominal organs, and various tumors and localized inflammations had long been part of standard medical literature – especially for the signs known to the ancients – postmortem observations on how these disorders looked and where they were located occasioned fairly frequent reports. Curiosity, too, about possible organic sites for certain clinical conditions, like angina pectoris or hydrophobia, inspired practitioners to perform postmortems that might help to explain, if not to make physically "external," such dangerous or peculiar diseases.[52]

From at least the early eighteenth century, medical authors had proclaimed that "opening the bodies of those, the state and progress of whose diseases we have observed before death" gave useful information for knowledge of disease in the living. London lecturers on physic regularly repeated this Boerhaavian maxim.[53] *Doing* autopsies, however, was a rather different matter from simply acknowledging their value. Among London hospital men, indeed, nowhere was the occupational distinction between physicians and surgeons in the construction of medical knowledge more apparent than in who actually performed postmortems. In case after case in the medical press, elite physicians turned to surgeons to assist them after the patient died. William Heberden, Sr., typifies the erudite, clinically oriented Fellow of the Royal College of Physicians who sought the appropriate expert. Having literally been left a corpse in a will to inspect for the cause of angina pectoris, in 1772 Heberden "procur[ed] that experienced and accurate anatomist, Mr. J. Hunter, to open the body."[54]

51 Susan C. Lawrence, "Anatomy and Address: Educating Medical Gentlemen in Eighteenth-Century London," in *The History of Medical Education in Britain*, ed. Vivian Nutton and Roy Porter (Amsterdam: Rodopi, 1995).
52 William Heberden, "Some Account of a Disorder of the Breast," *Medical Transactions of the Royal College of Physicians* 2 (1772): 59–69; William Heberden, "A Letter to Dr. Heberden, concerning the Angina Pectoris; and Dr. Heberden's Account of the Dissection of one, who had been troubled with that Disorder," *Medical Transactions of the Royal College of Physicians* 3 (1785): 1–11; John Wall, "A Letter from Dr. Wall to Dr. Heberden on the same Subject," *Medical Transactions of the Royal College of Physicians* 3 (1785): 12–24; John Haighton, "A Case of Hydrophobia," *London Medical Journal* 6 (1785): 361–5; Alexander Marcet, "A Case of Hydrophobia, with An Account of the Appearances after Death," *Transactions of the Medical and Chirurgical Society* 1 (1809): 132–56; Richard Satterley, "Case of Hydrophobia," *Medical Transactions of the Royal College of Physicians* 4 (1813): 348–70. For a detailed discussion of pathological anatomy in London after 1815, especially the changes attributed to the French, see Maulitz, *Morbid Appearances*.
53 James, *The Modern Practice of Physic*, 1: 2; William Saunders, Lectures on the Theory and Practice of Physic, 1788, 67, St. Thomas's Hospital Medical School MS.
54 Heberden, "A Letter to Dr. Heberden," 7–8; see also, Michael Morris, "An Account of a fatal Disease of the Stomach . . . with a Relation of the Appearances on opening the Body, by Mr. Henry Watson, FRS and Surgeon to the Westminster Hospital," *Medical*

From the 1790s on, several hospital physicians (primarily Licentiates) portrayed themselves more closely collaborating with surgeons over interesting cases at autopsy, but nonetheless deferring to the surgeon's expertise with the knife. In the unusual "Case of a Blue Girl," the subject of a clinical lecture at Guy's in 1805, for example, Dr. Alexander Marcet remarked that "the body having been opened, and the dissection carefully conducted by my colleague Mr. Astley Cooper, we observed the following appearances, which were immediately recorded."[55] Benjamin Brodie, in his own notes of hospital work, matter-of-factly described dissections on physicians' cases that he was asked to do, particularly by his colleague Dr. George Pearson, another quite active lecturer and author.[56]

Matthew Baillie was the only London hospital physician who regularly used his own hands to demonstrate the importance of anatomical knowledge and postmortem observations.[57] Baillie, trained in anatomy by his uncles, William and John Hunter, had the peculiar privilege of going off to Oxford to study physic in 1779, while continuing to assist William Hunter with his anatomy lectures at the Great Windmill Street Theatre. He inherited William's business in 1783 and took over his uncle's anatomical lectures; at the same time, he proceeded along the road to his election as physician to St. George's (1787), his Oxford MD (1789), and his FRCP (1790). In his lectures, and then in his *Morbid Anatomy of Some of the Most Important Parts of the Human Body* (1793), particularly in its second edition of 1797, Baillie reiterated the promise of postmortems for both diagnostic precision (even if too late to help the patient) and clinical practice. Such observations *could* lead the practitioner "to detect some marked difference, by which the disease may be distinguished in the living body."[58] And

Observations and Inquiries 6 (1784): 408–15; Morris simply asked Watson to perform the postmortem; the physician did not attend it.

55 Alexander Marcet, "Case of a Blue Girl, with Dissection," *Edinburgh Medical and Surgical Journal* 1 (1805): 414; Marcet, "A Case of Hydrophobia," 132–56; George Pearson, "An Account of a Division of the Liver, occasioned by a fall," *Medical Transactions of the Royal College of Physicians* 3 (1785): 337–84; Gilbert Blane, "History of a Case of Disease in the Brain, with an Account of the Appearances upon examination after Death, and some general Observations on Complaints of the Head," *Transactions of the Society for the Improvement of Medical and Chirurgical Knowledge* 2 (1800): 192–212, esp. 196, 203; and see Alexander Marcet, Hospital Practice and other miscellaneous cases and practical observations begun 13 April 1804, eg. pp. 138, 218, 233, Royal College of Surgeons (RCS) MS 67.e.9.

56 See, for example, Benjamin Brodie, Cases and Dissections (1807–11), 20, 39, 189, MS 31, St. George's Hospital Medical School Library.

57 The only other hospital physician I have discovered who performed his own postmortem observations was John Yelloly, LRCP, physician to the London from 1807 to 1818, in a very specific investigation he pursued. John Yelloly, "Observations on the Vascular Appearance in the Human Stomach, which is frequently mistaken for inflammation of that organ," *Transactions of the Medical and Chirurgical Society* 4 (1813): 371–424.

58 Matthew Baillie, *Lectures and Observations on Medicine* (London: Taylor, 1825), 83; the lectures printed here are the introductory discourses on anatomy that Baillie presented at Great Windmill Street in 1785; Alvin E. Rodin, ed., *The Influence of Matthew Baillie's Morbid Anatomy: Biography, Evaluation and Reprint* (Springfield, IL: Thomas, 1973), 9–11.

Baillie stressed some particulars, including palpation to discover whether the spleen were enlarged, that other physicians adopted.[59]

Matthew Baillie's work was a startling exception to the correct behavior expected of elite physicians, especially those with Oxford degrees. Other hospital physicians shared his interest in morbid appearances, started out learning anatomy as surgeons, and even mastered anatomical language enough to make precise descriptions of diseased parts, but did not perform autopsies. But Baillie was the only one who lectured on anatomy and ran a major anatomical school for sixteen years after becoming an elite physician.[60] He practiced as a physician at St. George's and in an expanding private practice at the very same time that he maintained considerable familiarity with anatomical knowledge and a surgeon's skills with dissecting tools. Thus, in the context of his dual career, Baillie was the only hospital physician in London for whom *not* asking a surgeon to conduct autopsies on interesting cases was socially and professionally necessary for his reputation – as a distinguished anatomist rather than as a distinguished physician.

In the process of making clinical knowledge, post-mortem observations became a familiar – if not routine – way to conclude the natural history of a condition when the case ended in death. By the end of the eighteenth century, hospital men rarely complained about not being able to open the body of a charity patient if they had reason to do so, although they reported that the families and friends of private patients still expressed reluctance, even after appeals about the importance of the autopsy for its contribution to knowledge.[61] Just how easy it was for hospital staff to demand postmortems on the hospital dead, however, remains obscure. According to Hampton Weeks, at least, Astley Cooper, surgeon to Guy's, was willing to resort to subterfuge and deception when he wanted a particular corpse. In 1802, Cooper lied about knowing the "friends' " wishes for

59 Baillie, *Morbid Anatomy*, 2nd ed., in Rodin, *Influence*, 194; Bree, "On Painful Affections of the Side," 84–101.
60 In 1799–1800, Baillie sold the Great Windmill Theatre, retired from St. George's, and devoted himself to lucrative practice. Baillie continued his interest in morbid anatomy, and remained quite active in the Society for the Improvement of Medical and Chirurgical Knowledge but published only a few studies of pathological appearances after he ceased teaching anatomy; see William Munk, *Roll of the Royal College of Physicians of London*, 2nd ed., 4 vols. (London: Royal College of Physicians, 1878), 2: 402–8, for the standard account of his life. Matthew Baillie, "On the Embalming of Dead Bodies," *Transactions of the Society for the Improvement of Medical and Chirurgical Knowledge* 3 (1812): 7–24; "Three Cases of inflammation of the Inner Membrane of the Larynx and Trachea," *Transactions of the Society for the Improvement of Medical and Chirurgical Knowledge* 3 (1812): 275–90; *Lectures and Observations on Medicine* (London: Taylor, 1825). This volume is a posthumous printing which, according to Munk, Baillie limited to 150 copies for his friends.
61 "Syllabus of a Course of Lectures on the Principles of Surgery," *European Magazine* (Oct. 1782): 247; Haighton, "A Case of Hydrophobia"; Wells, "On Rheumatism of the Heart," *Transactions of the Society for the Improvement of Medical and Chirurgical Knowledge* 3 (1812): 390; Everard Home, "Supplement to the Account of Mr. Hunter's Method of Operating for Popliteal Aneurism," *London Medical Journal* 8 (1787): 127.

the disposition of a body. Hampton and the others involved were "very merry about it" when Cooper opened a woman for whom "Mr. Pohill, a great Tobacconist" and "a governor of this Hospital" had expressly "sent word that she shd. not be inspected."[62]

Hampton's gossip about Cooper offers a sharp reminder that what medical men published about their clinical observations and their methods of investigation were not necessarily accurate accounts of either their performances or their behind-the-scenes manners. But, as I have already argued, the stories they wrote for the press were as much about the display of appropriate behavior as they were about clinical facts. Hospital physicians and hospital surgeons had a professional investment – as "pure" practitioners – to keep internal diseases and external disorders distinct, no matter how blurry the boundaries between them often were. And protecting that investment meant preserving, at least in the compositions they crafted, the decorum expected of elite practitioners and charitable men.

MEN OF SCIENCE: THE LURES OF EXPERIMENT

Clinical medicine, despite all the hopeful talk of accurate observation, induction, prudent trials, and detailed postmortems, remained (and remains) recalcitrant to universal agreement that it was, or could become, a "science." Eighteenth-century clinicians regularly reminded themselves and others that medicine – as a *practice* – was an "art," no matter how much knowledge of nature a medical man had.[63] For William Saunders, when orating on "the Improvement of Medicine," medicine was not, and could not be, a science. It would never have such rigor, not only because "it is difficult to subject a living Body to the test of Experiment," but also because diseases themselves could not be induced in ways to subject them to experimental investigation. He made these claims not on moral grounds, but by appealing to "the diversity of the human constitution" and its differing responses "when placed in similar situations & exposed to the action of the same occasional causes."[64] For Saunders, as for others, natural history provided a metaphor for rational observation, but "science" de-

62 Hampton Weekes to his father, 17 Feb. 1802, in Ford, ed., *A Medical Student*, 130.
63 Medicus, "Does a Minute Knowledge of Anatomy Contribute Greatly to the Discrimination and Cure of Disease?" *Edinburgh Medical and Surgical Journal* 5 (1809): 67–70; William Heberden, *Commentaries on the History and Cure of Diseases*, ed. and trans. William Heberden, Jr. (London: T. Payne, 1802), 7–8; Theodore M. Brown, "From Mechanism to Vitalism in Eighteenth Century English Physiology," *Journal of the History of Biology* 7 (1974): 211–16; Judy Sadler, "Ideologies of 'Art' and 'Science' in Medicine: The Transition from Medical Care to the Application of Technique in the British Medical Profession," in *The Dynamics of Science and Technology*, ed. Wolfgang Krohn, Edwin T. Layton, Jr., and Peter Weingart (Dordrecht: D. Reidel, 1978), 180–1.
64 William Saunders, Oration on the Improvement of Medicine, given 27 Jan. 1790, at the Crown and Anchor Tavern, RCP MS 529, n.p.

manded experiments of the sort that chemists did, where similar situations produced similar responses in neatly causal relationships.

Using experimental projects as a way to make medicine more like "science" required practitioners to do what *nonmedical* men did as "science," just as medical men earlier in the century had had to absorb the more general principles of natural history and natural philosophy familiar to well-educated gentlemen in order to make medicine suitably philosophical. The energy that twenty or so hospital men and their colleagues put into experimental work in surgery, chemistry, and physiology from the 1770s marks, in part, their hope to produce results using methods and materials detached from the complexities of clinical experience. At the same time, *doing* experimental science also distinguished such practitioners from those who could not, or would not, master the methods, knowledge, and patience required for investigations beyond the passive observations of events at the bedsides of the sick.

In their accounts of the experimental sciences, hospital physicians and surgeons maintained the same distinctions between their areas of expertise that they showed in their choice of lecturing topics and in their clinical practices. Physicians lectured on chemistry and did experimental chemistry, surgeons lectured on anatomy and physiology and did experimental surgery and physiology.[65] George Pearson, for instance, physician to St. George's, taught chemistry at his own laboratory outside the hospital. He was an early convert to Lavoisian chemistry and for one of his many projects wrote a *Translation of the Table of Chemical Nomenclature,* which contained wonderful tables on the various naming systems that chemists proposed for elements and compounds.[66] Similarly, John Hunter taught anatomy and the principles of surgery for years while publishing on comparative anatomy and making experiments to observe the blood's role

65 Adair Crawford, in contrast, did not lecture on chemistry after becoming physician to St. Thomas's in 1783. He had written the first edition of his *Experiments and Observations on Animal Heat and the Inflammation of Combustible Bodies,* while still in Edinburgh – where he learned his chemistry under William Irvine – and spent his free time in London working on the second, expanded edition of his volume, which appeared in 1788; see his *Experiments and Observations on Animal Heat, and the Inflammation of Combustible Bodies,* 2nd ed. (London: J. Johnson, 1788); Golinski, *Science as Public Culture,* 47. For the broader context of Crawford's work, see June Goodfield, *The Growth of Scientific Physiology* (London: Hutchison, 1960), 81–6; Everett Mendelsohn, *Heat and Life: The Development of the Theory of Animal Heat* (Cambridge, MA: Harvard University Press, 1964); Frederic L. Holmes, *Lavoisier and the Chemistry of Life* (Madison: University of Wisconsin Press, 1985).
66 George Pearson, *A Translation of the Table of Chemical Nomenclature, Proposed by De Guyton, formerly De Morveau, Lavoisier, Bertholet, and de Fourcroy, with Explanations, Additions and Alterations,* 2nd ed. (London: J. Johnson, 1799), preface; Golinski, *Science as Public Culture,* 149. Pearson converted to Lavoisian chemistry, yet he certainly distanced himself from Lavoisier in other ways. At least that is how I read his curious reference to "the immortal, and ever to be deplored, Lavoisier" in his "Experiments and Observations, tending to show the Composition and Properties of Urinary Concretions," *Philosophical Transactions* 88 (1798): 17.

in inflammation and healing.[67] Astley Cooper lectured on surgery when conducting his surgical experiments; Benjamin Brodie taught anatomy when he decided to do vivisectional research "on the influence of the brain on the generation of animal heat."[68] Charles Bell revealed the close connections between lecturing and actually doing experimental science when, as he later put it, he was "casting about for something to make new of" while teaching anatomy in 1807. His investigation into the difference between the motive and sensory nerve roots in the spinal cord required that he use his deft dissecting skills on animals during his vivisectional experiments.[69]

When elements of their experimental projects required skills outside their appropriate areas of expertise, physicians and surgeons consulted with each other just as they did when practicing medicine.[70] When John Yelloly, physician to the London, wanted to see Galen's experiment on the decussation of nerves in the brain stem, he asked Astley Cooper to perform it on a dog; when Dr. William Saunders wanted vivisectional experiments done for his book on the liver, he relied upon John Haighton to do them.[71] Similarly, the surgeons Everard Home and Benjamin Brodie belonged to

67 Stephen J. Cross, "John Hunter, the Animal Economy, and Late Eighteenth Century Physiological Discourse," *Studies in the History of Biology* 5 (1981): 1–110; John Hunter's work has been discussed at length in various biographies. See, as well: Jane M. Oppenheimer, "John and William Hunter and Some Eighteenth Century Scientific Moods," in *Essays in the History of Embryology* (Cambridge: Cambridge University Press, 1967), 308–19. Hunter became a far more significant figure in the history of surgery and science in the nineteenth century than he was during his lifetime. See Stephen J. Jacyna, "Images of John Hunter in the Nineteenth Century," *History of Science* 51 (1983): 85–108.

68 Benjamin Brodie, "The Croonian Lecture, on Some Physiological Researches Respecting the Influence of the Brain on the Action of the Heart, and on the Generation of Animal Heat," *Philosophical Transactions* 101 (1811): 36–48, and "Further Experiments and Observations on the Influence of the Brain on the Generation of Animal Heat," *Philosophical Transactions* 102 (1812): 378–93.

69 Quoted from a letter from Charles Bell to his brother, printed in the 1966 reprint edition of Charles Bell, *Idea of a New Anatomy of the Brain* (London: Dawsons, 1811), vi; Paul F. Cranefield, *The Way In and the Way Out: François Magendie, Charles Bell and the Roots of the Spinal Nerves* (Mount Kisco, NY: Futura, 1974); John Lesch, *Science and Medicine in France: the Emergence of Experimental Physiology, 1790–1855* (Cambridge, MA: Harvard University Press, 1984), 175–7.

70 In the early nineteenth century, some physicians and surgeons who ended up with hospital posts in London studied each others' sciences, as well. See, for example: Astley Cooper, Benjamin Travers in the *Dictionary of National Biography (DNB)*; Timothy Holmes, *Sir Benjamin Collins Brodie* (New York: Longmans, Green & Co., 1898), 31–4, 39; John Flint South, *Memorials of John Flint South*, comp. Charles Lett Feltoe (London: J. Murray, 1884), 23–4, 42, 58–60, 114; Benjamin Travers, Charles Aston Key, and John Flint South – all elite surgical pupils – also signed up for physicians' practice at Guy's: see Register of Physicians' Pupils, Guy's Hospital Medical School; Augustus B. Granville, *Autobiography*, ed. Pauline B. Granville, 2 vols. (London: H. S. King, 1874), I: 326–7; Pamela Bright, *Dr. Richard Bright (1789–1858)* (London: Bodley Head, 1983), 69–75.

71 John Yelloly, "A Case of Tumour in the Brain, with Remarks on the Propagation of Nervous Influence," *Transactions of the Medical and Chirurgical Society* 1 (1809): 197; William Saunders, *A Treatise on the Structure, Economy and Diseases of the Liver*, 3rd. ed. (London: W. Phillips, 1803), ix–x, 43–9.

the Animal Chemistry Club because they appreciated chemists' knowledge about tests for various substances in the blood, lymph, and urine for use in some of their vivisectional experiments.[72]

Reading the narratives that hospital physicians and surgeons wrote about their experiments, like reading their case histories, thus suggests the ways that medical practitioners positioned themselves in relation to the world they experienced. Their accounts show not only the nuances of collabora- tive behavior among elite medical men – part of the social culture of experimental science – but also their beliefs about what properly done science looked like – part of the intellectual culture of natural knowledge. From this perspective, performing an experiment was just one part of its significance. Transforming the experience into a rational, well-ordered narrative of its design, instrumentation, and results was what made its data into "facts" that others accepted, and those "facts" into grounds for others to believe the authors' interpretation of them.

An analysis of hospital men's accounts thus belongs to the complex history of "objectivity" in science and medicine that scholars are beginning to map for Western culture.[73] Modern faith in objectivity largely derives from the attributes it gives to certain kinds of knowledge; if objective, information is supposed to be impartial, neutral, verifiable, apolitical, and value free. Objective statements are *safe,* for, if appropriately constructed, they inscribe not only what *is* – not what might be or ought to be – but also what is (ideally) accessible to mutual agreement among a universalized humankind. They are safe because controversies in science – by defini- tion – hinge only on the production and narration of experiential "facts"; debates over their moral, theological, or political implications are relegated to nonscience, to personal religious commitments, to social agendas, to, in short, culture and human imperfections.

To bestow neutrality, impartiality, and verifiability upon matters of fact, however, requires a historically specific community consensus about just how observations get spoken about and written down in order to demon- strate their objectivity.[74] In eighteenth- and early-nineteenth-century Lon-

72 Home, "Experiments to Prove."
73 See, in addition to sources on the rhetoric of science cited in n. 74, Lorraine Daston and Peter Galison, "The Image of Objectivity," *Representations* 40 (1992): 81–128; Daston, "Marvelous Facts and Miraculous Evidence in Early Modern Europe," *Critical Inquiry* 18 (1991): 93–124. I am indebted to the insights Daston presented on "enlightened facts" at the History of Science Society annual meeting, Santa Fe, New Mexico, 13 Nov. 1993. For the feminist critique of "objectivity" that has inspired (directly or indirectly) so much of the refined attention to language in science, see Evelyn Fox Keller, "Spirit and Reason at the Birth of Modern Science," in her *Reflections on Gender and Science* (1985), 43–65, and the classic, Caroline Merchant's *The Death of Nature.*
74 In recent years, historians and philosophers have probed the ways that "experiments" make knowledge in science. Investigators construct experiments within a complex web of assumptions about the natural world, about the reliability and limitations of their tech-

don, hospital men participated in the ongoing construction of "objective" science and its incorporation into medicine through their accounts of experiments as members of larger communities of scientists and practitioners. They did so by writing with an undisguised commitment to a descriptive empiricism that literally demonstrated safe science. The significance of hospital men's research, especially that published in medical journals and the *Philosophical Transactions,* lies in the overwhelming message that experimental science could appear to be culturally benign. Done properly, it was factual, not speculative; pragmatic, not philosophical; theologically neutral, not threatening. It was appropriately written for communities of men of science and medicine, not for radical philosophers or conservative theologians: written, indeed, for men like Hampton Weekes, the student who opened this chapter, not for the unenlightened and uninitiated.

Physicians and clinical chemistry

Chemistry's long association with medicine, as both a practical ancillary discipline for studying the materia medica and a source of physiological metaphors, had firmly established this science as an appropriate subject for medical gentlemen to follow. Chemists promoted their discipline as a rational and practical science, one bound to appeal to those from the salon as well as the shop. London physicians seeking the cachet of science for their work needed to look no further for an appropriate subject worthy of their time for lecturing or experimental projects. Most of the hospital physicians who performed chemical experiments, however, were Licentiates of the Royal College of Physicians, not Oxbridge Fellows. Investigators like George Fordyce of St. Thomas's, George Pearson of St. George's, and Alexander Marcet of Guy's had studied in Edinburgh and brought their enthusiasm for the rapidly changing science with them to London. There they were sustained not only by lively circles of chemists in the metropolis, but also by the excitement that chemical studies inspired in the towns of provincial England and across the Continent.[75]

niques and instruments, and about how to read the matters of fact generated by their manipulations. Geoffrey Cantor, "The Rhetoric of Experiment," in *The Uses of Experiment: Studies in the Natural Sciences,* ed. David Gooding, Trevor Pinch, and Simon Schaffer (Cambridge: Cambridge University Press, 1989), 159–80; Alan G. Gross, *The Rhetoric of Science* (Cambridge, MA: Harvard University Press, 1990); Bruno Latour, *Science in Action: How to Follow Scientists and Engineers through Society* (Milton Keynes, UK: Open University Press, 1987), esp. 21–62; Dudely Shapere, "On Deciding What to Believe and How to Talk about Nature," in *Persuading Science: The Art of Scientific Rhetoric,* ed. Marcello Pera and William R. Shea (Canton, MA: Science History Publications, 1991), 89–90, 98–100.

75 Golinski, *Science as Public Culture;* idem, "Peter Shaw: Chemistry and Communication in Augustan England," *Ambix* 30 (1983): 21; Lester King, *The Medical World of the Eighteenth Century* (Chicago: University of Chicago Press, 1958; reprint, 1971), 59–62, 77–8; Trevor Levere, "Dr. Thomas Beddoes at Oxford: Radical Politics in 1788–1793 and the Fate of the Regius Chair in Chemistry," *Ambix* 28 (1981): 61–9.

Chemistry's prestige and promise as an experimental discipline destined to improve human knowledge of, and control over, the natural world, lent these physician–chemists a language of utility that buoyed their projects. Through hands-on experimental chemistry – *not* speculative armchair chemistry – ambitious Licentiates distinguished themselves from the image of the overly learned and bookish physicians produced by England's universities. Throughout the eighteenth century, elite physicians pursued chemically related topics particularly in their work on the materia medica, on the analysis of bladder stones and other bodily concretions, the composition of therapeutic waters, and articles of diet.[76] A few, notably the busy clinician George Fordyce, made forays into the commercial and manufacturing promise of chemical analysis and products later in the eighteenth century.[77]

Far more distinctive and overt applications of chemical ideas and techniques to medical concerns, however, occurred during the 1780s to 1810s, when a handful of physicians tried using new techniques of chemical analysis on the body's fluids to attempt to discover their connections to health and disease. Historians have paid considerable attention to the success that

76 George Pearson, "An Account of the Preparation and Use of the Phosphorated Soda," *London Medical Journal* 9 (1788): 393–405; Adair Crawford, "On the Medicinal Properties of the Muriated Barytes," *Medical Communications* 2 (1790): 301–60; Augustus Brande [apothecary to the Queen], "Observations on the Angustura Bark," *London Medical Journal* 11 (1790): 38–46; George Pearson, "Experiments and Observations Tending to Show the Composition and Properties of Urinary Concretions," *Philosophical Transactions* 88 (1798): 15–46; William Babington and William Allen, *A Syllabus of a Course of Chemical Lectures read at Guy's Hospital* (London, 1802); Maurice P. Crosland, *Historical Studies in the Language of Chemistry* (New York: Dover Publications, 1978), 196, 200–1; Clark, *Royal College of Physicians*, 2: 642–5; Noel G. Coley, "Physicians and the Chemical Analysis of Mineral Waters in Eighteenth-century England," *Medical History* 26 (1982): 123–44. In the 1770s and 1780s, the discoveries of the different "airs" within the atmosphere reinspired those locating the cause of diseases in environmental conditions. Several historians have discussed the ways that such science vitalized reformers' calls for ventilation around the sick and led to various improvements in the circulation of air in hospitals. London hospital men supported these renovations, although they rarely engaged in investigating these applications of chemical beliefs and reformist ideals. See John Latham, *A Plan of a Charitable Institution to be established on the Sea Coast* (London, 1791); James Carmichael Smyth, "Process for determining the Effect of the Nitric Acid in Destroying Contagion," *Tilloch's Philosophical Magazine* 2 (1798): 68–73. For airs, environment and hospital reform, see John Howard, *An Account of the Principal Lazarettos in Europe* (Warrington, 1789); John Woodward, *To Do the Sick No Harm: A Study of the British Voluntary Hospital System to 1875* (London: Routledge and Kegan Paul, 1974); Roy Porter, *Doctor of Society: Thomas Beddoes and the Sick Trade in Late-Enlightenment England* (London and New York: Routledge, 1992); Simon Schaffer, "States of Mind," 233–90.
77 George Fordyce, *Elements of Agriculture and Vegetation* (Edinburgh, 1765; 3rd ed., London, 1779); idem, "New Method of Assaying Copper Ores," *Philosophical Transactions* 70 (1780): 30–41; William Hamilton, physician to the London 1787–1807, and lecturer on chemistry at the hospital from 1788, quickly produced the first English translation of Berthollet's *Eléments de l'art de la teinture* 2 vols. (Paris, 1791) as *Elements of the Art of Dyeing*, 2 vols. (London, 1791); Musson and Robinson, *Science and Technology*, 360–5; William Hyde Wollaston, MD Cambridge and FRCP 1795, retired from practice and devoted himself to chemistry; he discovered the malleability of platinum and made a fortune. Munk, *Roll*, 2: 438–9.

morbid anatomists had in localizing the manifestations of disease in visible changes of organs and tissues. In their chemical work, however, physicians made similar efforts to "see" significant alterations in body fluids. From the perspective of the later history of organic chemistry, their projects were hopelessly premature.[78] At the time, nevertheless, physician–chemists had considerable faith that chemical traces of morbid action surely would appear if only the proper means could be devised to find them. William Thomas Brande, a chemistry lecturer and close collaborator of Everard Home and Benjamin Brodie, for instance, eagerly tried "electrical decomposition" of blood serum using the voltaic pile, imitating Humphry Davy's renowned achievements in discovering new elements, unfortunately with no useful results.[79]

Linking chemical experiments to clinical experience offered physician–chemists a way to make medicine a science through its direct application to clinical practice.[80] George Pearson, physician to St. George's, made a detailed examination into pus, for example. His project illustrates the way some hospital men worked hard to exploit chemistry's pragmatic potential. Pus, after all, was an overwhelmingly familiar and plentiful substance in hospital and private practice, and had a wide variety of diagnostic implications. His primary goal was to be able to distinguish "purulent matter" from mucus in expectorated material, as it was a crucial signal of inflammation in the respiratory organs and often confused with more benign excretions in the early stages of disease. He failed to discover chemical tests for these important substances, but did lay out more refined visual ways to differentiate pus from mucus and further elaborated on the diagnosis of pulmonary disorders by placing types of pus and mucus into a range of clinical categories.[81]

78 See, for instance, D. C. Goodman, "The Application of Chemical Criteria to Biological Classification in the Eighteenth Century," *Medical History* 15 (1971): 44; Frederic L. Holmes, "Elementary Analysis and the Origins of Physiological Chemistry," *Isis* 54 (1963): 59, 65. In his *Birth of the Clinic*, for example, Foucault remarked that the "new" Paris clinicoanatomists rejected chemistry: "It did not function as a technical extension of their gaze." (p. 167); John Lesch discusses, in contrast, how a pragmatic, experimental, and "clinical" chemistry figured significantly among physicians in his *Science and Medicine in France: the Emergence of Experimental Physiology, 1790–1855* (Cambridge, MA: Harvard University Press, 1984).

79 William Thomas Brande, "Chemical Researches on the Blood, and Some other Animal Fluids," *Philosophical Transactions* 102 (1812): 99.

80 For other examples of clinical chemistry, see Thomas Skeete, "Case of a considerable Effusion of Bile into the cavity of the Abdomen," *London Medical Journal* 6 (1785): 274–88; Fryer, "Case of Extravasation of Bile into the Cavity of the Abdomen, from Rupture of the Liver or Gall-Bladder," *Transactions of the Medical and Chirurgical Society* 4 (1813): 330–4, esp. the editors' note, p. 334; George Pearson, "An Account of a Singular Cure of a Dropsy," *Medical Transactions of the Royal College of Physicians* 3 (1785): 319–24; William Babington, "A Case of Exposure to the Vapour of Burning Charcoal," *Transactions of the Medical and Chirurgical Society* 1 (1809): 83–98.

81 George Pearson, "Observations and Experiments on Pus," *Philosophical Transactions* 100 (1810): 294–317; for similar chemical investigations of diabetic fluids, see John Rollo, *An*

Investigations into the composition of other morbid fluids took place when practitioners had similar access to body products produced in clinical circumstances propitious to performing analyses. Alexander Marcet's collaboration with Astley Cooper on spina bifida, for instance, displays the fortuitous conjunction of clinical opportunity, elite consultations, and professional expertise. Their accounts, in a paired set of articles in the *Transactions of the Medical and Chirurgical Society*, reveal how the physicians – Marcet, among others – who consulted on his cases urged Cooper to describe his anatomical and clinical observations on spina bifida, as he then did in detail. Marcet, in his article, thanked "that able and indefatigable inquirer [Cooper]" for giving him the samples of spinal fluid he subjected to chemical study. Marcet determined that the fluid of spina bifida, like that of the other "species of dropsy" he went on to examine using material from other patients, came from the serum of the blood. What significance, if any, he attached to this conclusion, however, Marcet did not share with his readers.[82]

Experimental chemistry promised to make medicine scientific by improving clinical diagnosis and pointing to possible treatments. In these accounts, the rhetorical force of "experiment" relied, of course, on chemistry's success as the new science of the Enlightenment. Utilitarian; fairly accessible through lectures, books, and modest amounts of equipment (at least for some procedures, such as analyzing pus); and, with the increasing use of more precise measurement, neatly quantitative, the new chemistry could give medicine a much needed method for scientific certainty without embroiling its champions in speculative controversies.[83] That it did not produce particularly useful results was entirely beside the point for the hopeful physician–chemists who pursued safe science by describing their experiments in meticulous detail.

Account of Two Cases of Diabetes Mellitus, with Some Observations on the Nature of Sugar by William Cruickshank, 2 vols. (London: C. Dilly, 1797) [N.B. The Cruickshank of this work was a chemist, *not* the anatomist William Cumberland Cruikshank of Great Windmill Street.]; Matthew Baillie, "An Account of a Case of Diabetes, with an Examination of the Appearances after Death," *Transactions of the Society for the Improvement of Medical and Chirurgical Knowledge* 2 (1800): 70–89; William Henry, "Experiments on the Urine Discharged in Diabetes Mellitus," *Transactions of the Medical and Chirurgical Society* 3 (1811): 130–1; William Hyde Wollaston, "On the Non-existence of Sugar in the Blood of Persons labouring under Diabetes Mellitus," *Philosophical Transactions* 101 (1811): 96–105; Alexander Marcet, "Reply of Dr. Marcet on the same Subject," *Philosophical Transactions* 101 (1811): 106–9; John Bostock, "Observations on Diabetes Insipidus," *Transactions of the Medical and Chirurgical Society* 3 (1812): 113–4.

82 Astley Cooper, "Some Observations on Spina Bifida," *Transactions of the Medical and Chirurgical Society* 2 (1811): 322–39; Alexander Marcet, "A Chemical Account of Various Dropsical Fluids," *Transactions of the Medical and Chirurgical Society* 2 (1811): 340–381, quotation p. 340.

83 Jacob Berzelius, "General Views of the Composition of Animal Fluids," *Transactions of the Medical and Chirurgical Society* 3 (1812): 198–276. Berzelius contributed this essay at Alexander Marcet's request. Berzelius had worked with Marcet on a visit to London. Berzelius put the attitude of the London physician–chemists well when they discussed secretions of

Surgeons and experimental surgery and physiology

Whereas physicians turned to chemistry for experimental methods that could incorporate science into medicine, hospital surgeons applied the skills they used in practice – dissecting and operating – to perform experiments that linked surgery to science. Natural philosophers and physicians had put these skills to use when studying natural history, comparative anatomy, and physiology for centuries, of course. Aristotle and Galen served as their major sources for classical legitimacy and surgeons as their sources for techniques and labor.[84] During the eighteenth century, elite surgeons and anatomists increasingly devised their own investigative projects that made comparative anatomy and physiology into *their* sciences. Such projects both connected surgeons to a respected learned tradition and displayed their expertise with scalpels and saws.

As I have noted, observing surgeons did a great deal of postmortem dissecting to study normal and pathological structures. Experimental surgeons, in contrast, performed vivisections on animals. These demanded the character and hands of skilled *operators:* the ability to stay calm when inflicting pain, the deftness to cut precisely, and the competence to achieve postoperative survival. Just describing the experiments themselves thus served to demonstrate surgical expertise to both medical and lay readers, no matter what particular problem the surgeon addressed. Displaying expertise in this way, however, carried a possible cultural penalty, for doing animal vivisection started to signify a lapse in moral sensibility among some circles during the later eighteenth century. Andreas-Holger Maehle has shown that the gentleman "of feeling" – who emerged in midcentury novels and essays – reacted with anger to the deliberate cruelty to animals embodied in medical men's methods.[85] Dr. James Sims, in his address to

the fluids by organs or constituents in the blood: "Avoiding vain conjectures on a subject which perhaps will ever remain a mystery, let us determine from the knowledge we already possess the chemical nature of the materials of their products" (234). See also St. Bartholomew's Medical and Philosophical Society, Minutes, 30 June 1810; Guy's Hospital Physical Society, Minutes, 27 Dec. 1806, 7 Mar. 1807, for interest in clinical–chemical analysis.

84 F. J. Cole, *A History of Comparative Anatomy from Aristotle to the Eighteenth Century* [1949] (New York: Dover Publications, 1975). That anatomical dissection as a method of investigation dominated physiology was later seen as a reason why physiology lagged in its development as a separate science. See, for example, Pauline Mazumdar, "Anatomical Physiology and the Reform of Medical Education," *Bulletin of the History of Medicine* 57 (1983): 230–46; Gerald L. Geison, "Social and Institutional Factors in the Stagnancy of English Physiology," *Bulletin of the History of Medicine* 46 (1972): 30–58. But see also Nellie B. Eales, "The History of the Lymphatic System, with Special Reference to the Hunter–Monro Controversy," *Bulletin of the History of Medicine* 29 (1974): 280–94; Lloyd G. Stevenson, "Anatomical Reasoning in Physiological Thought," in *The Historical Development of Physiological Thought*, ed. Paul F. Cranefield and Chandler M. Brookes (New York: Hafner, 1959), 27–37; Lesch, *Science and Medicine in France*, 13–30.

85 Andreas-Holger Maehle, "Literary Responses to Animal Experimentation in Seventeenth and Eighteenth Century Britain," *Medical History* 34 (1990): 27–51; Richard D. French,

the Medical Society of London in 1774, for instance, roundly condemned "the anatomist" who experimented on "a faithful guard or affectionate companion." "Observe," Sims commanded, "the savage pleasure with which he relates the result, because it happens to support some peculiar fancy of his own, or destroy that of his antagonist."[86]

Many hospital practitioners did not indulge in experimental physiology, or any experimental projects at all, and may well have agreed with such sentiments. Yet, within the pages of the *Philosophical Transactions,* only John Haighton, lecturer on physiology at Guy's and avid vivisectionist, evinced any concern for over-indulgence in animal experiments among the handful of hospital men who wrote about them. When experimenting on the regeneration of nerves in dogs in the 1790s, he refused to pin down "the precise point" when the nerves he cut could once again function. This, he noted, "would require the sacrifice of more animals than a question of mere curiosity could justify."[87] Knowing the line between accumulating sufficient evidence to establish that nerves could regenerate (at least in a few dogs) and "mere curiosity," of course, implicitly separated Haighton from others less astute.

The other hospital surgeons and lecturers who used experimental vivisections, such as William Cruikshank, Astley Cooper, Benjamin Brodie, and Everard Home, dealt with their sensibilities by ignoring them in their published accounts. They avoided making comments like Haighton's, I believe, precisely because such feelings did not belong in scientific reports. To include them, even tangentially, opened their methods and their morals to possible debate and criticism based upon their own qualms about their procedures. Instead, the value and legitimacy of their work remained implicit: whatever vivisections they performed were necessary and valuable for advancing knowledge. This assumption underlies both of the principal applications of vivisectional techniques that hospital men pursued. The first, experimental surgery, connected the researcher to pragmatic problems in operative procedures and showed surgeons using science in the service of patient care. The second, experimental physiology, connected

Anti-Vivisection and Medical Science in Victorian Society (Princeton, NJ: Princeton University Press, 1975), 15–25; Robert J. Frank, Jr., *Harvey and the Oxford Physiologists: Scientific Ideas and Social Interaction* (Berkeley: University of California Press, 1980), discusses animal experimentation in the seventeenth century.

86 Sims, *A Discourse on the Best Method of Prosecuting Medical Enquiries,* 83; a more general critique of overindulgence in anatomical studies in London appeared in Medicus, "Does a Minute Knowledge of Anatomy Contribute Greatly to the Discrimination and Cure of Diseases?" *Edinburgh Medical and Surgical Journal* 5 (1809): 67–70.

87 Haighton, "An Experimental Inquiry Concerning the Reproduction of Nerves," 196; see, too, idem, "An Attempt to Ascertain the Powers concerned in the Act of Vomiting, by Experiments made in April, 1787," and "Two Experiments on the Mechanism of Vomiting, Supplementary to a Paper lately read before this Society," *Memoirs of the Medical Society of London* 2 (1789): 250–61, 512–16, where Haighton offers few reasons for his vivisections, even though James Sims was then president of the Society.

the inquiring surgeon to ongoing questions among learned men and showed science in the service of professional prestige.

Considering the rhetorical and practical benefits of trying new operative techniques on animals before performing them on humans, surprisingly few of London's hospital surgeons actually mention that they did so.[88] The one well-known instance was John Hunter, who studied ways to tie arteries in the 1770s and 1780s in order to treat aneurysms in patients' arms and legs. Until that point, the standard surgical treatment was amputation. Hunter argued that vessels with aneurysms could be tied off, preserving the limb while giving the patient relief from the threat of a sudden rupture of the aneurysmal sac and bleeding to death. To be convincing, he had to establish that smaller arteries expanded to take over blood flow when a major vessel was constricted and eventually severed. He demonstrated this phenomenon in animal trials and explained the sufficiency of the collateral circulation with a suitably theoretical discourse on physiological action. Hunter's investigation led to several successful operations on human patients and the expansion of his techniques by his successors.[89]

The surgical experiments that appeared in the medical press in the early 1800s dealt strictly with questions about tying arteries and blood flow, for reasons that are still unclear to me.[90] A few of Astley Cooper's reports, in fact, illustrate the rhetorical potential that experimental surgery had for justifying risky practice. In his work, "experiment" took on a significant role as an element within a specific case history. In 1809, Cooper published a paper in the *Transactions of the Medical and Chirurgical Society* about tying one of the carotid arteries in a male patient, who had a carotid aneurysm, in Guy's Hospital. (Since the carotid supplies the head, amputation was not an option.) Cooper mentioned, almost in passing, that he "had many years ago made the experiment of tying these vessels [both carotid arteries] in

---

88 Just why London's surgeons did not do more work with animals in their search for operative expertise requires further research; I suspect that the surgeons who concentrated on conditions with specifically human pathological characteristics (bladder stone, diseases of the testis, cancers), as hospital men did, would not have seen "normal" animals as particularly relevant to their concerns. Toby Gelfand, in his *Professionalizing Modern Medicine*, mentions that surgeons in Paris at midcentury used animals to try their procedures. Anita Guerrini's ongoing work on animal dissection in the seventeenth and early eighteenth centuries promises to be an important contribution to this issue. Anita Guerrini, "Animal Tragedies: The Moral Theater of Anatomy, 1660–1750," paper presented to the History of Science Society, Santa Fe, New Mexico, 12 Nov. 1993.

89 Lloyd Allen Wells, "Aneurysm and Physiologic Surgery," *Bulletin of the History of Medicine* 44 (1970): 411–24.

90 Benjamin Travers (surgeon at St. Thomas's) and William Lawrence (surgeon at St. Bartholomew's), for instance, returned to the problem of arterial ligatures, seeking ways to get an artery to heal closed, not to necrose and break open around the compression. Benjamin Travers, "Observations on the Ligature of Arteries and the Causes of Secondary Hemorrhage," *Transactions of the Medical and Chirurgical Society* 4 (1813): 435–65; William Lawrence, "A New Method of Tying the Arteries in Aneurism, Amputation and other Surgical Operations," *Transactions of the Medical and Chirurgical Society* 6 (1815): 156–208.

the dog" to check the effect on "the functions of the nervous system." The results showed no "visible effect." A preparation from "this dog," he continued, "has long been preserved in the collection at St. Thomas's Hospital" to illustrate how the brain was supplied with sufficient blood by other arteries.

Yet Cooper had not offered this experimental support in an earlier paper in the *Transactions* (1806) about the *first* trial he had made to tie the carotid. He convinced a woman who entered Guy's briefly but then went home of the "probability of a fatal termination of the disease" so as to procure her consent to the operation. Because her case had "terminated unsuccessfully," Cooper quite obviously used his experimental success in the dog at the outset of the second paper to support his claim that the operation *would* work. That he was correct, with the man "discharged cured . . . without any diminution of his mental or corporeal powers" gave the surgeon "a degree of pleasure which compensated for the disappointment I felt in the issue of the former."[91] Cooper's experimental surgery served a vital persuasive function precisely because it made the animal the subject of the real experiment, not the humans on whom the technique was later used. Here the "experiment" justified Cooper's heroic – and successful – procedure and legitimized his decision to operate on the male patient at Guy's after the death of the poor woman.

Perhaps other elite surgeons were reluctant to write up accounts like Cooper's in part because experimental surgery was *too* narrowly clinical and case oriented, suitable only for medical audiences. In contrast, experimental physiology provided many more opportunities for surgeons to become "men of science," particularly for members of the Royal Society. The Society's Croonian lectureship, discussed in Chapter 7, offered a prominent platform for elite medical men to display their erudition and skills on the subject of "muscular motion." Between the 1770s and 1810s, surgeons gave most of the Croonian lectures and used them regularly to report on projects involving vivisectional experiments. They addressed specific questions already laid out in the physiological literature, moreover, which connected them to the larger worlds of learning among gentlemen scientists and natural philosophers. Benjamin Brodie's study of the effect of the brain on the heart's action and on animal heat (the Croonian lecture for 1811), for instance, depended upon observations reported by William Cruikshank in 1795 and by Bichat in his *Récherches physiologiques sur la vie et la mort*. Brodie's elaborate experimental design amply displayed the surgeon's dissecting dexterity and his knowledge of learned physiological

91 Astley Cooper, "Second Case of Carotid Aneurism," *Transactions of the Medical and Chirurgical Society* 1 (1809): 223; idem, "A Case of Aneurism of the Carotid Artery," *Transactions of the Medical and Chirurgical Society* 1 (1809): 1–10. The first case was read on 29 June 1806; the second on 21 Feb. 1809.

principles: he removed the heads of rabbits and dogs, and, with appropriate ligatures to prevent them from bleeding to death, kept the animals alive through "artificial respiration" with bellows while he took their body temperatures.[92]

Brodie's papers for the Royal Society, along with those by Everard Home, William Cruikshank, and John Haighton, show anatomist–surgeons deeply involved in research questions that had nothing directly to do with surgical practice. The experiments on animal heat, the functions of the spleen, the possible regeneration of nerves, and reproduction in rabbits that these men performed promised no immediate payoffs for patient care. Yet it is precisely because such projects addressed topics of broader interest that they were suitable for readers of the *Philosophical Transactions*. And appealing to members of the Royal Society gave these surgeons the status of "men of science" so coveted by hospital men and lecturers – and so unobtainable by ordinary surgeon–apothecaries.

Experiments and narratives

Below the surface, each hospital man's account of his experiments contained much more than the details of his project and his relationships to other investigators. Such accounts showed the proper ways that medical

92 Benjamin Brodie, "The Croonian Lecture, on Some Physiological Researches Respecting the Influence of the Brain on the Action of the Heart, and on the Generation of Animal Heat," *Philosophical Transactions* 101 (1811): 36–48; idem, "Further Experiments and Observations on the Influence of the Brain on the Generation of Animal Heat," *Philosophical Transactions* 102 (1812): 378–93; idem, Physiological Experiments and Observations, 1810, 1811, MS 40 and Physiological Observations and Experiments, 1811–16, MS 41, St. George's Hospital Medical School Library. Goodfield, in *The Growth of Scientific Physiology*, 93–8, quotes extensively from Brodie; and see Mendelsohn, *Heat and Life*, 168–9; Max Neuburger, *The Historical Development of Experimental Brain and Spinal Cord Physiology before Flourens*, ed. and trans. Edwin Clarke (Baltimore: Johns Hopkins University Press, 1981), 232–6. See also Everard Home, "On the Structure and Uses of the Spleen," *Philosophical Transactions* 97 (1807): 45–54; idem, "Further Experiments on the Spleen," *Philosophical Transactions* 98 (1808): 133–42; idem, "Experiments to Prove that Fluids Pass Directly From the Stomach to the Circulation of the Blood, and From Thence Directly into the Cells of the Spleen, the Gall Bladder and the Urinary Bladder, without going Through the Thoracic Duct," *Philosophical Transactions* 101 (1811): 163–70; idem, *Lectures on Comparative Anatomy, in which are explained the preparations in the Hunterian Museum*, 2 vols. (London: G. and W. Nicol, 1814), 1: 224–44; see also St. Bartholomew's Medical and Philosophical Society Minutes, 2 Mar. 1808, 23 Jan. 1810, for evidence that Home's work was discussed among pupils and practitioners; William Cruikshank, "Experiments on the Nerves, Particularly on their Reproduction; and on the Spinal Marrow of Living Animals," *Philosophical Transactions* 85 (1795): 177–89; idem, "Experiments in which, on the Third Day after Impregnation, the Ova of Rabbits were found in the Fallopian Tubes; and on the fourth Day after Impregnation in the Uterus itself; with the first Appearance of the Foetus," *Philosophical Transactions* 87 (1797): 197–215; John Haighton, "An Experimental Inquiry Concerning the Reproduction of Nerves," *Philosophical Transactions* 85 (1795): 190–201; idem, "An Experimental Inquiry Concerning Animal Impregnation," *Philosophical Transactions* 87 (1797): 159–96.

men should write science for publication. Reporting on many experiments, for instance, offered readers repeated cases of the same causes producing the same effects. The ways that authors reconstructed their experiments on paper, moreover, revealed the researcher's active presence or omniscient absence as he made knowledge. Each hospital man's publications were thus small episodes in the ongoing process of expressing objectivity. These practitioners, in ways still insufficiently appreciated by historians, were among the hundreds of obscure people in the eighteenth and nineteenth centuries who removed revealing self-awareness from descriptions of doing science.

To enhance the veracity of their observations and the inevitability of their conclusions, experimenters such as William Cruikshank (anatomy lecturer at Great Windmill Street), John Haighton, Everard Home, and Benjamin Brodie kept up a litany of repeated experiments. "I divided the spinal marrow of a rabbit . . . I then secured the blood vessels in the neck and removed the head . . . ; I repeated the experiment on a middle-sized dog . . . ; The experiment was repeated on a rabbit . . . ; The experiment was repeated on a dog of small size."[93] In the same way that practitioners marshaled multiple case histories to establish facts of disease and treatment, these investigators detailed selected experiments in serial order to lead the reader to unmistakable conclusions. And these, of course, were supposed to be transparently obvious.[94] "Nerves are not only capable of being united when divided, but . . . *the new formed substance is really and truly nerve.*"[95] "1. The influence of the brain is not directly necessary to the action of the heart. . . . 4. When the air respired is colder than the natural temperature of the [headless] animal, the effect of respiration is not to generate, but to diminish animal heat."[96]

"I forbear to enter into any speculative inquiries," Benjamin Brodie concluded his article on death by poisons, "as it is my wish, in the present communication, to record such facts only, as appear to be established by actual experiment."[97] Brodie detailed his "actual" experiments with care. "One drop of the essential oil of bitter almonds was applied to the tongue of a young cat. She was instantly seized with violent convulsions; then lay on one side motionless, insensible, breathing in a hurried manner." The animal was apparently dead, Brodie continued, "but, on opening the thorax, the heart was found acting regularly eighty times a minute . . . and it continued to act for six or seven minutes afterward." In the next experiment, "I injected into the rectum of a cat half an ounce of water, with two

93 Brodie, "The Croonian Lecture," 37, 38, 39, 41.
94 Gross, *The Rhetoric of Science*; Shapere, "On Deciding What to Believe," 89–103.
95 Haighton, "An experimental Inquiry," 200; emphasis original.
96 Brodie, "The Croonian Lecture," 48.
97 Brodie, "Experiments and Observations," 207.

drops of the essential oil." The same effect occurred after a longer period. Then Brodie recounted his personal experience. "I dipped the blunt end of a probe into the essential oil, and applied it to my tongue, meaning to taste it, and having no suspicion that so small a quantity could produce any of its specific effects on the nervous system. . . . I experienced a very remarkable and unpleasant sensation, which I referred chiefly to the epigastric region, but the exact nature of which I cannot describe." He tried small quantities a few more times, but with no better insights on how to describe the effect of bitter oil of almonds. From the evidence of his sensations and the two trials on the cats, "we may conclude that this poison acts on the brain through the medium of the nerves, without being absorbed into the circulation."[98]

In just one part of his paper, Brodie evoked the omniscient investigator (the oil "was applied"), the active experimenter ("I injected"), the clinical reporter ("I experienced"), and the unseen networks of practitioner–researchers ("we may conclude"). Using the passive voice distanced him from being the cause of the next events, the dramatic effect of the poison. Yet using the first person allowed Brodie (as it had allowed authors in the preceding centuries) to establish the logic of his experimental manipulations and the credibility of subsequent observations. Using the first person to describe his own sensations, moreover, let Brodie make them into useful data. Using the collective pronoun incorporated the community into the logic of his deductions from his sensations and observations. He was not alone.

In its use of multiple voices and perspectives, Brodie's work illustrates a moment in the long, uneven transition from locating credibility in the narrator's actions to placing facticity in the direct perception of nature's responses to stimulation by invisible (human) hands.[99] Brodie's deft use of quite plain, descriptive narrative for his experiments on animals and on himself, furthermore, reveals a moment when those different voices served the same ends: a detachment from the emotional experience of vivisection and a divorce from the moral and metaphysical implications of experimental investigation. Yet Brodie's multiple voices also reveal the continuing tensions between reporting personal, subjective experience and making external, objective descriptions. Brodie included his own ("unpleasant") sensations, I believe, because subjective feelings of pain and discomfort provided irreplaceable data for the practicing surgeon seeking diagnostic symptoms from his patients. In this context, however, stating his subjec-

---

98 Benjamin Brodie, "Experiments and Observations on the Different Modes in which Death is Produced by Certain Vegetable Poisons," *Philosophical Transactions* 101 (1811): 183–4.
99 I am *not* claiming chronological or geographical uniqueness for the use of multiple "voices" in scientific accounts by any means. See Peter Machamer, "The Person-Centered Rhetoric of Seventeenth-Century Science," in *Persuading Science,* ed. Pera and Shea, 143–57.

tive feelings actually demonstrated what he did not – *could* not – say about the convulsing cats. To state explicitly that the poison was "unpleasant" for the cats would introduce the moral questions about vivisection and the metaphysical speculations about animal consciousness that the objective (safe) observer needed to erase from the practice of science.

I have offered an extensive example of Brodie's prose to illustrate the seemingly *little* ways that language worked to transfer elite medical men's private activities into public contributions to objective, factual knowledge. Between the mid-1770s and early 1820s, hospital men had significant reasons – whether conscious or not – to adopt and promote a narrative style shorn of philosophical introspection, reasons that thus helped to cement detachment to properly done science. During these decades, defining "living powers" as embedded in material substances, superadded to matter, or coexisting with matter had once again become a potent theological issue. Materialism, with the problem of the existence of the soul (what could the soul be? how could it act?) and potential atheism, lay on one hand, while giving matter active powers, and hence a possible argument for pantheism (was God everywhere?), lay on the other.[100] This distressing spectrum, which had plagued philosophers and churchmen for centuries, reached a new level of public and popular awareness in the late eighteenth century.

Simon Schaffer and Jan Golinski have persuasively argued that the success of free-market lecturing brought both electrical displays and Enlightenment chemistry to ever larger circles of "uneducated" people and, in the process, gave common folk dangerous ideas about natural powers, self-improvement, and participation in politics. In the 1790s, the polemical association of the French Revolution, secular rationalism, excessive materialism, and atheism further linked physiological abstractions to questions about natural and social order.[101] In the early 1800s and 1810s, the conservative response to revolution abroad and unrest at home, coupled with the bitter war against Napoleonic France, spurred a resurgence in loyal sentiments to God and country, and a renewed dedication among the mainstream clergy and middle classes to a bucolic natural theology. Against

---

100 John Henry, "The Matter of Souls: Medical Theory and Theology in Seventeenth-Century England," in *The Medical Revolution of the Seventeenth Century*, ed. Roger French and Andrew Wear (Cambridge: Cambridge University Press, 1989), 87–113, has an excellent discussion of these issues for the seventeenth century. For the later eighteenth century, see Schofield, *Mechanism and Materialism*. Much of the discussion of forces, matter theory, and their religious implications after the 1760s has centered on Joseph Priestly and the notion of rational dissent. For a useful introduction, see Isaac Kramnick, "Eighteenth Century Science and Radical Social Theory: The Case of Joseph Priestley's Scientific Liberalism," *Journal of British Studies* 25 (1986): 1–30 and Maurice P. Crosland, "The Image of Science as Threat: Burke versus Priestley and the 'Philosophical Revolution'," *British Journal of the History of Science* 20 (1987): 277–307.
101 Simon Schaffer, "Natural Philosophy and Public Spectacle in the Eighteenth Century," *History of Science* 21 (1983): 1–43; Golinski, *Science as Public Culture*, 8–10.

this larger backdrop, chemists and vivisectionists like George Pearson, Alexander Marcet, and Benjamin Brodie seem exceptionally dull. Neither John Haighton nor Benjamin Brodie, for example, discussed the larger issues involved in studying the nerves and their place in physiological processes. They offered neither references to "vital powers" nor hints that nerves carried aetherial substance or electrical fluid. And they certainly did not mention the location, meaning, organization, or characteristics of "life," which more philosophical men pondered when considering the uses and function of nerves.[102]

Describing the way that the blood changed color, apparently in its usual way, during its passage through the lungs in decapitated rabbits kept "breathing" with bellows as their bodies got colder and gradually died led Brodie to conclude that the brain was necessary to maintain "animal heat." This observation could have supported a wide range of theoretical positions about the role of the blood in living things, about animal heat, and about how nerves served as pathways between the brain and the body. But Brodie's position cannot be read from the article itself. Was he a materialist, seeing living powers as mere by-products of the organization of matter? Was he a devout high Anglican, seeing his results as further evidence for the wisdom and necessity of an ever-active Creator? Was he neither? Did he care? We do not know, and neither did the people who read his articles. We, like other readers who knew nothing about his personal life or the opinions he expressed in private conversations, may speculate on his beliefs, his politics, or the state of his soul. But he is, and was, safe from our certainty.

Brodie's science, like George Pearson's in his study of the chemical properties of pus or Alexander Marcet's in his article on the composition of the fluid of spina bifida, created and legitimized a narrative of experiment devoid of wonderment and free of risk. Most hospital researchers followed this path, especially in the pages of medical journals and the *Philosophical*

---

102 London lecturers on physic routinely introduced overarching rhetorical concepts of "powers" (of various sorts) to students; at least from the 1780s, moreover, surgeons – especially John Hunter – did too. For the most part, however, lecturers avoided drawing any implications at all from their discussions of matter and powers. Of course their concepts probably stemmed from their philosophical and theological assumptions (even if not articulated) and certainly had philosophical and theological consequences. The important point to remember, I believe, is that other people had to make such leaps from the material as presented in lecture. See: John Hunter, Notes of lectures, n.d., 2 vols. MS 8–9, 1: 39–40, St. George's Hospital Medical School Library; Charles Brandon Tyre, A Rational of Surgery collected from the lectures of John Hunter, 1785, 3 vols., MS 11–13, 1: 5, St. George's Hospital Medical School Library; George Fordyce, "Natural History of the Human Body" and "On Diseases in General" in Lectures on Medicine, 1788, vol. 3, n.p., MS St. Thomas's Hospital Medical School Library; William Saunders, Lectures on Physic, 1788, 3–4, 55–6, MS St. Thomas's Hospital Medical School Library; Astley Cooper, Lectures on Surgery, 1808, 6–11, St. Thomas's Hospital Medical School Library.

Transactions of the Royal Society. Because they were members of the medical elite who were at once teachers, clinicians, and men of science, their caution was central to maintaining the social and intellectual status quo at the very same time they could appear to be active, innovative, and dedicated contributors to new knowledge using the newest methods. Progressive yet conservative, scientific yet circumspect, these men stayed securely ensconced in their positions of institutional and cultural authority. To be otherwise, as William Lawrence discovered, was dangerous.

DANGEROUS DISPUTES

A notably nasty dispute at the Royal College of Surgeons between two hospital surgeons, William Lawrence and John Abernethy, in the late 1810s provides a fitting denouement for this chapter. A parable of science, speculation, and status, this episode brings my arguments about the emergence of a medical community in London, the implications of safe science, and the importance of appropriate behavior among elite practitioners to life – and to a close. It illustrates three crucial points. First, the conventions of "objective" language, those attempts to make science safe through un-adorned descriptions of matters of fact, were always tenuous. Second, "safe" was always relative to audience. What could be said *within* the medical community in early-nineteenth-century London took on different implications when judged by lay outsiders. What seemed appropriate for professional discussion and disagreement became dangerous when made broadly public. Third, elite practitioners always paid a price for the cultural and social status that supported their professional and intellectual authority. Most of the physicians and surgeons to London's hospitals were probably oblivious to the cost of conformity, having easily adopted the dominant values and beliefs of the secure middling and upper classes for their own. But if called upon to make a choice? Lawrence's decision – like that of Astley Cooper described at the outset of this chapter – reveals the compro-mises required not only to become an elite hospital practitioner, but also to stay one.

In 1816, the Royal College of Surgeons appointed William Lawrence to give the series of lectures on comparative anatomy required for the newly opened Hunterian museum at the College. At thirty-three, Lawrence had all the signs of a rising member of the elite: Fellow of the Royal Society, assistant surgeon at St. Bartholomew's, demonstrator for John Abernethy's anatomy course at the hospital, a member of the Council of the Medical and Chirurgical Society, and author of a book and several articles. John Abernethy, his former master and current colleague, had already arrived. At fifty-two, Abernethy was full surgeon at St. Bartholomew's, Fellow of the Royal Society, member of the Council of the Medical and Chirurgical

Society, and Professor of Anatomy from 1814 to 1817 at the Royal College of Surgeons, where he had been elected to the inner sanctum – the ruling Council – in 1810.

In tribute to his hero, John Hunter, Abernethy enthused in his lectures on the "vital principle" he saw central to Hunter's anatomy, physiology, and surgery; indeed, Abernethy went a long way toward articulating and extending Hunter's vision. On the platform at the Royal College of Surgeons, Abernethy expressed the views he had been teaching for years, although in a more grandiose way.[103] When Lawrence took to *his* podium at the College, he took the same liberty that Abernethy did to expand upon the meaning of physiological concepts and methods. Lawrence used his discussion of comparative anatomy in part as an opportunity to summarize the way that men like Home, Brodie, Cooper, and Yelloly had proceeded in *doing* experimental physiology with vivisection, if not in thinking about its philosophical basis in material or vital forces. Like the Continental authors he admired – especially Bichat and Cuvier – Lawrence thought the guiding assumption to investigate living processes was obvious:

> I say, *physiologically speaking:* and beg you to attend particularly to this qualification: because the theological doctrine of the soul, and its separate existence, has nothing to do with this physiological question [of "life"] but rests on a species of proof altogether different. These sublime dogmas [the immortality of the soul] could never have been brought to light by the labors of the anatomist and physiologist. An immaterial and spiritual being could never have been discovered in the blood and filth of the dissecting room.[104]

In his critique of the Hunterian adherence to vital powers that Abernethy held so dear, moreover, Lawrence denied their usefulness as explanatory principles. *His* "species of proof" argued that principles that failed to explain anything were clearly not *necessary* ones – be they vague vital powers, soul, or mind added to observable matter.[105] He chose – in the lecture theater of the Royal College of Surgeons – to address a possible

103 John Abernethy, *An Inquiry into the Probability and Rationality of Mr. Hunter's Theory of Life* (London: Longman, Hurst, Rees, Orme and Brown, 1814); *Physiological Lectures, exhibiting a General View of Mr. Hunter's Physiology, and of his Researches in Comparative Anatomy* (London: Longman, Hurst, Rees, Orme and Brown, 1817); these were later reprinted, with Abernethy's Hunterian Oration and an essay on Gall and Spurzheim, in *Physiological Lectures, addressed to the Royal College of Surgeons* (London: Longman, Hurst, Rees, Orme and Brown, 1821).

104 William Lawrence, *Lectures on Physiology, Zoology and the Natural History of Man* (London: Benbow, 1822), 7; part of this passage was also quoted in Goodfield-Toulmin, "Some Aspects of English Physiology: 1780 -1840," 300.

105 Figlio, "The Metaphor of Organization," 34–42; William Lawrence was certainly not original with such views, expressed in various ways from the seventeenth century on. For a London man's earlier explicit point that evoking the "living principle . . . explains nothing," see James Sims, *A Discourse on the Best Method of Prosecuting Medical Enquiries, delivered before the Medical Society of London, 18 January 1774* (London: J. Johnson, 1774), 65.

interpretation of what contemporary research methods meant. In taking this step, Lawrence marched right into the rhetorical domain of those concerned about the slippery slope from implicit materialism, to atheism, to radical action against church and state.

In the next year, 1817, Abernethy used his lectures at the Royal College of Surgeons to revile such "Sceptics" openly and plainly. While he did not mention Lawrence by name, his vehemence left no one in doubt that his principal target was his own younger colleague. Abernethy spelled out the danger of Lawrence's supposedly materialistic views, claiming that the "thinking people" of England "consider the probable ends of conduct from its beginning," and that denying the active presence of an immaterial, beneficent vital life force "inculcates opinions tending to subvert morality, benevolence, and the social interests of mankind." Anyone who starts on this path "deserves the severest reprobation from every member of our profession, because his conduct must bring it into distrust with the public."[106] Announcing his opinions in Surgeons' Hall certainly stirred his audience; but publishing them, as he did that year, opened Abernethy's plaint to a much wider circle of critics. Indeed, the Cambridge-based Rev. Thomas Rennell (among others) took up Abernethy's charges about the danger of materialist views – that is, Lawrence's – and introduced the issue to the public through his sermons and published comments. Lawrence responded by preparing his 1817 lectures for the press, noting in his preface that "had the author [Abernethy] been content with pronouncing his attack from the chair of the College, I should have been satisfied with defending myself in the same place. The publication of his charge has made it necessary for me to publish my reply."[107]

At this point, with the quarrel at the College becoming embarrassingly well known, the governors of Bridewell and Bethlem hospitals, where Lawrence was a full surgeon, decided to suspend him from office.[108] Faced with such tangible effects of public suspicion, Lawrence chose to retreat. Lawrence seemingly preferred – willingly or not – success to science. He withdrew his published lectures from the printer and resigned as lecturer at the Royal College of Surgeons. A few years later, in 1822, Lawrence took the printers who pirated his text to court to try to suppress its unauthorized publication. In the ironic result, the Chief Justice, Lord Eldon, upheld his previous opinion that no author had property in blasphemous or seditious works. He agreed that Lawrence's lectures undermined Scripture, so the surgeon lost the case. Once judged dangerous, of course, the very material that Lawrence felt obliged to try to restrict became very popular indeed.

It is significant that no murmurs of concern slipped into the governors'

---

106 Abernethy, *Physiological Lectures* (1817), 52–3.
107 Lawrence, *Lectures on Physiology*, 1. The prefatory letter containing this quotation was signed at the "College of Physicians 8 Feb. 1819."
108 Desmond, *The Politics of Evolution*, 121.

minutes at St. Bartholomew's between 1816 and the mid-1820s. In May of 1824, just over two years after Lord Eldon heard the case, the charity's governors, including a smattering of earls, gentlemen, and men of the cloth, appointed Lawrence as full surgeon in an uncontested election.[109] Any lingering stain of blasphemy apparently did not bother those about to entrust Lawrence with the care of the poor or the teaching of young practitioners. Lawrence, however, then flirted with medical reform, supporting Thomas Wakley in starting the *Lancet* and attending meetings critical of the Royal College of Surgeons, another potentially dangerous move for his career. He gave this amusement up as well, and, shortly thereafter, his peers – including John Abernethy – elected him to the Court of Assistants (1828) at the Royal College of Surgeons. Lawrence settled down nicely, eventually attending Queen Victoria and dying – in 1867 – with a brand-new knighthood.

The dispute between Lawrence and Abernethy makes a lively story of physiology, power, and apparent persecution. It aptly conveys how religious and political concerns intertwined with natural philosophy and medical science in Britain in the tense decade after the Napoleonic wars. In the attention that historians have given this episode, Abernethy represents the conservative, backward, and stubborn elite surgeon determined to keep England safe from French materialism, while Lawrence stands for the young progressive, trying to open England to the French moderns. Lawrence usually appears as rather tactless for challenging Abernethy's views at the Royal College of Surgeons, and a bit of a coward for distancing himself from his claims.[110] And perhaps he was. Yet, in 1816, when the fracas began, the medical community openly supported both a modestly speculative Hunterian approach to physiology and an observational Baconian vision for making good medical knowledge. Both Abernethy's and Lawrence's reputations were rooted in clinical experience, in teaching, in participation in medical societies, in publication for professional audiences, and in the ineffable mantle of hospital authority. And both of them expressed and subsequently polarized physiological positions familiar to anyone who already knew their work, including members of the College's Council.[111] However escalated through intemperate language and public

109 Journal of the Board of Governors, 19 May 1824, St. Bartholomew's Hospital Archives, Ha1/17 (1815–26); the post of assistant surgeon then opened had three candidates, two of whom had been Abernethy's apprentices, and one of whom, Eusebius Arthur Lloyd, won the election.

110 Goodfield-Toulmin, "Some Aspects of English Physiology," 308, 319; Desmond, *The Politics of Evolution*, 117, 120.

111 Abernethy later claimed that Lawrence, as a student, had constantly scoffed at John Hunter's ideas. That may have bothered Abernethy, but if he voiced his concern as a member of the Council of the Royal College of Surgeons on Lawrence's appointment, it clearly did not deter his peers; Abernethy, postscript to his *Hunterian Oration, for the Year 1819* (London: Longman, Hurst, Rees, Orme and Brown, 1819), 59. For explicit

display, their disagreements began in a safe place, within the lecture theater of their own corporate body. It was only after the *publication* of Abernethy's and Lawrence's lectures, with their even more pointed criticism of each other, that serious trouble began for Lawrence. The nonmedical press reviewed them; the Rev. Rennell (and others) *read* them; in the end Lord Eldon judged the *text* to be blasphemous.[112]

So this story now offers a different lesson from the one other historians have presented. Both Abernethy and Lawrence knew the medical community, knew their colleagues, pupils, patients, and friends. Lawrence then displayed, albeit in tendentious terms, the vision of medical science as it was already *done* among his peers. Many of them, like Benjamin Brodie, eschewed appeal to mind, soul, or ephemeral vital powers as they went about observing and experimenting, even if they may have believed that immaterial vital forces were necessary to living things. Lawrence exposed some of the possible implications of undertheorized science, but I doubt very much that either ordinary surgeons or John Abernethy was taken by surprise. What Lawrence misjudged was not his surgical audience, but the power of lay opinion when fueled by Abernethy's published comments, even as he took his own pages to the printer.

What could be said safely within the newly emerging medical community could not withstand assaults from church or state when it challenged the foundations of moral and social order. Being a "man of science" put Lawrence in the right London circles of practice and professional influence, but only appropriate behavior and rhetorical style could keep him there. Whether he planned to or not, Lawrence had tested the boundaries around

expressions of Lawrence's earlier views, see especially his "Account of a Child, Born without a Brain," *Transactions of the Medical and Chirurgical Society* 5 (1814): 210, 214: "Not content with exercising his mental faculties on what comes under the operation of his senses, and exploring the instructive scenes of nature, man is ever disposed to enter the regions of imagination, and to give to the beings of his fancy, whom he first clothes with all the attributes of perfection, the designs and actions which accord only with his own shortsightedness and ignorance. He is as positive about what goes on in this unseen region, as if he directed all the operations himself, and can tell you very precisely what does, and does not harmonize with the wisdom of the Creator, which turns out at last to be the exact representation of his own knowledge or prejudices. . . . It is enough that the thing happens: whether nature has any design in these formations or not, we leave undetermined, until we are informed of some data on which a decision may be grounded" (210). Later, on p. 214, Lawrence states: "The simple truth is, that man, considered at the epoch of his first formation, is merely a secretion from the vessels of the ovary." Such opinions could indeed have offended those concerned with the theological implications of "physiological" methods.

112 Goodfield-Toulmin, "Some Aspects of English Physiology," 315–19. Lawrence's first lectures, in 1816, sparked Abernethy to call his former apprentice a skeptic in his 1817 lecture. Yet the anonymous reviewer of the *Annals of Medicine and Surgery* 1 (1817): 385–8, came up with no stronger words than that Lawrence's lectures were "like his other performances . . . utterly devoid of originality." The lecture on "Life," the reviewer noted calmly, was "almost all taken from some continental works upon physiology and zoology" (pp. 385–6).

"freedom of inquiry and speech" in philosophico-medical matters and discovered them at his heels.[113] With a prudent retreat, he regained his place and all the daily authority granted to a London lecturer, a hospital surgeon at St. Bartholomew's, and, within a few years' time, a member of the Council of the Royal College of Surgeons.

The significance of the way that hospital men made medical knowledge between the 1760s and 1810s rests in the way they constructed their experiences within communities of practitioners and men of science. Hospital posts were necessary to their authority as clinical observers, lecturers, and experimenters, yet never sufficient, in and of themselves, for their status as elite physicians and surgeons. Throughout the eighteenth century, the customs of hospital elections, ward rounds, and consultations demanded that physicians practice as "pure" physicians and surgeons practice as "pure" surgeons. On hospital wards, they simultaneously demonstrated to their students and to each other the ways that concepts and methods from physic and surgery overlapped, while maintaining the appropriate distinctions between their areas of expertise.

I have argued that the distinctions between physicians and surgeons, the ones played out every week in every metropolitan hospital, profoundly shaped the ways that staff men could make new knowledge. When presenting accounts of clinical cases, elite practitioners had to display the manners and marks of elite practice: judicious consultations with physicians or surgeons when "internal" and "external" conditions overlapped; deference of physicians to surgeons when it came time for inspection of the corpse; and references to well-to-do private patients as well as to the poor. They advanced clinical knowledge through prudent "experiments" on their patients, yet reported on trials made in homes as well as in the hospitals, blurring the boundaries between private and public practice even as they claimed that public practice gave them the extensive, witnessed experience that other medical men could not have. No matter how much hospital physicians and surgeons talked to each other about what they saw, their professional manners maintained the conceptual differences between constitutional disorders, whose causes could not be anatomically located, and specifically organic diseases, whose presence appeared unmistakably at autopsy.

I have further argued that the distinctions between physicians and surgeons extended to their areas of scientific expertise. The hospital men who lectured on one of medicine's ancillary disciplines – chemistry and anatomy – divided these neatly between physicians and surgeons. The small number of staff men who pursued experimental projects, moreover, consistently respected these boundaries. Physicians used chemistry, especially the new chemistry of the later eighteenth and early nineteenth centuries, to try to "localize" signs of constitutional disorders in bodily fluids. Surgeons used their operating skills to pursue questions in experimental surgery and physiology, performing vivisections on animals in projects welcomed both in the medical press and at meetings of the Royal Society. Their choices, in short, defined them as active men of science in ways that supported their areas of medical expertise, and vice versa. They did science not as a decorative avocation, but as a constituent part of who they were as both serious medical men *and* presentable gentlemen.

Lastly, I have argued that expectations about suitable behavior for elite practitioners supported their adherence to descriptive narratives when they wrote up their science for the press. The hospital physicians and surgeons I have discussed in this chapter by no means invented the conventions that marked "objective" prose or the cultural value placed upon descriptive narratives as contributions to the stockpile of facts. But they adopted and perpetuated these conventions and values precisely because being uncontroversial maintained their positions as dignified, cautious, and prudent practitioners. As influential men in medical circles – when teaching, attending meetings of medical societies, or publishing papers in medical journals – hospital practitioners thus encouraged a particular style of science within medicine. Writing ostensibly simple accounts of observations of patients, corpses, chemical experiments, or animal vivisections, these men offered useful additions to knowledge, not enlargements upon speculative philosophy. How conscious medical men were of this strategy – men like Brodie, that is, not Astley Cooper, William Lawrence or John Abernethy – is a moot point, for its results lie mutely in page after page of medical and scientific journals.

On the surface, the descriptive, "objective" science I have emphasized here seemed stable and secure. But that is the common illusion of all narratives of matters of fact. Both William Lawrence and John Abernethy exposed the polemical assumptions and implications that some simple "facts" were hiding, an exposé that troubled outsiders and made Lawrence's science blasphemous. Yet I believe that the emergence of a medical community around medical societies and the medical press, the role that experimenting surgeons had at the Royal Society, and the increasing influence of hospital men over students and other practitioners during the preceding decades were precisely what made Lawrence's lectures both possible and threatening. He spoke, he thought, to his professional colleagues and peers. Abernethy, royally annoyed by Lawrence's opinions and the supposedly demoralizing influence they could have on students, printed his vituperative response and cast it before the public. Hospital men *were* gaining significant authority, and, from Abernethy's perspective, they had to use it to uphold elite interests or lose the political and social support from the upper ranks that helped to keep the traditional corporations (like the new Royal College of Surgeons) in power.

For their power and prestige were threatened. By the mid-1820s the generation of hospital men elected in the 1790s to 1810s were coming under attack from their former students and dissatisfied colleagues, both for their old-fashioned methods and for their elitist attitudes. These stories belong to other historians, who have traced the nineteenth-century moves and motives of radical anatomists trained in Paris, of general practitioners unhappy with the Apothecaries' Act and feeble licensing laws, of clinicians wielding stethoscopes, and of microscopists gesturing at cells and tissues. The new generation, with its new actors, agendas, and methods, portrayed the hospital elite as foes and old fogies, images that some historians have perpetuated. Yet that elite had been long in the making, and ever precarious. Over the course of the eighteenth century, hospital physicians and surgeons had to construct their authority and maintain their status over and over again. By the 1820s hospital men, both as individuals and as a group, came under bitter criticism precisely because they had finally made it: a hospital post was supposed to signify that the man who held it had legitimate claims to authority and deserved respect. And because hospital men *had* made it, and, in the process had incorporated clinical observations and experimental research into the work that active hospital men were supposed to do, new men could criticize them, and their inadequacies, more openly.

Hospital posts acquired this meaning because complex sources of cultural and intellectual authority had first intertwined in hospital men themselves. Many of these practitioners donated their charitable service, taught on the wards, lectured to classes of pupils, observed numerous cases among the poor, and practiced extensively among the rich. They published, went to medical society meetings, performed experiments, promoted safe science and minded their manners. *All* of that – inextricably mixed – created the modern profession of medicine, where hospital consultants loom over medical students, lecture podiums, ordinary practitioners – and, of course, patients.

CONCLUSION

In 1776, Joseph Hooper, a London surgeon and man-midwife, published a short case history in *Medical Observations and Inquiries*. A female midwife had called him to see a woman who was a few months pregnant. The midwife was disturbed, Hooper wrote, because she was unable to "feel the mouth of the womb." He proceeded to examine the patient *per vaginum*. At that moment, Hooper reported, "I immediately recollected what Dr. Hunter had said in his public lecture upon the subject of the inverted uterus." While making the inspection, Hooper continued, "the woman, with expressions of much joy, said she could make water." Hooper helped her to relieve her distended bladder and, following what he learned from William Hunter's course, manipulated the uterus back into its proper position.[1]

Hooper decided to tell this story – and it was his story, for no doubt the midwife and the patient had their own versions – to medical readers. He depicted himself, of course, as a clever and competent practitioner, certainly more knowledgeable than the midwife. Yet he also chose to ascribe his knowledge to William Hunter's lectures. Here he not only revealed his regular education, but also borrowed Hunter's authority and expertise. Hooper's flash of memory and insight (even if contrived) illustrates just how ordinary practitioners both accepted and established lecturers' influence and reputations. Throughout my work, I have argued that stories like Hooper's reveal a great deal about the construction of medical authority in eighteenth-century London. My book has centered on the significance of all those small, day-to-day acts that collectively and cumulatively defined just who made "good" knowledge and how they did so.

London's rich resources for a case study in urban medical culture prompted me to reflect upon the ways that eighteenth-century medical knowledge, medical training, hospitals, clinical experience, natural philos-

---

1 Joseph Hooper, "The Case of a Retroverted Uterus," *Medical Observations and Inquiries* 5 (1776): 104.

ophy, and public science intersected, both historically and conceptually. At its core, this book argues that the articulation of medical epistemology and clinical perceptions, the appropriation of the hospital as a site for teaching and research, and the formation of a broadly based medical community were inseparable elements in the transition from early modern to modern Western medicine. They are inseparable precisely because this transition fundamentally involved a shift in the grounds for, and location of, medical authority, and medical authority depended, and still depends, on multiple factors acting simultaneously. "Authority," from this perspective, only makes sense when it is actually put to use in relationships between individuals, for only then is a person's claim accepted, ignored, or challenged, and his or her orders obeyed or resisted.

In early modern medicine, which I now characterize in the most sweeping terms, medical practitioners had authority – that is, patients and other practitioners accepted their claims and followed their treatments – very much on a case by case basis. Few generalizations work; that is one reason why describing medical practice as an open marketplace is such a useful metaphor. Aristocrats saw learned physicians, but they also consulted irregulars and dosed themselves with preparations made in their own kitchens. Middling sorts in cities called for licensed surgeons, but they also bought elixirs in shops and had their barbers bleed them. At a bookseller's, impressive Latin medical texts likely shared shelf space with vernacular medical manuals and recipe books. Aspiring physicians studied university-approved books for their disputations, read others recommended by their tutors, and often learned to practice by practicing; surgeons and apothecaries followed a single master, perhaps reading texts, too, but primarily learning what the senior man had learned from his master and through his experience. Medical authority – at least from the perspective of early-eighteenth-century London – was *everywhere*.

In any particular encounter between a practitioner and a patient, then, the reasons why the patient might have believed and obeyed the medical man reads like a list of sociological and psychological items for analysis. Social status: Who had the higher rank, and hence the customs of social deference to call into play? Kinds of knowledge: Who valued what texts contained? what experience taught? what mother always said? Degree of dependence: Was the person sick enough just to do what the practitioner determined? desperate enough to deny his practitioner's caution? Or was the practitioner so eager for a fee that he would cater to the patient's every whim? I could go on. The point is that medical certification, be it a medical degree from Oxford or membership in the Worshipful Society of Apothecaries, was only one item on this list, and only one small part of the total judgment an early modern patient made when deciding to obey her medical adviser.

Modern medicine, to indulge in more sweeping – but useful – generalizations, works quite differently. The sources of authority have narrowed and stabilized. Standardized medical education and training, with proper examinations and degrees, produce competent doctors. Accreditation and peer review of universities, medical schools, and hospital programs maintain those standards and determine what constitutes good knowledge, good practice, and successful demonstration of medical skills. Laws regulate who can practice mainstream medicine, and with what privileges, and where, and when. An ill person's choice of a doctor and decision to follow his or her advice to take a medication, have an operation, or change diet still depend, of course, on many personal elements. Some of these are the personal attributes of the practitioner, such as class, race, gender, family background, and local reputation. But these now nuance the practitioner's authority; they do not – on their own – establish it apart from proper medical credentials. Noncompliance, instead, is usually attributed to the patient's ignorance and idiosyncrasies, rather than to his or her rational choice of what are now – by definition – alternative practitioners, such as herbalists and faith healers. Ill and injured people may criticize their medical practitioners and resist their suggestions, but we all know who has, and is, the "real" authority. Medical authority is now *localized* in quite specific people.

The transition from early modern to modern medicine, then, was a very long and gradual process of localization. And the localization of medical authority in hospital physicians and surgeons was a fundamental part of this change, one that was essentially complete in London by the 1820s. I have argued in this book that this localization occurred as various sources of social, pedagogical, and intellectual authority coalesced in hospital men and then in the hospital post itself. All of these sources of authority, moreover, worked through relationships between people. Within the hospitals, the interactions among lay governors, medical governors, staff men, pupils, and patients determined the ways that the hospital became an institution for teaching as well as caring, with the patients becoming objects of clinical scrutiny as well as of charitable obligation. Within and around the hospitals, the interactions among hospital physicians and surgeons, other elite practitioners, ordinary practitioners, nonhospital lecturers, and pupils gradually constructed a medical community in which hospital men had considerable prominence. Outside the hospitals, the interactions of hospital men, members of the Royal Society, the ruling members of the Royal College of Physicians, and the Company, later Royal College, of Surgeons, and well-to-do patients configured the ways that hospital practitioners behaved, approached natural knowledge, and wrote about their clinical work and their science.

From this broad perspective, the men who became the physicians and surgeons to the London hospitals in the first decades of the eighteenth century conferred whatever social and professional prestige they already had on their hospital posts. Since clinical responsibilities and knowledge were already clearly divided between physicians and surgeons in the hospitals, as they were between the traditional corporate bodies and elite urban practitioners, hospital service imposed and maintained the conventional differences between these occupations. In this sense, both by being elected by lay governors of the middling and upper ranks and by their weekly practice on the wards, hospital men had to identify with, and to behave like, the established medical elites. Part of this identification included adopting (if one did not already have them) gentlemanly manners and gentlemanly avocations, including the pursuit of natural history and natural philosophy. The works of those who decided to make written contributions to knowledge, from short case histories in the *Philosophical Transactions* to learned monographs, quite literally displayed – and, I argue, had to display – hospital men's social and intellectual status among their contemporaries. Their authority, then, depended on the multiple sources that I have said characterized early modern medicine.

The gradual appropriation of the hospitals for clinical teaching, however, increased the influence that hospital men had over other practitioners. The expansion of ward instruction at all of the London hospitals built upon the traditional customs of apprenticeship and personal tutoring. It was the increasing number of short-term paying pupils, however, that slowly reduced the adequacy of apprenticeship for sufficient clinical experience to train a regular medical man. Ward teaching transformed the private relationship between master and apprentice, with its emphasis on personal loyalty, craft skills, and moral responsibility, to the public relationships among hospital administrators, clinicians, and medical students. Similarly, it was the number and diversity of inexpensive, flexible lecture courses that opened up academic medicine to ordinary surgeons and apothecaries. Independent courses allowed aspiring practitioners to pursue the subjects that they thought would benefit them most professionally and personally. Medical lectures, like ward-walking, made teaching and learning medical knowledge into a public activity. Advertised in the daily papers, accessible to anyone who could pay, and open to questioning by members of the audience, lectures revealed just what confident practitioners decided constituted correct theory and good treatments. Hospital men both responded to and developed the markets for ward-walking and private lecturing. Through their teaching, hospital physicians and surgeons simultaneously enhanced their own authority as knowledgeable men and helped to construct a medical community around these shared educational experiences.

During the second half of the eighteenth century, as ward-walking became more popular and the governors at four of the seven hospitals built lecture theaters for their staff men to use, individual hospital physicians and surgeons continued to take their personal reputations and prestige to their hospital posts. At some point between the 1780s and the 1810s, I believe that the hospital post itself began to bestow authority upon the man who held it. Having a hospital post *meant* that a man was a gentleman, that he practiced as a "pure" physician or a "pure" surgeon, that he was likely to obtain an FRS if seriously interested in knowledge of the natural world, and that, if he offered lectures, students would attend them. It meant, as well, that he would most likely conform to the opinions of his well-to-do patients, to the policies of the ruling councils of the Royal College of Physicians and the Royal College of Surgeons, and that, if he pursued projects in science – especially in chemistry and physiology – he would do so safely. Only with such expectations attached to the posts themselves does the bitter criticism that reformers heaped upon hospital men in the 1820s make sense. They had authority not simply as individuals, but as individuals connected to institutions – the general hospitals – that affected the lives of many ordinary surgeons, surgeon–apothecaries, and non-Oxbridge physicians. When the Royal College of Surgeons started to require hospital practice for its membership diploma in 1812, and the Apothecaries' Examiners demanded proof of hospital experience to acquire the Licentiate after the Apothecaries' Act passed in 1815, the modern links between formal certification and hospital training were forged. To become a regular practitioner literally meant that a student had to pay attention to hospital practitioners for at least six months. He could hate it, disagree with hospital practice, and dispute clinicians' opinions, but he had to do it. Although apprentices still respected their masters, and patients still sought treatments from druggists and irregulars, the new policies at Surgeons' Hall and Apothecaries' Hall officially localized medical authority in hospital men, completing a process begun over a century earlier.

The authority that hospital men acquired from their lecturing, their appropriation of London's hospitals for clinical teaching, and their prominence in medical societies was, to a large extent, authority over the shape and expression of good medical knowledge. In their published clinical work, hospital men used their positions to claim extensive experience among the sick. While they certainly wrote about hospital patients, including discussions of clinical trials made on ward cases and of postmortem appearances on hospital autopsies, they did not focus exclusively on their experience among the poor. I have argued that hospital men needed to write about private patients in order to demonstrate their elite clientele. But their choices also had significant consequences for clinical perceptions, particularly when case histories appeared as articles in periodicals.

When practitioners first began to write up descriptions of interesting ill and injured people for publication in the *Philosophical Transactions,* they made clinical observations of patients into discrete accounts of matters of fact, akin to reports of objects and experiences in natural history and natural philosophy. While patients had been treated as clinical "objects" in texts at least from the time of the Hippocratic writings, separating these descriptions from the larger context of medical books expanded the pool of patients whose noteworthy conditions could be written up in a single article, not just kept as possible data for a monograph or collection. With their decisions to write about the well-to-do along with the poor, hospital men, like other elite practitioners, effectively made *all* patients, public and private, into clinical objects. Thus, although it may have been socially and psychologically easier for some practitioners and their pupils to objectify the poor unknowns on hospital wards, I believe that the invention of the case history article in the eighteenth century had deeper consequences. These demonstrated, over and over again, that clinicians could see their patients simultaneously as subjects, as ill people to be cared for, and as objects, as diseased flesh or disordered mechanisms to be watched, analyzed, and dissected. This double vision is crucial for a practitioner's bedside authority, when he brings the abstractions of science to bear on the suffering individual.

Separating cases from larger texts, moreover, turned *any* observing practitioner into a potential participant in the advancement of knowledge. This belief not only underlay the expansion of medical periodicals in the eighteenth and nineteenth centuries, but also further defined the community of regular medical men. They were the ones – not part-time irregulars and quacks – who knew how to compose case histories, how to read them, and how to appreciate the particulars of clinical variations and innovative treatments. Writing case histories, moreover, literally embodied and legitimized the cultural value given to descriptions of observations. The repeated publication of short, descriptive case histories constantly reinforced the notion that good medical knowledge came from relatively passive observation of what happened during a patient's illness, injury, recovery, or autopsy, not from armchair speculation about disease.

The short narratives of clinical experience that began in the *Philosophical Transactions* and then dominated medical periodicals were, if written with appropriate circumspection, extremely safe contributions to the advancement of knowledge. I have deliberately used "safe" to express the way that certain topics, clinical methods, and ways of writing supported a practitioner's social and occupational status, and hence helped to preserve his authority. "Safe," in this context, by no means implies that medical men did not engage in controversies, mutual criticism, and outright name-calling, especially during priority disputes and discussions of medical reform. Being disputatious or offensive served some practitioners' ambitions to be noticed, despite the risk of alienating patients and other practitioners.

And, indeed, some medical men made mistakes, and were publicly humiliated or privately impoverished because of them. But very few hospital men fell that far from grace. Most, because of their family background, medical training, or social aspirations, probably did not have to think twice about staying safe, and taught what they had been taught, wrote about predictably interesting cases, and introduced new ideas and techniques into practice with snail-paced caution. Hospital men who published nothing – the ones it is easiest to overlook, of course – may have been the safest of them all.

Several hospital men, nevertheless, enjoyed making more immediate and noticeable efforts to improve medicine. And to them belonged the subtle forms of safe science. With very few exceptions, active hospital researchers in the late eighteenth and early nineteenth centuries wrote unadorned, descriptive accounts of their scientific observations and experiments. In these – using that potent tool, omission – they avoided connecting what they were doing in chemistry and physiology to the political, philosophical, and theological implications these sciences had in some contemporary circles. Exactly why most of the hospital surgeons and physicians who cast themselves as men of science primarily chose to describe their work, and not to speculate upon its larger meanings, remains unknown. And that is the point of safe science. Even with the narrator an active participant in his story, as many practitioners were when dealing with patients and experimental apparatus, an author could write as though completely detached from his feelings, his beliefs, and his opinions. In this sense, hospital men were integrally involved with the entrenchment of objectivity – those ways that we come to believe that facts have meanings that are independent of cultural context – into modern science and medicine. The "objectivity" of modern science, in turn, powerfully localizes authority in the people who make it, legitimize it, and teach it, because such people are seen as merely the channels through which the truth of nature gets decoded and speaks.

In the early 1820s, when my story ends, many parts of modern medicine were obviously yet to come. The decline of private teaching, the rise of laboratory-based biomedicine, and the legislation of rigorous licensing for medical practitioners were just some of the next episodes, full of new actors and changing social forces, that continued to localize medical authority in the people who belonged to quite specific institutions, followed established ways of knowing, and fell under the penumbra of the law. But subsequent transformations of London's medical world in the nineteenth century took place within a profession already dominated by hospital men. Over the course of the eighteenth century, hospital physicians and surgeons in London established their authority to make good medical knowledge and to teach it in institutions devoted to care of the sick poor. With their pupils, fellow lecturers, and other practitioners, they collectively created a medical community and established themselves as its professional elite. They participated in constructing and legitimizing the clinician's modern double vision, which sees patients – all patients, public or private – simultaneously as ill people and as clinical objects. They helped to make science safe. Hospital men still do all of these things, along with the scientists, university professors, and licensing examiners who make new doctors – our doctors – every day.

Appendix I.   London Hospital Men, 1700-1815

I.A.   Physicians, surgeons, and accoucheurs elected to Guy's, St. Thomas's, St. Bartholomew's, the London, the Westminster, St. George's, and the Middlesex

Name	Hospital	Post	Elected Asst	Elected Full	Died or resigned
Abernethy, John	St. Bartholomew's	Surgeon	1787	1815	1827
Adams, Thomas	St. Thomas's	Physician		1749	1759
Ainslie, Henry	St. Thomas's	Physician	1795	1795	1800
Akenside, Mark	St. Thomas's	Physician	1759	1759	1770
Alexander, Benjamin	London	Physician		1765	1768
Amyand, Claudius	Westminster	Surgeon		1721	?
	St. George's	Surgeon		1733	1738
Andree, John	London	Physician		1740	1760
Askew, Anthony	St. Bartholomew's	Physician		1754	1774
Austin, William	St. Bartholomew's	Physician		1786	1793
Babington, William	Guy's	Physician	1795	1802	1811
	Guy's	Physician	1811		1813
Baillie, John	St. George's	Physician		1735	1744
Baillie, Matthew	St. George's	Physician		1787	1800
Baker, Robert	Guy's	Surgeon		1727	1733
Baker, Thomas	St. Thomas's	Surgeon		1739	1768
Baker, William	Westminster	Surgeon		1749	1754
Bancroft, Edward	St. George's	Physician		1808	1811
Barclay, JohnRobertson	St. George's	Physician		1785	1800
Barker, John	Westminster	Physician		1746	1748
Barrowby, William	St. Bartholomew's	Physician		1750	1752
Bateman, Joseph	St. Thomas's	Surgeon		1704	?
Bathurst, Richard	Middlesex	Physician		1754	1756
Batt, John Thomas	St. George's	Physician		1746	1762
Bayford, David	St. George's	Surgeon	1773		1778
Baylies, William	Middlesex	Physician		1764	1766
Belchier, John	Guy's	Surgeon		1736	1768
Bell, Charles	Middlesex	Surgeon		1814	1836
Biddulph, Francis	St. Bartholomew's	Physician		1793	1794
Bigg, Anthony	St. Bartholomew's	Surgeon	1749		1750
Bigg, Thomas	St. Bartholomew's	Surgeon	1728	1737	1745
Birch, John	St. Thomas's	Surgeon		1784	1815
Blackburne, William	Westminster	Physician		1791	1794
Blane, Sir Gilbert	St. Thomas's	Physician		1783	1795
Blanshard, Wilkinson	St. George's	Physician		1766	1770
Blicke, Charles	St. Bartholomew's	Surgeon	1779	1787	1815
Blizard, Sir William	London	Surgeon		1780	1833
Blizard, Thomas	London	Surgeon		1795	1820
Booth, Montague	Middlesex	Surgeon		1752	1753
Bradley, Thomas	Westminster	Physician		1794	1813
Brickenden, John	Westminster	Physician		1766	1775
Brisbane, John	Middlesex	Physician		1758	1773
Brodie, Benjamin Collins	St. George's	Surgeon	1808	1822	1840
Bromfield, Charles	St. George's	Surgeon	1778		1780

Name	Hospital	Post	Elected Asst	Elected Full	Died or resigned
Bromfield, William	St. George's	Surgeon		1744	1780
Brooke, Thomas	Westminster	Physician		1757	1766
Broxolme, Noel	St. George's	Physician		1733	1735
Brudenell, Exton	Middlesex	Accoucheur		1747	1749
Buchan, Alexander Peter	Westminster	Physician	1813		1821
Budd, Richard	St. Bartholomew's	Physician		1780	1801
Bull, Henry	St. Bartholomew's	Surgeon	1722	1727	1728
Burgess, John	St. George's	Physician		1774	1787
Burton, Simon	St. George's	Physician		1733	1735
Buxton, Isaac	London	Physician		1807	1822
Cade, Salusbury	St. Bartholomew's	Physician		1708	1720
Carlisle, Sir Anthony	Westminster	Surgeon		1793	1840
Cartwright, Richard	Middlesex	Surgeon		1806	1825
Caulet, John Gideon	St. Bartholomew's	Physician		1784	1786
Chafey, James	Middlesex	Surgeon		1763	1793
Chandler, George	St. Thomas's	Surgeon		1783	1822
Cheselden, William	St. Thomas's	Surgeon	1718	1718	1738
	Westminster	Surgeon		1724	1733
	St. George's	Surgeon		1733	1738
Cholmeley, James	Guy's	Physician	1804	1811	1837
Church, Randolph	St. Bartholomew's	Surgeon	1720		1722
Clarke, Matthew	Guy's	Physician		1731	1754
Clephane, John	St. George's	Physician		1751	1758
Cline, Henry	St. Thomas's	Surgeon		1784	1812
Cline, Henry, Jr.	St. Thomas's	Surgeon		1812	1820
Coatsworth, Caleb	St. Thomas's	Physician	1694	1715	1729
Coningham, John	London	Physician		1743	1749
Cooke, John	London	Physician		1785	1807
Cooper, Andrew	Guy's	Surgeon		1725	1732
Cooper, Astley Paston	Guy's	Surgeon		1800	1825
Cooper, Thomas	Middlesex	Accoucheur		1763	1769
Cooper, William	Guy's	Surgeon		1783	1800
Cotes, Charles	Westminster	Physician		1733	1739
Cowell, Benjamin	St. Thomas's	Surgeon		1749	1768
Cox, Daniel	Middlesex	Physician		1746	1749
Coxe, William	Westminster	Physician		1750	1757
Craddock, Hasel	Guy's	Surgeon		1732	1736
Crane, Stafford	St. Bartholomew's	Surgeon	1748	1755	1784
Crawford, Adair	St. Thomas's	Physician		1783	1795
Crichton, Sir Alexander	Westminster	Physician		1794	1804
Croft, Francis	Guy's	Surgeon		1725	1727
Currey, George C.	St. Thomas's	Physician	1802	1816	1823
Curry, James	Guy's	Physician	1802	1802	1819
Dargent, James	Westminster	Physician		1762	1788
Dawson, Ambrose	St. George's	Physician		1745	1760
Dawson, Thomas	London	Physician		1764	1770
	Middlesex	Physician		1759	1761
Denman, Thomas (MD)	Middlesex	Accoucheur		1769	1783
DeUrban, John (MD)	Middlesex	Accoucheur		1760	1763

Appendix I.A. (*cont.*)

Name	Hospital	Post	Elected Asst	Elected Full	Died or resigned
Dickens, Ambrose	Westminster	Surgeon		1721	1733
	St. George's	Surgeon		1733	1738
Dickenson, William	St. Thomas's	Surgeon		1714	1719
Dickson, Thomas	London	Physician		1759	1784
Didier, Andrew	Middlesex	Physician	1755	1756	
Dobyns, John	St. Bartholomew's	Surgeon	1719	1725	1730
Dodd, Pierce	St. Bartholomew's	Physician		1725	1754
Dodson, Henry	London	Surgeon	1744		1753
Douglas, John	Westminster	Surgeon		1721	?
Douglass, William	Middlesex	Physician		1750	1752
Earle, Henry	St. Bartholomew's	Surgeon	1815	1827	1838
Earle, James	St. Bartholomew's	Surgeon	1770	1784	1815
Eaton, John	Middlesex	Physician		1749	1751
Else, Joseph	St. Thomas's	Surgeon		1768	1780
Feake, Charles	Guy's	Physician		1744	1762
Fearon, Devey	Middlesex	Physician		1803	1807
Ferne, James	St. Thomas's	Surgeon		1705	?
Ford, James	St. George's	Physician		1786	1793
Fordyce, George	St. Thomas's	Physician		1770	1802
Forster, Thompson	Guy's	Surgeon		1790	1824
Fox, Joseph	London	Physician		1789	1800
Frampton, Algernon	London	Physician		1800	1840
Franck, James	Guy's	Surgeon		1768	1783
Freke, John	St. Bartholomew's	Surgeon	1725	1729	1755
Gataker, Thomas	Westminster	Surgeon		1754	1760
	St. George's	Surgeon		1760	1769
Gay, Robert	St. Bartholomew's	Surgeon		1719	1728
Girle, John, Sr.	St. Thomas's	Surgeon		1710	?
Girle, John, Jr.	St. Thomas's	Surgeon		1731	1749
Gisborne, Thomas	St. George's	Physician		1757	1781
Gower, Charles	Middlesex	Physician		1801	1822
Green, William	St. Bartholomew's	Surgeon	1722	1728	1737
Greene, Edward	St. Bartholomew's	Surgeon	1698	1710	1728
Grieve, James	St. Thomas's	Physician		1762	1773
Griffiths, John	St. George's	Surgeon		1796	1822
Griffiths, Thomas	St. Bartholomew's	Surgeon	1750		1761
Grindall, Richard	London	Surgeon	1750		1797
Gunning, John	St. George's	Surgeon	1760	1765	1798
Gunning, John, Jr.	St. George's	Surgeon		1800	1823
Hadley, John	St. Thomas's	Physician	1760	1760	1764
Hall, Abraham	St. Thomas's	Physician		1733	1749
Hamilton, Richard	Middlesex	Surgeon		1746	1750
Hamilton, William	London	Physician		1787	1807
Hamon, John	Middlesex	Physician		1789	1793
Harrison, John	London	Surgeon		1740	1753
Harvey, Ludford	St. Bartholomew's	Surgeon	1784	1807	1824
Hawkins, Caesar	St. George's	Surgeon		1735	1774
Hawkins, Charles	St. George's	Surgeon	1773	1774	1792
	St. George's	Surgeon		1798	1800

Name	Hospital	Post	Elected Asst	Elected Full	Died or resigned
Hawkins, George	St. George's	Surgeon		1780	1783
Hawkins, Pennell	Middlesex	Surgeon		1747	1756
Hawley, James	Westminster	Physician		1739	1750
Haworth, James	St. Bartholomew's	Physician		1802	1823
Hayes, Sir John M.	Westminster	Physician		1793	1794
Headington, Richard C.	London	Surgeon	1797	1799	1831
Healde, Thomas	London	Physician		1770	1789
Heathfield, Robert	Westminster	Surgeon	1746	1749	1755
Heberden, William, Jr.	St. George's	Physician		1793	1803
Heineken, Hermann	Middlesex	Physician		1749	1750
Hervey, James	Guy's	Physician		1779	1802
Hewitt, William	St. George's	Surgeon		1744	1760
Hibbins, James	London	Physician	1746	1748	1750
Hicks, George	Westminster	Physician		1775	1792
Hinckley, Henry	Guy's	Physician		1756	1779
	Middlesex	Physician		1752	1756
Hoadley, Benjamin	Westminster	Physician		1736	?
	St. George's	Physician		1736	1746
Holland, Samuel	Middlesex	Physician		1801	1806
Holland, Richard	Westminster	Physician		1725	1730
Home, Everard	St. George's	Surgeon	1787	1793	1827
Howard, Samuel	Middlesex	Surgeon		1759	1810
Huck, Richard (See Saunders, Richard Huck)					
Hume, Thomas	Westminster	Physician		1810	1813
Humphreys, Abraham W.	Westminster	Surgeon		1760	1770
Hunter, John	St. George's	Surgeon		1768	1793
Hutton, Addison	St. George's	Physician		1736	1742
Jebb, Sir Richard	Westminster	Physician		1754	1762
	St. George's	Physician		1762	1769
Joberns, John	Middlesex	Surgeon		1801	1832
Jodrell, Sir Paul	London	Physician		1786	1787
Jones, Walter	London	Surgeon		1746	?
Jurin, James	Guy's	Physician		1725	1731
Justamond, John Obadiah	Westminster	Surgeon		1770	1786
Keate, Robert	St. George's	Surgeon	1800	1813	1853
Keate, Thomas	St. George's	Surgeon	1787	1792	1813
Keir, William	St. Thomas's	Physician		1780	1783
Kennedy, Hugh Alexander	Middlesex	Physician		1759	1782
Keylmay, Robert	St. Bartholomew's	Surgeon	1710	1720	1725
Knight, Gowin	Westminster	Physician		1748	?
Knox, Robert	Middlesex	Physician		1769	1782
Krohn, Henry	Middlesex	Accoucheur		1769	1798
Laird, James	Guy's	Physician	1813	1819	1824
Latham, John	Middlesex	Physician		1789	1793
	St. Bartholomew's	Physician		1793	1802
Latham, Peter Mere	Middlesex	Physician		1815	1824
Lawrence, William	St. Bartholomew's	Surgeon	1813	1824	1865
Layard, Mr.	Middlesex	Accoucheur		1747	1747

Appendix I.A. (*cont.*)

Name	Hospital	Post	Elected Asst	Elected Full	Died or resigned
Letherland, Joseph	St. Thomas's	Physician		1736	1759
Leeds, Samuel	London	Physician		1768	1769
Levett, Henry	St. Bartholomew's	Physician		1707	1725
Lister, William	St. Thomas's	Physician	1790	1795	1817
Long, William	St. Bartholomew's	Surgeon	1784	1791	1807
Lucas, William, Jr.	Guy's	Surgeon		1799	1824
Lucas, William, Sr.	Guy's	Surgeon		1773	1799
Lynn, William	Westminster	Surgeon	1787	1788	1834
Maddocks, James	London	Physician		1770	1786
Magie, William	Guy's	Physician		1754	1756
Manaton, Francis William	St. Bartholomew's	Surgeon	1745		1749
Marcet, Alexander	Guy's	Physician	1802	1804	1819
Martin, George	St. Thomas's	Surgeon		1768	1784
Maton, William George	Westminster	Physician		1800	1809
Matthews, John	St. George's	Physician		1781	1783
Mayo, John	Middlesex	Physician		1788	1803
Mayo, Paggen William	Middlesex	Physician		1793	1801
Mead, Richard	St. Thomas's	Physician		1703	1715
Merriman, Samuel (MD)	Middlesex	Accoucheur		1809	1826
Middleton, David	St. George's	Surgeon		1733	1765
Millan, Daniel	Middlesex	Surgeon		1746	?
Milman, Francis	Middlesex	Physician		1777	1789
Milner, Thomas	St. Thomas's	Physician	1751	1759	1762
Minors, Daniel	Middlesex	Surgeon		1779	1801
Minors, Isaac	Middlesex	Surgeon		1753	1779
Moffat, James	Middlesex	Surgeon		1759	1765
Monro, Donald	St. George's	Physician		1758	1786
Morel, William Richard	Westminster	Surgeon		1788	1823
Morris, George Paulet	Westminster	Physician		1788	1810
Morris, Michael	Westminster	Physician		1761	1791
Morton, Charles	Middlesex	Physician		1750	1754
Muckleston, W. H.	St. George's	Physician		1783	1787
Munckley, Nicholas	Guy's	Physician		1748	1770
Neale, George	London	Surgeon		1753	1797
Nevinson, Charles	St. George's	Physician		1800	1825
Nourse, Edward	St. Bartholomew's	Surgeon	1731	1745	1761
Oldfield, John	Guy's	Physician		1725	1748
Paris, John Ayrton	Westminster	Physician		1809	1813
Pate, Robert	St. Bartholomew's	Physician		1752	1762
Paul, Joseph	St. Thomas's	Surgeon		1741	1760
Paul, Josiah	St. Thomas's	Surgeon		1715	?
Pearson, George	St. George's	Physician		1787	1828
Pemberton, Christopher	St. George's	Physician		1800	1808
Pepper, William	St. Thomas's	Surgeon	1701	1702	?
Pepys, Lucas	Middlesex	Physician		1769	1775
Peters, Charles	St. George's	Physician		1735	1746
Petit, John Lewis	St. George's	Physician		1770	1774
	St. Bartholomew's	Physician		1774	1780
Petty, William	London	Surgeon		1743	1753

Name	Hospital	Post	Elected Asst	Elected Full	Died or resigned
Phillips, James	St. Bartholomew's	Surgeon		1730	1749
Pierce, James	Guy's	Surgeon		1744	1745
Pitcairn, David	St. Bartholomew's	Physician		1780	1793
Pitcairn, William	St. Bartholomew's	Physician		1749	1780
Pitts, Edmund	St. Bartholomew's	Surgeon	1760	1784	1791
Plumtre, Henry	St. Thomas's	Physician		1718	1736
Poignand, Louis	Middlesex	Accoucheur		1798	1809
Poole,	Middlesex	Physician		1746	1746
Pott, Percivall	St. Bartholomew's	Surgeon	1745	1749	1787
Powell, Richard	St. Bartholomew's	Physician		1801	1824
Price, Charles	Middlesex	Physician		1807	1815
Price, John	Westminster	Surgeon	1733	1735	?
Pyle, John	Westminster	Surgeon	1735	1746	1788
Pyle, William	Westminster	Surgeon		1733	?
Ramsden, Thomas	St. Bartholomew's	Surgeon	1791		1813
Rawlinson, John	St. Thomas's	Physician		1773	1780
Reeve, Thomas	St. Thomas's	Physician		1740	1760
Relph, John	Guy's	Physician		1789	1804
Reynolds, Henry Revell	Middlesex	Physician		1773	1777
	St. Thomas's	Physician		1777	1783
Richardson, Edward	London	Physician		1764	1765
Risoliere, Gabriel	London	Surgeon	1752	1763	1763
Roberts, Edward	St. Bartholomew's	Physician		1794	1834
Ross, David	St. George's	Physician		1733	1757
Russell, Alexander	St. Thomas's	Physician	1759	1760	1768
Sandys, Henry	St. George's	Surgeon	1760		1762
Satterley, Richard P.	Middlesex	Physician		1806	1815
Saunders, Richard Huck	Middlesex	Physician		1766	1768
	St. Thomas's	Physician		1768	1777
Saunders, William	Guy's	Physician		1770	1802
Sayer, Robert	Middlesex	Physician		1747	1751
Scrafton, Richard	St. Bartholomew's	Surgeon	1737		1738
Sharp, Samuel	Guy's	Surgeon		1733	1757
Sharp, William	St. Bartholomew's	Surgeon	1755		1778
Sheldon, John	Westminster	Surgeon		1786	1788
Skeete, Thomas	Guy's	Physician		1788	1789
Smith, Hugh	Middlesex	Physician		1756	1764
Smith, Nathaniel	St. Bartholomew's	Surgeon	1714		1723
Smith, Thomas	St. Thomas's	Surgeon		1760	1784
Smyth, James Carmichael	Middlesex	Physician		1775	1789
Southey, H. H.	Middlesex	Physician		1815	1827
St. Andre, Nathaniel	Westminster	Surgeon		1723	1750
Stuart, Alexander	Westminster	Physician		1719	1733
	St. George's	Physician		1733	1736
Silvester, Sir John	London	Physician		1749	1764
Symons, Joshua	St. Thomas's	Surgeon		1728	1731
Tanner, Joseph	St. Thomas's	Surgeon	1719	1719	?
Tessier, George Lewis	Westminster	Physician		1725	1733
	St. George's	Physician		1733	1735

Name	Hospital	Post	Elected Asst	Elected Full	Died or resigned
Thomlinson, Robert	Guy's	Physician		1764	1788
Thompson, Henry	London	Surgeon	1752	1763	1780
Townsend, John	St. Bartholomew's	Surgeon	1739		1748
Travers, Benjamin	St. Thomas's	Surgeon		1815	1841
Turner, Thomas	St. Thomas's	Physician	1800	1802	1816
Tuthill, George Leman	Westminster	Physician		1813	1835
Tyson, Richard, Sr.	St. Bartholomew's	Physician		1725	1749
Tyson, Richard, Jr.	St. Bartholomew's	Physician		1762	1784
Vaughan, Henry (Sir Henry Halford)	Middlesex	Physician		1793	1800
Vaux, George	London	Surgeon		1795	1797
Villeneau, John	Middlesex	Surgeon		1745	1751
Villeneau, Thomas	Middlesex	Surgeon		1746	1747
Vincent, John Painter	St. Bartholomew's	Surgeon	1807	1816	1847
Wadsworth, Thomas	St. Thomas's	Physician		1715	1733
Wagstaffe, William	St. Bartholomew's	Physician		1720	1725
Walker, William	St. George's	Surgeon		1783	1796
Wallace, James	Westminster	Surgeon		1755	1762
Waring, John	St. Thomas's	Surgeon		1780	1783
Warner, Joseph	Guy's	Surgeon		1745	1790
Warren, Pelham	St. George's	Physician		1803	1816
Warren, Richard	Middlesex	Physician		1756	1758
	St. George's	Physician		1760	1766
Wasey, William	Westminster	Physician		1720	1733
	St. George's	Physician		1733	1745
Watkinson, John	St. Thomas's	Physician		1783	1783
Watson, Henry	Middlesex	Surgeon		1751	1762
	Westminster	Surgeon		1762	1793
Watson, Robert	Westminster	Physician		1752	1754
Way, Lewis	Guy's	Surgeon		1757	1773
Webb, Joseph	St. Bartholomew's	Surgeon	1729		1749
Webb, Richard	St. Bartholomew's	Surgeon	1755		?
Wells, William Charles	St. Thomas's	Physician	1795	1800	1817
White, Anthony	Westminster	Surgeon	1806	1823	1849
White, Thomas	London	Surgeon	1795	1797	1799
Whitehead, John	London	Physician		1784	1784
Whiting, John	St. Thomas's	Surgeon		1738	?
Whittier, Tristam	Westminster	Physician		1813	1820
Wigan, John	Westminster	Physician		1733	1737
Wilbraham, Thomas	Westminster	Physician		1739	1761
Wilkie, James	Westminster	Surgeon		1724	1733
	St. George's	Surgeon		1733	?
Wilmott, Edward	St. Thomas's	Physician		1729	1740
Witham, Henry	Middlesex	Surgeon		1797	1814
Wollaston, Charlton	Middlesex	Physician		1757	1758
	Guy's	Physician		1762	1764
Wreden, John	St. George's	Surgeon		1734	?
Wright, Richard	St. George's	Physician		1769	1785
Wyatt, John	Middlesex	Surgeon		1765	1797

Appendix I.A. (cont.)

Name	Hospital	Post	Elected Asst	Elected Full	Died or resigned
Yelloly, John	London	Physician		1807	1818
Young, Robert	St. Bartholomew's	Surgeon	1749	1761	1784
Young, Thomas	St. George's	Physician		1811	1829
Young, William	Middlesex	Surgeon		1750	1758

Sources: *St. Bartholomew's*: Sir Norman Moore, *The History of St. Bartholomew's Hospital*, 2 vols. (London: C. A. Pearson, 1918); Victor C. Medvei and John L. Thornton, eds., *The Royal Hospital of Saint Bartholomew, 1123-1973* (London: St. Bartholomew's Hospital, 1974); *St. Thomas's*: Frederick G. Parsons, *The History of St. Thomas's*, 3 vols. (London: Methuen & Co., 1932-6); *Guy's*: Hector C. Cameron, *Guy's Hospital, 1726-1948* (London and New York: Longmans, Green, 1954); Samuel Wilks and G. T. Bettany, *A Biographical History of Guy's Hospital* (London: New, Ward, Lock, Bowden & Co., 1892); *The Westminster*: J. G. Humble and Peter Hansell, *Westminster Hospital, 1716-1766* (London: Pitman Medical, 1966); John Langdon-Davies, *Westminster Hospital: Two Centuries of Voluntary Service, 1719-1948* (London: John Murray, 1952); *St. George's*: Joseph Blomfield, *St. George's, 1733-1933* (London: Published for St. George's Hospital by the Medici Society, 1933); William E. Page, "Some Account of St. George's Hospital and School," *St. George's Hospital Reports* 1 (1866): 1--24; George C. Peachey, *The History of St. George's Hospital (1733-1753)* (London: J. Bale, Sons & Danielsson, 1910); *The London*: A. E. Clark-Kennedy, *The London: A Study in the Voluntary Hospital System*, 2 vols. (London: Pitman Medical, 1962); E. W. Morris, *A History of the London Hospital*, 3rd ed. (London: Arnold, 1926); *The Middlesex*: Hilary Aidan St. George Saunders, *The Middlesex Hospital, 1745-1948* (London: Parrish, 1949); Sir William J. Erasmus Wilson, *The History of Middlesex Hospital during the First Century of Its Existence, Compiled from the Hospital Records* (London: John Churchill, 1845). William Munk, comp. *Roll of the Royal College of Physicians of London*, 2nd. ed., 4 vols. (London: Royal College of Physicians, 1878); *Dictionary of National Biography*, various editions. In addition to these published sources, I surveyed staff elections recorded in the hospitals' governors' minute books to check and to correct the names of staff men and dates of their appointments. See Chapter 2, esp. nn. 95 and 98, for references to these manuscript sources.

I.B. Number of positions for staff physicians and surgeons at the general hospitals, c. 1700-1825

Hospital	Physicians		Surgeons	
	Full	Assistant	Full	Assistant
St. Bartholomew's	3	0	3	3
St. Thomas's	2 3 (1718+)	1 (1751-60)	3 1 (1790+)	1 (1701/1718-9)
Guy's	2 (1726-44) 3 (1744+)	1 (1740s?) 1 (1795+)	2 (1726-44) 3 (1744+)	1 (1821)
Westminster	3	0	3	1 (1735-46) 1 (1787-8) 1 (1806-3)
St. George's	4	1 (1800)	4	1-2 (1760-1813)
London	3	1 (1744)	3	2 (1744-63) 3 (1795-7)
Middlesex	3[a]		4 (1752-93) 3 (1793+)	
Totals				Total
1755	22	1	23	5	51
1800	22	3	22	4	51

[a]Plus one physician-accoucheur
Sources: Appendix I.A.

I.C. Physicians elected to the general hospitals: Fellows, Licentiates, and nonmembers, 1700-1820

	FRCP	LRCP	LRCP after election	Non-RCP during service	Total
1700-19[a]	5 (71%)		1 (17%)		6
1720-39[b]	23 (85%)		3 (11%)	1 (4%)	27
1740-59[c]	18 (40%)	5 (11%)	15 (33%)	7 (16%)	45
1760-79	16 (46%)	16 (46%)	1 (3%)	2 (6%)	35
1780-99	16 (41%)	17 (44%)	3 (8%)	3 (8%)	39
1800-19	25 (71%)	10 (29%)			35
Total	103 (55%)	48 (26%)	23 (12%)	13 (7%)	187

Note: FRCP includes only those physicians who had the Fellowship on election or obtained it as their first membership in the RCP. Licentiates raised to the Fellowship by special grant late in their careers are not included; LRCP includes only those with a Licentiate date before or during the calender year of their election; "LRCP after election" includes only those with a Licentiate date in a calender year after their election; "Non-RCP" includes all physicians who never obtained the LRCP or FRCP, either through choice, exclusion, or sudden death.
[a]St. Thomas's, St. Bartholomew's, and the Westminster (1719).
[b]St. Thomas's, St. Bartholomew's, the Westminster, Guy's (1726), and St. George's (1734).
[c]St. Thomas's, St. Bartholomew's, the Westminster, Guy's, St. George's, the London (1740) and the Middlesex (1745).
Sources: Appendix I.A.

I.D. Physicians elected to each hospital, 1700-1820: Fellows, Licentiates, and non-RCP

	St. Bartholomew's (pre-1700)	St. Thomas's (pre-1700)	The Westminster (1719)	Guy's (1726)	St. George's (1734)	The London (1740)	The Middlesex (1745)
1700-39							
FRCP	5(100%)	6(100%)	7 (8%)	3(100%)	8 (80%)	--	--
LRCP			2 (2%)		1 (10%)	--	--
Non-RCP					1 (10%)	--	--
Total	5	6	9	3	10	--	--
1740-69							
FRCP	5 (83%)	6 (55%)	4 (40%)	5 (63%)	8 (73%)	2 (18%)	6 (26%)
LRCP	1 (17%)	5 (45%)	5 (50%)	2 (25%)	3 (27%)	6 (55%)	13 (57%)
Non-RCP			1 (10%)	1 (12%)		3 (27%)	4 (17%)
Total	6	11	10	8	11	11	23
1770-1820							
FRCP	8 (89%)	5 (42%)	6 (55%)	1 (13%)	10 (77%)	2 (22%)	10 (83%)
LRCP	1 (11%)	6 (50%)	5 (45%)	7 (87%)	2 (15%)	7 (78%)	2 (17%)
Non-RCP		1 (8%)			1 (8%)		
Total	9	12	11	8	13	9	12

Appendix I.D. (cont.)

	St. Bartholomew's (pre-1700)	St. Thomas's (pre-1700)	The Westminster (1719)	Guy's (1726)	St. George's (1734)	The London (1740)	The Middlesex (1745)
Totals							
FRCP	18 (90%)	17 (59%)	17 (57%)	9 (47%)	26 (76%)	4 (20%)	16 (46%)
LRCP	1 (5%)	11 (38%)	12 (40%)	9 (47%)	6 (18%)	13 (65%)	15 (43%)
Non-RCP	1 (5%))	1 (3%)	1 (3%)	1 (5%)	2 (6%)	3 (15%)	4 (11%)
Total	20	29	30	19	34	20	35

Note: FRCP includes only those physicians who had the Fellowship upon election, or obtained it as their first membership in the RCP. Licentiates raised to the Fellowship by special grant late in their careers are not included; LRCP includes those obtained a Licentiate before or after election; Non-RCP includes all physicians who never obtained the LRCP or FRCP, either by choice, exclusion, or sudden death.

Sources: Appendix I.A, I.C.

I.E. Hospital Surgeons[a] on the Court of Assistants[b] of the Company of Surgeons (1745-1800) and Royal College of Surgeons (1800-20)

Year	St. Bartholomew's	St. Thomas's	The Westminster	Guy's	St. George's	The Middlesex	The London	Total Hospital	Others
Company									
1745	4	1	2	-	-	-	1	7	13
1750	5	2	-	-	1	-	2	10	11
1760	5	2	-	2	3	-	1	13	8
1770	3	1	1	2	3	-	1	11	10
1780	5	1	2	3	-	2	1	14	7
1790	3	-	2	3	4	3	1	16	5
RCS									
1800	3	3	-	4	2	1	1	14	7
1810	5	3	-	1	3	1	1	14	7
1820	2	2	1	3	3	1	1	13	8

Note: William Cheselden was surgeon to St. Thomas's (1718-38), the Westminster (1724-33), and St. George's but was counted only once, as surgeon to St. Thomas's; Ambrose Dickens was surgeon to the Westminster (1721-33) and St. George's (1733-38) but was counted only once, as surgeon to the Westminster; Henry Watson was surgeon to both the Middlesex (1751-62) and the Westminster (1762-93) but was counted only as surgeon to the Westminster.

[a] The figures include Assistants who had retired from their hospital posts.

[b] The Court of Assistants of the Company of Surgeons and the Royal College of Surgeons had 21 members. When a departure and a new admission to the Court fell in the sampled years, the status of the surgeon elected was counted.

Sources: Cecil Wall, *The History of the Surgeons' Company* (London, 1937), 212-21. Zachary Cope, *The History of the Royal College of Surgeons of England* (London, 1959), 341. Hospital identifications based on Appendix I.A.

APPENDIX II
LONDON HOSPITAL PUPILS, 1725–1820

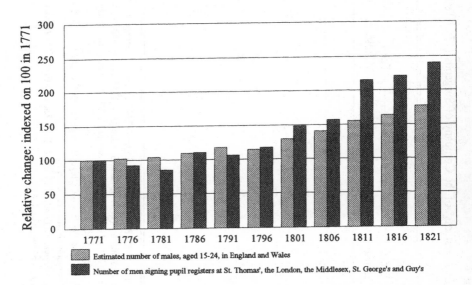

II.A. Population growth and hospital pupils, 1771–1821, indexed on 1771 at 100. *Sources:* For hospital pupils, see II.C–II.G. Population estimates from E. A. Wrigley and R. S. Schofield, *The Population History of England, 1541–1871: A Reconstruction* (Cambridge, MA: Harvard University Press, 1981).

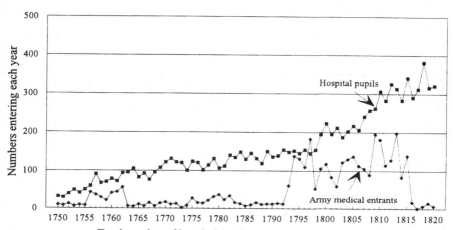

II.B. Hospital pupils and army medical entrants, 1750–1820. *Sources:* For hospital pupils, see II.C–II.G; army medical entrants from Alfred Peterkin and William Johnson, comps., *Commissioned Officers in the Medical Services of the British Army, 1660–1960,* 2 vols. (London: Wellcome Historical Medical Library, 1968).

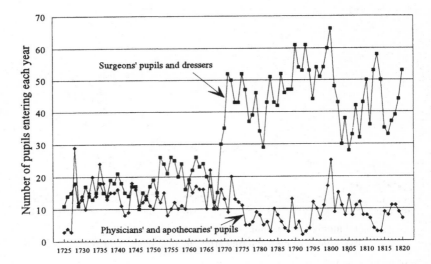

II.C. St. Thomas's Hospital: Entering pupils, 1725–1820 *Sources:* St. Thomas's Hospital Medical School Library, Pupil Registers. (Each volume is listed according to the designation given on the binding or title page). Apothecaries' Pupils, 1753–1759/Surgeons' and Apothecaries' Pupils, 1760–1768; Dressers, 1796–1833 [Surgeons' and Apothecaries']; Physicians' Pupils, 1729–1832; Pupils, 1775–1799 [Surgeons']; Pupils, 1799–1833 [Surgeons']; Pupils: St. Thomas's and Guy's; 1768–1801 [Surgeons']; St. Thomas's Hospital, Pupils: St. Thomas's and Guy's; Register of Pupils and Dressers: Pupils 1723–1775, Dressers 1750–1796 [Surgeons' and Apothecaries']; Register of Surgeons' Dressers and Pupils Entering to the Medical Practice, 1788–1812.

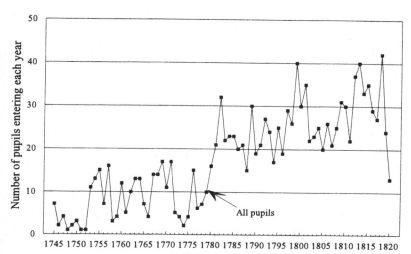

II.D. The London Hospital: Entering pupils, 1745–1820. *Sources:* London
Hospital, House Committee Minutes, 1741–1817, LH/A/5/1–16, District
Archives, Tower Hamlets Health Authority; London Hospital Medical
College Registers, 1740–1860, MC/S/1/1–3.

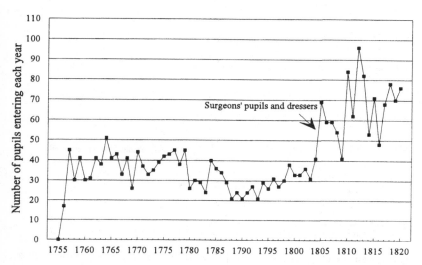

II.E. St. George's Hospital: Entering pupils, 1756–1820. *Sources:* Register
of Pupils and House Officers, 1756–1837, St. George's Hospital Medical
School Library.

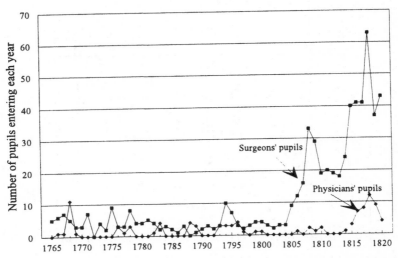

II.F. The Middlesex Hospital: Entering pupils, 1765–1820. *Sources:* Register of Physicians' Pupils, 1766–1840; Register of Surgeons' Pupils, 1763–1845, Middlesex Hospital Archives, Middlesex Hospital.

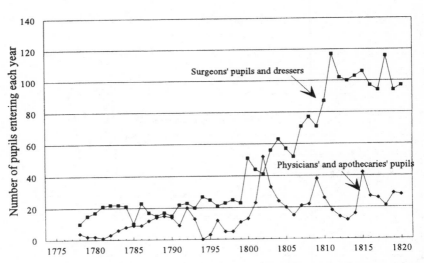

II.G. Guy's Hospital: Entering pupils, 1778–1820. *Sources:* Entry Books of Physicians' and Surgeons' Pupils and Dressers, 4 vols., 1778–1845; General Entry of Pupils, 3 vols., 1805–1840, Secretary's Office, Guy's Hospital Medical School.

Appendix III.   London medical lectures, 1700–1820

The following table lists all the medical men who lectured in London between 1700 and 1820 on anatomy, practical anatomy (dissection), surgery, chemistry, materia medica, physic (or, later, medicine), midwifery, and hospital cases (clinical lectures). Each individual is listed in chronological order by the year of his first known lecture. The dates of each lecturing career are approximate in many cases. All individuals listed as partners, with their years of collaboration, are also given separately. Finally, selected addresses have been included. Where the lecturer had more than one advertised location over his career, the date of the given address has been noted.

Key

*   The lecturer held a position at a dispensary or lying-in charity, or was a physician-accoucheur to the lying-in ward of the Middlesex hospital during some or all of the years in which he offered courses.

**   The lecturer was a physician or surgeon to a general London hospital during at least some of the years he offered courses.

/   Large gaps in the years in which the lectures were given are apparent from the available sources.

italic Indicates that the person is only known to have lectured, or lectured at a particular location, from references other than newspaper advertisements.

Name	Subject	Known dates	Partners	Selected locations
Wilson, George	Chemistry	1700-6		Elaboratory, Well Yard
Rolfe, George	Anatomy	1701-6/1713		
Robertson, James	Chemistry	1704-?		
Douglas, *James*	Anatomy	1706-?		
Smith, Nathanial**	Anatomy	1708		Surgeons' Hall
Cheselden, William**	Anatomy	1710?-22	F. Hauksbee (1720-2)	Crane Court, Fleet St.

Appendix III (*cont.*)

Name	Subject	Known dates	Partners	Selected locations
"T.C."	Physick	1710		
Bright, Edward	Chemistry	1711/1715		Laboratory, White Fryers
Stringer, Samuel	Chemistry	1713, 1715-?		Laboratory, White Fryers (1715)
Figuel, Mr?	Anatomy & Surgery	1715		St. Martin's St.
*Symons, Joshua***	Anatomy	1717-?		
Douglas, John (I)	Anatomy & Surgery	1719-22		Fetter Lane (1719)
St. André, Nathaniel**	Anatomy	1719-26		Northumberland Court, Charing Cross
White (of Oxford)	Chemistry	1721-22		Elaboratory, New St., between Shoe and Fetter Lanes
Coltheart, Peter	Surgical Operations	1721-24		Bedford Court, Covent Garden
Quincy, John	Pharmacy	1722-?		Laurence Hill, Cannon St. (1722)
Strother, Edward	Materia Medica	1722/1724		
Maubray, John	Midwifery	1724		
Wilsford, T.	Anatomy	1724		Fenchurch St.
Ranby, John	Anatomy & Surgery	1725-?		King St., Bloomsbury
Robinson, Nicholas, MD	Physick	1725?/1743		
Macculloch, Peter	Anatomy	1726-1736		Golden Square (1728)
Sargeant, John	Popular Anatomy	1726-?		
Nicholls, Frank, MB	Anatomy & Physiology	1727/1729/ 1730-6/ 1739-41		Druggists, Old Fish St. (1730) Lincoln's Inn Fields (1738)
Pead, Jonathan	Chemistry	1727-?		
Graeme, William	Physick	1728-?		
Nourse, Edward**	Anatomy & Surgery	1729-41		Aldersgate St. (1729)
Shaw, Peter	Chemistry	1731-2/1734		
Chovet, Abraham	Anatomy & Surgery	1733-6		Leicester Sq. (1735)
Hawkins, Caesar**	Anatomy & Surgery	1735-6		Pall Mall Court (1735)
Bromfield, William**	Anatomy & Surgery	1735-50	Sherwood (1747-?)	Hart St., Covent Garden (1746)
Chapman, Edmund	Midwifery	1736/1738		

Name	Subject	Known dates	Partners	Selected locations
Lewis, William	Chemistry	1736-46		Elaboratory, Fetter Lane (1739)
Pemberton, Henry, MD	Chemistry	1738-9/1745		Gresham College, Bishopsgate St.
Griffiths, T[homas]**	Midwifery & Surgery	1739-41		Sadler Hall Ct., Cheapside
Manningham, Richard, MD	Midwifery	1739-?		
Hewitt, William**	Anatomy & Surgery	1740/1743/ 1746-9		Leicester Fields, St. Martin's Lane
Schaw, William, MD	Physick	1740-?		
Parsons, James	Midwifery	1741-?		
*Pott, Percival***	Anatomy & Surgery	1741/1765/ 1783+		*St. Bartholomew's?* (1767)
Vitrack, Mr.	Anatomy & Dissection	1741-?		
Smellie, William	Midwifery	1742-57		Wardour St., Soho
*Girle, John***	Anatomy	1743-?		*St. Thomas's*
*Sharp, Samuel***	Anatomy	1743-?		*St. Thomas's or Guy's* (?)
Lawrence, Thomas	Anatomy & Physiology	1743/1746-50		Essex St., Strand (1750)
Freeman, John	Anatomy & Surgery	1744-5		Warwick Ct, Holborn
Ingram, Dale	Anatomy & Surgery	1744?-60		Fenchurch St. (1756)
Hunter, William, MD	Anatomy	1746-83	Hewson (1765-71), Cruikshank, W. (1775-83)	Theatre of Anatomy, Great Windmill St. (1767+)
James, Robert	Physick	1746		Hart St., Covent Garden (1746)
Lobb, Theophilus	Physick	1747-50		Bagnio Ct, Newgate St.
Sherwood, Mr.	Practical Anatomy	1747-?	Bromfield** (1747-?)	
*Harrison, John***	Surgery?	1749		*London Hospital*
Moffat, James**	Anatomy & Surgery	1749-65		Great Queen St., Lincoln's Inn (1760)
Douglas, John (II)	Anatomy & Surgery	1752-8		Miles Lane, Cannon St. (1753)
Didier, Andrew**	Materia Medica	1753-5		Apartments of the Navy Surgeons, Covent Garden
	Physick	1753-5		
Exton, Brudenell, MD*	Midwifery	1753-5		Frith St., Soho

Appendix III (cont.)

Name	Subject	Known dates	Partners	Selected locations
Greive, James, MD**	Chemistry	1753		Mr. Hodgson's Laboratory, Bartholomew Close
Kelly, Christopher, MD*	Midwifery	1753-60		Broad Pavements, St. Martin's Lane
Lucas, Charles, MD	Chemistry	1753		Great Room, Exeter Exchange, Strand
MacDonough, Felix, MD	Midwifery	1753-7		Bury St., St. James
Minors, Isaac**	Anatomy & Surgery	1753-63		Warwick Ct., Holborn (1753)
Crawford, Hugh	Midwifery	1754-5		Near the Haymarket
Morris, Michael, MD**	Chemistry	1754-7		Laboratory, Stable Yard, Great Ryder St. (1754)
Orme, David, MD	Midwifery	1754-80	Lowder, W. (1775-80)	Theatre, St. Saviour's Churchyard, Southwark (1775+)
Risoliere, Gabriel**	Anatomy & Surgery	1754-5	Thomson, H.** (1754-5)	Newman's Court, Cornhill
Thomas, N[oah?], MD**	Materia Medica	1754-5		Leicester Fields
Thomson, Henry**	Surgery	1754-60	Risoliere** (1754-5)	*London Hospital* (?1759); Paternoster Row (1760)
Mackenzie, Colin, MD	Midwifery	1755-72		St. Saviour's Churchyard, Southwark (1763+)
Martin, John	Midwifery	1755		Bow St., Covent Garden
Watson, Henry**	Anatomy	1755/1760-6		Southwark (?)
Jentry, Mr.	Anatomy & Surgery	1757		Fetter Lane, Fleet St.
Smith, Hugh, MD**	Physick	1757/1760-8		Proposals from available from Mincing Lane in 1760; *Middlesex Hospital* (1757? 1766?)
Monro, Donald, MD**	Physick	1758		Leicester Square
Bengough, Mr.:?	Midwifery	1759		Wardour St., Soho
Harvie, Dr.	Midwifery	1760-9		Theatre, No. 12 Mark Lane, Fenchurch St. (1777)
Maclaurin, Robert	Anatomy	1760-83	Blizard, W.* (1778-81)	Walbrook
Marryat, Dr.	Physiology	1760		
Fordyce, George, MD**	Chemistry	1761-1800		Laboratory, Theobalds Court (1761-3)
	Physick	1763-1800		Patterson's, in Essex St., Strand (1765)
	Materia Medica	1765-1800		House, Essex St., Strand (1775-1800)
	Clinical Lectures	1780-3		St. Thomas's Hospital
Wallis, George	Medicine	1762/1793		
Bayford, David**	Anatomy & Surgery	1763-8		Great Russell St., Bloomsbury (Proposals from, 1763)

Appendix III (*cont.*)

Name	Subject	Known dates	Partners	Selected locations
Krohn, Henry, MD*	Midwifery	1763-5/ 1785-97		Lecture Room, No.17 Bartholomew Close, and House, Southhampton St., Strand (1788)
Cooper, [William?], MD*	Midwifery	1764-6/1768		Northumberland St., Charing Cross
St. Thomas's surgeons (?)	Anatomy & Surgery	1765-6	Thomas Baker, Benjamin Cowell, &/or Thomas Smith	Theatre, St. Thomas's Hospital
Hewson, William	Anatomy	1765-72	Hunter, W. (1765-71)	Theatre of Anatomy, Great Windmill St. (1767+)
Saunders, William, MD**	Chemistry	1765-88	Keir, W.* (1778-82)	No.13 Red Lion Court (1766)
	Materia Medica	1766-9/ 1783-5/ 1790-2		Theatre, Guy's Hospital (all lectures 1770+)
	Physick/Medicine	1768-98	Babington** (1797-8)	
	Clinical Lectures	1770-1800	Keir** (1783) Relph** & Hervey** (1790-4/1797) Babington** (1800)	Guy's Hospital (all lectures 1770+)
Devalangin, [Francis?], MD	Physick	1766-8		Mr. Rose's, Maze Pond, Southwark (1766)
Leake, John, MD*	Midwifery	1766-91		Craven St., Strand (to 1789); Parliament St. (1790-1)
Else, Joseph**	Anatomy	1768-80		Theatre, St. Thomas's Hospital
Neale, George**	?Surgery	1768-?		*London Hospital?*
Awister, Dr.	Chemistry	1769		
Horsley, Mr/Dr.	Anatomy & Surgery	1769/1771/ 1777/1783		No. 4 Rathbone Place (1777)
Alexander, Dr.	Putrid Diseases	1770		Bedford St., Covent Garden
Denman, Thomas*	Midwifery	1770-80	Osborn (1770-80)	Queen St., Golden Square (1772+)
Osborn, William, MD	Midwifery	1770-80/ 1791-1803	Denman* (1770-80) Clarke, J. (1791-1803)	Queen St., Golden Square (1772+)

Name	Subject	Known dates	Partners	Selected locations
Hunter, John**	Surgery	1770-93	Home, E.** (1788-93)	Jermyn St. (1770); Great Windmill Street (1776-7)
	Practical Anatomy	1785-93	Home, E.** (1788-93)	28 Haymarket (1778-82); 13 Castle St., Leicester Fields (1783+)
Logan, Dr.	Physick [not given]	1770		High Holborn, Bloomsbury Square
Rowley, Mr.	Midwifery	1770-1		
	Surgery	1771		
Clark, Mr. (surgeon)	Anatomy & Surgery	1771-2		No. 197 Temple Bar, Fleet St.
Maddocks, James, MD**	Medicine	1772-85		Hotel, No. 5 Capel Court, near the Bank (1772)
	Materia Medica	1774		House, No. 6 Capel Court (1774)
	Physic & Surgery	1775/1776/ 1779		Theatre, London Hospital (all lectures 1782+)
	Clinical Lectures	1783		London Hospital
Higgins, Bryan, MD	Chemistry	1774-6/1780 1788		Chemical Elaboratory, Greek St., Soho (1775)
Andree, Mr.	Anatomy & Surgery	1775		No. 17 Little Knightrider St., Doctors Commons
Falconer, Magnus	Anatomy & Surgery	1775-7		Theatre, No. 27 Craven St., Strand
Cruikshank, William	Anatomy	1775-91	Hunter, W. (1775-83)	Theatre of Anatomy, Great Windmill St. (all lectures 1775+)
	Anatomy & Physiology	1792-9	Baillie** (1783-98) Wilson (1799)	
	Practical Anatomy	1785-99	Baillie** (1785-98) Wilson (1799)	
Lowder, William, MD	Midwifery	1775-80/ 1794-1800	Orme (1775-80) Haighton (1794-1800)	Theatre, St. Saviour's Churchyard, Southwark (1775-80, 1794-1800); Theatre, Guy's Hospital (1794-1800)
Hunt, Mr.	Surgery	1776		Percy St., Rathbone Place
Sheldon, John**	Anatomy & Surgery	1777-86	Blackall (1778-9)	Theatre, Great Queen St., Lincolns Inn Fields
Blackall, [Andrew?]	Anatomy & Surgery	1778-80	Sheldon (1778-9)	Anatomical Theatre, Thavies Inn (1780)
Blizard, William**	Anatomy & Surgery	1778-85/ 1794-1800	Maclaurin (1778-81) Blizard, T.** (1795-1800)	Theatre, No. 12 Mark Lane, Fenchurch St. (1778-82); Anatomical Theatre, London Hospital (1783+)

Appendix III (*cont.*)

Name	Subject	Known dates	Partners	Selected locations
Blizard, William** (*cont.*)	Anatomy & Physiology	1785-93	Orange (1788-93)	
	Surgery	1788-98		London Hospital
	Clinical Observations	1802-7	Blizard, T.** & Headington.** (1802-3) Blizard, T.** (1805-7)	
Keir, William, MD**	Chemistry	1778-83	Saunders** (1779-82)	No. 7 Adam St., Adelphi (1779-80), and Guy's Hospital (1778-83)
Cline, Henry, Sr.**	Clinical Lectures	1783	Saunders** (1783)	Guy's and St. Thomas's Hospitals
	Anatomy & Surgery	1780-1811	Cooper, A.** (1799-1811)	Theatre, St. Thomas's Hospital
Baillie, Matthew, MD**	Anatomy	1783-98	Cruikshank (1783-98)	Theatre of Anatomy, Great Windmill St.
	Practical Anatomy	1785-98	Cruikshank (1783-98)	
Bland, Robert	Midwifery	1783		St. Alban's St.
Cooke, John, MD**	Chemistry	1783-5		Theatre, London Hospital
	Physic	1788-1812	Roget, P.M.* (1812)	Theatre of Anatomy, Great Windmill St. (1810-12)
	Clinical Cases	1790-3/ 1800	Hamilton, W.* (1790-3/ 1800)	London Hospital
Hall, John*	Surgery, Anatomy	1783-8		Anatomical Theatre, Broad St., Soho
	Midwifery	1790-1	Squire, J.* (1790-1)	
Healde, Thomas, MD**	Materia Medica	1783-5		Theatre, London Hospital
*Justamond, J. O.***	Surgery	1783		*Macclesfield St., Soho*
Pearson, John*	Surgery	1783-1803		Golden Square
*Simmons, Samuel F., MD**	Clinical Lectures	1783		*Westminster General Dispensary*
*Wilson, Andrew, MD**	Diseases of Children	1783		*Beaufort Buildings*
Young, Mr.	Anatomy & Surgery	1783		Theatre, Great Marlborough St.
Dennison, Richard, MD*	Midwifery	1785-1810	Squire, J.* (1800-7) Dennison, B. (1809)	Theatre, London Hospital (1785-1810), and Theatre No. 13 St. Pauls Chain, St Pauls Churchyard (1800)
Kentish, Dr.	Physick & Chemistry	1785		
Lister, William, MD**	Chemistry	1785		Theatre, Guy's Hospital

Appendix III (*cont.*)

Name	Subject	Known dates	Partners	Selected locations
Walsh, Philip P., MD*	Midwifery	1785		Theatre, Great Queen St.
Black, William, MD	Physick	1787		*17 Harley St.*
Hamilton, William, MD**	Chemistry	1788-1806	Frampton, A.** (1800) Yelloly** (1805-6)	Theatre, London Hospital
	Clinical Cases	1790-3/1800	Cooke, J.**s (1790-3/1800)	London Hospital
	Medicine	1791		Broad St., Royal Exchange (1791)
	Materia Medica	1792-3		
Home, Everard**	Surgery	1788-1815	Hunter, J.** (1788-93)	Lecture Room, No. 13 Castle St. (1795); No. 42, Great Windmill St. (1815)
Orange, Samuel	Anatomy & Physiology	1788-93	Blizard, W.** (1788-93)	Theatre, London Hospital (all lectures 1788+)
Skeete, Thomas, MD**	Materia Medica	1788		Theatre, Guy's Hospital
Thynne, Andrew, MD*	Midwifery	1788-1813	Gooch, R. (1813)	Theatre, Water Lane, Fleet St. (1788); Medical Theatre, St. Bartholomew's Hospital
Babington, William, MD**	Chemistry	1790-1816	Allen (1802-3/1806) Allen & (1807-16) Marcet**	Theatre, Guy's Hospital (all lectures 1790+)
	Materia Medica	1794/1797	Saunders** (1797-8)	
	Medicine	1797-1816	Curry, J.** (1802-16)	
	Clinical Lectures	1800/1805-7	Saunders** (1800) Curry** & (1805-7) Marcet**	Guy's Hospital
Fox, Joseph, MD**	Materia Medica	1790-1	Cooke** (1790-1)	Theatre, London Hospital (1790-1)
	Clinical Cases	1790-1		
	Medicine	1797-8	Bradley** (1797-8)	
Hervey, James, MD**	Clinical Lectures	1790-4/1797	Saunders** & Relph** (1790-4/1797)	Lecture Room, No. 21 Great Eastcheap (1797-8)

Appendix III (*cont.*)

Name	Subject	Known dates	Partners	Selected locations
Marshall, Andrew, MD	Anatomy	1790-2		Thavies Inn, Holborn (1790-93)
	Anatomy & Surgery	1793-9		Anatomical Theatre, Bartlett's Court, Holborn (1791-9)
	Practical Anatomy	1793-9		
Relph, John, MD**	Clinical Lectures	1790-4/1797	Saunders** & Hervey** (1790-4/1797)	
Squire, John, MD*	Midwifery	1790-1/	Hall, J. (1790-1)	Anatomical Theatre, Broad St., Soho (1790-1)
		1794-1815	Dennison, R. (1800-7)	No. 30 Ely Place, Holborn (1810-15)
Abernethy, John**	Anatomy & Physiology	1791-1820+		Theatre, St. Bartholomew's Hospital (all lectures 1791+)
	Surgery	1791-1820+		
Austin, William, MD**	Chemistry & Materia Medica	1791	Latham, J.** (1791)	Theatre, St. Bartholomew's Hospital
	Practice of Physic	1791		
Clarke, John, MD*	Midwifery	1791-1814	Osborn (1791-1803)	Queen St., Golden Sq. (1791-4); Dr. Clarke's House, New Burlington St. (1797-1803)
			Clarke, C. M. (1807-14)	Lecture Room, No. 10 Upper John St., Golden Sq. (1805-12)
Latham, John, MD**	Chemistry & Materia Medica	1791	Austin** (1791)	Theatre, St. Bartholomew's Hospital
	Physic	1794		
	Clinical Lectures	1798		
Haighton, John, MD*	Physiology	1792-1820	Blundell, J. (1816-20)	St. Bartholomew's Hospital
	Midwifery	1794-1820	Lowder, W. (1794-1800)	Theatre, Guy's Hospital (all lectures 1792+)
			Blundell, J. (1814-20)	
Pearson, George, MD**	Chemistry	1792-1815		Laboratory, Wilcomb St. (1792-1805)
	Physic	1792-1815		No. 9 Great George St, Hanover Sq. (1806-15)
	Materia Medica	1797-1812		
	Clinical Lectures	1792/1797-8/ 1805-12	Harrison, R. (1812)	St. George's Hospital

Appendix III (cont.)

Name	Subject	Known dates	Partners	Selected locations
Pole, T.*	Midwifery	1793-1800		No. 102 Leadenhall St (1793/1800); Medical Lecture Rooms, No. 21 Great Eastcheap (1798)
Bradley, Thomas, MD**	Medicine & Materia Medica	1794		Westminster Hospital (1794)
	Clinical lectures	1794	Crichton** & Morris** (1794)	Westminster Hospital (1794)
Carlisle, Anthony**	Medicine	1797-1806	Fox, J.** (1797-8)	Lecture Room, No. 102 Leadenhall St. (1799)
	Surgery	1794/ 1806-14	Lynn, W.** (1794)	Westminster Hospital (1794); Soho Square (1806)
Crichton, Alexander, MD**	Clinical Lectures	1794	Lynn, W.** (1794)	Westminster Hospital (1794)
	Physic	1794/ 1797-1803		Westminster Hospital (1794)
	Clinical Lectures	1794	Bradley** & Morris** (1794)	Westminster Hospital (1794)
	Materia Medica	1795-1803		Spring Gardens (1797)
	Chemistry	1795-1800		Laboratory & Lecture Room, No. 15 Clifford St., New Bond St.
Lynn, William**	Surgery	1794	Carlisle** (1794)	Westminster Hospital
	Clinical Lectures	1794	Carlisle** (1794)	Westminster Hospital
Powell, Richard, MD**	Chemistry	1794-95/ 1798-1803		Theatre, St. Bartholomew's Hospital (all lectures 1794+)
	Materia Medica	1799-1805		
	Medicine	1803-13	Roberts, E.** (1803-7)	
Squire, John, MD	Midwifery	1794-1815		No. 56 Great Queen St. (1794-8)
Wilson, James	Surgery	1794-99	Cruikshank (1799); Thomas, Mr. (1800-3); Brodie** (1807-10)	Argyle St., Hanover Square (1799)
	Anatomy & Surgery	1799-1820		Theatre of Anatomy, Great Windmill St. (1799+)

Appendix III (*cont.*)

Name	Subject	Known dates	Partners	Selected locations
Wilson, James (*cont.*)				
	Practical Anatomy	1799-1820	Bell (1812-20)	
			Cruikshank (1799)	
			Thomas, Mr. (1800-3)	
			Brodie** (1807-12)	
Blizard, Thomas**	Anatomy & Surgery	1795-1800	Blizard, W.** (1795-1800)	Theatre, London Hospital
	Surgical Cases	1803-7	Blizard, W.** (1802-7)	London Hospital
Cooper, Astley P.**	Surgery	1797-1820+		Theatre, St. Thomas's Hospital (1797-9)
	Anatomy & Surgery	1799-1818	Cline, H. Sr.** (1799-1811)	Theatre, Guy's Hospital (1800-3)
			Cline, H. Jr.** (1811-18)	Guy's and St. Thomas's Hospitals (1805+)
	Surgical Cases	1800-3		Guy's Hospital
Roberts, Edward, MD**	Medicine	1798-1807	Powell, R.* (1803-7)	Medical Theatre, St. Bartholomew's Hospital
	Clinical Lectures	1803		
Batty, Dr.	Midwifery	1799		Great Marlborough St.
Headington, Richard**	Anatomy & Surgery	1799-1820+	Frampton, Mr. (1803-16)	Theatre, London Hospital (all lectures 1799+)
	Practical Anatomy	1803-20+	Frampton, Mr. (1803-16)	
			Cobb, R. (1818)	
			Harkness, Mr. (1820)	
Brookes, Joshua	Surgery	1803-20		
	Anatomy & Surgery	1800-20+		Theatre of Anatomy, Blenheim St. (1800+)
	Practical Anatomy	1800-20+		
Carpue, Joseph*	Anatomy & Surgery	1800-20+		No. 50 Dean St. Soho (1805+)
	Practical Anatomy	1800-20+		
Chevalier, Thomas*	Surgery	1800-10		No. 20 South Audley St., Grosvenor Square
Curry, James, MD**	Medicine & Materia Medica	1800-19	Cholmely** (1807-19)	Theatre, Guy's Hospital (all lectures 1800+)
	Practice of Medicine	1803-19	Babington** (1803-16)	
			Cholmely** (1818-19)	

Appendix III (*cont.*)

Name	Subject	Known dates	Partners	Selected locations
Curry, James** (*cont.*)	Clinical Lectures	1806-7	Babington** & Marcet** (1806-7)	Guy's Hospital
Frampton, Algernon, MD**	Clinical Lectures	1800/1807	Cooke, J.** (1800)	London Hospital
	Materia Medica	1806		Theatre, London Hospital
Thomas, Mr.	Anatomy & Surgery	1800-3	Wilson, J. (1800-3)	Theatre of Anatomy, Great Windmill St.
	Practical Anatomy	1800-3	Wilson, J. (1800-3)	
	Surgery	1805-7		No. 12 Leicester Place
Macartney, James	Comparative Anatomy	1801-10		Theatre, St. Bartholomew's Hospital
Allen, William	Chemistry	1802-20	Babington** (1802-3/1806)	Theatre, Guy's Hospital (all lectures 1802+)
			Babington** & Marcet** (1809/1813/1816)	
			Marcet** (1817)	
			Bostock & Aiken (1820)	
Armiger, Mr.*	Practical Anatomy	1802-6/ 1811-12		Theatre, London Hospital (1802-6)
Frampton, Mr.	Anatomy & Surgery	1811-12		Theatre of Anatomy, Bartletts Court, Holborn (1812)
	Anatomy & Surgery	1802-16	Headington** (1802-16)	Theatre, London Hospital
	Practical anatomy	1802-16		
Badham, Charles, MD*	Chemistry	1803/1806-7		Laboratory and Lecture Room, No. 15 Clifford St., New Bond St.
Accum, Mr.	Practice of Physic	1806-7/1816		22 South Audley St. (1816)
	Chemistry	1805/1807/ 1812		Laboratory, No. 11 Old Compton St., Soho (1805)
Edwards, Richard, MD	Chemistry	1805-7		Theatre, St. Bartholomew's Hospital
Lawrence, William**	Practical Anatomy	1805-15		St. Bartholomew's Hospital

Appendix III (*cont.*)

Name	Subject	Known dates	Partners	Selected locations
Marcet, Alexander, MD**	Clinical Lectures	1805-7	Babington** & Curry** (1805-7)	Theatre, Guy's Hospital (all lectures 1805+)
		1816/1818	Cholmely** & Laird** (1816/1818)	
	Chemistry	1807-18	Babington** & Allen (1807-16) Allen (1817)	
Reid, John, MD*	Medicine	1805-12		No. 7 Cateaton St (1805); Grenville St., Brunswick Square (1806-12)
Taunton, Mr.*	Anatomy & Surgery	1805		Finsbury Dispensary
	Practical Anatomy	1805		
Yelloly, John, MD**	Chemistry	1805-7	Hamilton** (1805-6)	Theatre, London Hospital (all lectures 1805+)
	Physic	1816		
Gunning, John, Jr.**	Surgery	1806-8		No. 43 Conduit St., Hanover Sq. (1806-8)
Bell, Charles**	Anatomy & Surgery	1807-20	Wilson, J. (1811-20)	No. 10-11 Leicester Square (1807-10)
	Practical Anatomy	1809-20		Theatre of Anatomy, Great Windmill St. (1811+)
	Surgery	1809-20		
Boys, Dr.	Midwifery	1807		
Brodie, Benjamin C.**	Anatomy & Surgery	1807-10	Wilson, J. (1807-10)	Theatre of Anatomy, Great Windmill St. (1807-12)
	Practical Anatomy	1807-10		The Theatre, No. 42 Great Windmill St. (1814)
	Surgery	1809-20+		
Buxton, Isaac, MD**	Materia Medica	1807-8		Theatre, London Hospital (all lectures 1807+)
	Medicine	1808-13		
Cholmely, James, MD**	Medicine & Materia Medica	1807-20	Curry, J.** (1807-18) Back** (1820)	Theatre, Guy's Hospital (all lectures 1807+)
	Clinical Lectures	1816/1818	Marcet** & Laird** (1816/1818)	
	Practice of Medicine	1820		Guy's Hospital

Appendix III (*cont.*)

Name	Subject	Known dates	Partners	Selected locations
Clarke, Charles M.	Midwifery	1807-20+	Clarke, J.* (1807-14); Blagden, Mr. (1818-20)	No. 10 Saville Row, Burlington Gardens (1815)
Clough, Henry, MD*	Midwifery	1807-20		Lecture Room, No. 68 Berners St.
Hooper, Dr.	Physic	1807-14	Ager (1810-14)	Lecture Room, Cork St., Burlington Gardens (1807-13),
	Chemistry & Materia Medica	1807-14	Ager (1810-14)	Theatre of Mr. Brookes, Blenheim St. (1814)
Young, Thomas, MD**	Physic	1809-10		Middlesex Hospital
Adams, Joseph, MD*	Medicine	1810-16		No. 17 Hatton Gardens (1812)
Ager, Joseph, MD	Chemistry & Materia Medica	1810-20+	Hooper (1810-14)	Lecture Room, Cork St., Burlington Gardens
	Physic	1810-20+	Hooper (1810-14)	Theatre of Anatomy, Blenheim St. (1815+)
Anderson, Robert, MD	Chemistry	1810		Laboratory, No. 17 Frith St., Soho
Brande, William Thomas	Chemistry	1810-20		Theatre of Anatomy, Great Windmill St. (1810-12)
	Materia Medica	1810-12		The Theatre, No. 42 Great Windmill St. (1815); Royal Institution (1816)
Clutterbuck, Henry, MD*	Medicine	1810-20+		No. 1 Crescent, New Bridge St. (1810+)
	Materia Medica	1810-20+		General Dispensary, Aldersgate St. (1820)
	Chemistry	1810-20+		
	Clinical Lectures	1808/1816	Birkbeck, G. (1808)	General Dispensary, Aldersgate St.
Hopkins, J.*	Midwifery	1810-20+	Pearson, Mr. (1810-12); Hunter, Mr. (1816)	Lying-In Institution, Queen St., Westminster (1810+)
Hue, Clement, MD	Chemistry	1810-20+		Medical Theatre, St. Bartholomew's (1810+)
	Medicine	1814-20+		
Pearson, Mr.	Midwifery	1810-12	Hopkins, J. (1810-12)	Lying-In Institution, Queen St., Westminster (1810)
Ramsbotham, Francis, MD	Midwifery	1810-20+		No. 9 Old Jewry (1810-14); Theatre, London Hospital (1815+)
Reece, R. MD	Physic & Surgery	1810		Chemical & Medical Hall, Bedford St., Covent Garden
Roget, Peter M., MD*	Physic	1810-15	Cooke** (1812)	Theatre of Anatomy, Great Windmill St. (1812)

Appendix III (cont.)

Name	Subject	Known dates	Partners	Selected locations
Roget, Peter M. (cont.)	Materia Medica	1814		Medical Theatre, No. 42 Great Windmill St. (1814-15)
Tuthill, George L., MD**	Physic	1810-18		No. 13 Soho Square (1810+)
	Chemistry	1810-18		
Cline, Henry Jr.**	Anatomy & Surgery	1811-18	Cooper, A.** (1811-18)	Theatre, St. Thomas's Hospital
Dennison, Byam, MD	Midwifery	1812-14		Theatre, London Hospital
Harrison, R., MD	Clinical Lectures	1812	Pearson, R.* (1812)	St. George's
	Clinical pathology	1814		
	Therapeutics & Medical Jurisprudence	1814-15	Roget, P.M.* (1814)	Medical Theatre, No. 42 Great Windmill St.
Merriman, Samuel, MD*	Midwifery	1812-20	Ley* (1816-20)	Middlesex Hospital
Davis, David D., MD*	Midwifery	1814-20+		No. 29 George St., Hanover Square, and Taunton's Theatre, Hatton Garden (1818)
Davy, John, MD	Chemistry	1814		Medical Theatre, No. 42 Great Windmill St.
Gooch, Robert, MD	Midwifery	1814-20+		Theatre, St. Bartholomew's Hospital
Stewart, Dr.	Midwifery	1814		No. 38 Golden Square
Cooper, Mr.	Chemistry	1815-18		Laboratory, No. 76 Drury Lane (1815)
Shaw, Mr.	Practical Anatomy	1815-20	Bell** (1815-20)	Theatre of Anatomy, Great Windmill St.
Stanley, Mr.	Practical Anatomy	1815-20+	Abernathy** (1815-20+)	Medical Theatre, St. Bartholomew's Hospital (all lectures 1816+)
Blundell, James, MD	Physiology	1816-20+	Haighton (1816-20)	
	Midwifery	1814-20	Haighton (1814-20)	
Currey, George G., MD**	Medicine	1816-18		St. Thomas's Hospital (1817)
Foley, Dr.*	Midwifery	1816		61 Berners St.
Guthrie, George J.	Surgery	1816-20+		Royal Westminster Eye Infirmary Waiting Room (1817)
Latham, Peter M., MD**	Practice of Physic	1816-18	Southey** (1816-18)	Middlesex Hospital (1816)
	Materia Medica	1817	Southey** (1817)	
Phillips, Richard	Chemistry	1816-20+		Theatre, London Hospital
Southey, Henry H., MD**	Practice of Physic	1816-20	Latham, P.M.** (1816-8)	Middlesex Hospital (1816)

Appendix III (*cont.*)

Name	Subject	Known dates	Partners	Selected locations
Southey, Henry H. ** (*cont.*)	Materia Medica	1817/1820	Latham, P.M.** (1817) / Ashburner** (1820)	"Medical School," Middlesex Hospital (1820)
Thynne (son of Andrew?)	Midwifery	1816		9 Berners St.
Unwins, David, MD*	Medicine	1817-19		House (address not given)
Cleves, Dr.	Physic	1818-19	Gregory* (1818-19)	No. 14 Old Burlington St.
Cobb, R. Mr	Practical Anatomy	1818-19	Headington** (1818-19)	
Davies, Henry, MD*	Midwifery	1818-20	Cleves (1818-19)	Royal Westminster Eye Infirmary
Gregory, George, MD*	Physic	1818-19		No. 14 Old Burlington St.
Mayo, Herbert	Anatomy	1818-20+		Theatre of Anatomy, No. 18 Berwick St., Soho
Pettigrew, Mr.	Anatomy & Physiology	1818-20+		22 Spring Garden
Aiken, Arthur	Chemistry	1819-20	Bostock (1819) / Allen & Bostock (1820)	
Billing, Archibald, MD**	Materia Medica	1819-20+	Aiken (1819) / Allen & Aiken (1820)	Theatre, London Hospital
Bostock, John	Chemistry	1819-20		Theatre, Guy's Hospital (all lectures 1819+)
Conquest, Dr.*	Midwifery	1819-20		Royal Westminster Eye Infirmary
Emerson, Dr.	Materia Medica	1819		Theatre, London Hospital
Robinson, Benjamin, MD**	Medicine	1819-20+		St. Thomas's Hospital
Travers, Benjamin**	Surgery	1819		"Medical School," Middlesex Hospital
Ashburner, John, MD**	Chemistry	1820		"Medical School," Middlesex Hospital
	Materia Medica	1820	Southey** (1820)	
Grainger, Edward	Anatomy & Physiology	1820+		No. 13 St. Saviour's Churchyard, Southwark
Harkness, Mr.	Practical Anatomy	1820	Headington** (1820)	"Medical School," London Hospital
Power, Dr.	Midwifery	1820		No. 20 Argyll St., Oxford St., and near Guy's Hospital
Stephenson, Dr.	Midwifery	1820		No. 8 Gerrard St., Soho

Appendix III (*cont.*)

Sources: *The Champion, Daily Advertiser, Gazetteer and New Daily Advertiser, Lloyd's Evening Post, London Chronicle, London Daily Post, Daily Courant, Gazetteer and London Daily Advertiser, General Advertiser, London Evening Post, Post Boy, Postman, Public Advertiser, Morning Chronicle, St. James Chronicle, Times; Edinburgh Medical and Surgical Journal;* Donald Monro, *Treatise on Mineral Water* (1770); Samuel Foart Simmons, *Medical Register* (1783); "Sketch of the Life [of Hugh Smith]" in Hugh Smith, *Formulae Medicamentorum Concinnatae* (London: J. S. Barr, 1791); William Black, *Outline of a Course of Medical Lectures* (London, 1787) [cited in Macalpine and Hunter, *George III and the Mad-Business* (London: 1964), 305]; Kay, *Diary;* Shippen, *Diary;* House Committee Minutes, London Hospital; Minutes of the Weekly Board, Middlesex Hospital; Minutes of the Grand Committee, St. Thomas's Hospital, Greater London Record Office (GLRO) H1/ST/A6/7; Donald Monro, Lectures on Physick (1758), National Library of Medicine (NLM) MS B47; Henry Thomson, Notes on Surgery, taken from the lectures read . . . at the London Hospital, 1759, Royal College of Physicians (RCP) MS 254; Cooper, "Diary," Wellcome Institute for the History of Medicine (WIHM) MS 1856; George N. Clark, *A History of the Royal College of Physicians,* 3 vols. (Oxford: Clarendon Press for the Royal College of Physicians, 1962–72), 2: 770; *Dictionary of National Biography;* Nicholas Hans, *New Trends in Education in the Eighteenth Century* (London: Routledge & Kegan Paul, 1951), 150; William Munk, *Roll of the Royal College of Physicians,* 4 vols. (London: for the Royal College of Physicians, 1878); George Peachey, *A Memoir of William & John Hunter* (Plymouth, UK: William Brendon & Son, 1924); George Peacock, *Life of Thomas Young, MD FRS* (London: John Murray, 1855), 218–20; Appendix I.A. for positions in the general hospitals.

INDEX

Continued from the front of the book

The science of woman: Gynecology and gender in England, 1800–1929
ORNELLA MOSCUCCI
Quality and quantity: The quest for biological regeneration in twentieth-century France WILLIAM H. SCHNEIDER
Bilharzia: A history of imperial tropical medicine JOHN FARLEY
Preserve your love for science: Life of William A. Hammond, American neurologist BONNIE E. BLUSTEIN
Patients, power, and the poor in eighteenth-century Bristol MARY E. FISSELL
AIDS and contemporary society EDITED BY VIRGINIA BERRIDGE AND PHILIP STRONG
Science and empire: East Coast fever in Rhodesia and the Transvaal
PAUL F. CRANEFIELD
The colonial disease: A social history of sleeping sickness in Northern Zaire, 1900–1940 MARYINEZ LYONS
Mission and method: The early nineteenth-century French public health movement ANN F. LABERGE
Meanings of sex differences in the Middle Ages: Medicine, science, and culture
JOAN CADDEN
Public health in British India: Anglo-Indian preventive medicine, 1859–1914
MARK HARRISON
Medicine before the Plague: Practitioners and their patients in the Crown of Aragon, 1285–1345 MICHAEL R. MCVAUGH
The physical and the moral: Anthropology, physiology, and philosophical medicine in France, 1750–1850 ELIZABETH A. WILLIAMS
A social history of wet nursing in America: From breast to bottle
JANET GOLDEN

Printed in the United States
By Bookmasters